Computers
in the
Medical
Office

Fourth Edition

Code 1	Description	Amount	Type Description
		$46.00	Procedure charge
99201	OF--new patient, minimal	$62.00	Procedure charge
99202	OF--new patient, low	$86.00	Procedure charge
99203	OF--new patient, detailed	$124.00	Procedure charge
99204	OF--new patient, moderate	$162.00	Procedure charge
99205	OF--new patient, high	$24.00	Procedure charge
99211	OF--established patient, minimal	$38.00	Procedure charge
99212	OF--established patient, low	$52.00	Procedure charge
99213	OF--established patient, detailed	$76.00	Procedure charge
99214	OF--established patient, moderate	$115.00	Procedure charge
99215	OF--established patient, high	$140.00	Procedure charge
99381	Pr...	$145.00	Procedure charge
99382	...ars	$140.00	Procedure charge
99383	...ars	$175.00	Procedure charge
99384	...ears	$165.00	Procedure charge
99385	...years	$178.00	Procedure charge
99386	...0-64 years	$199.00	Procedure charge
99387	...y, 65 & up years		

Includes NDCMedisoft™ Advanced Student Data Disks

Version 9

Susan M. Sanderson

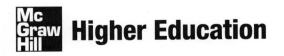

Mc Graw Hill Higher Education

Boston   Burr Ridge, IL   Dubuque, IA   Madison, WI   New York   San Francisco   St. Louis
Bangkok   Bogotá   Caracas   Kuala Lumpur   Lisbon   London   Madrid   Mexico City
Milan   Montreal   New Delhi   Santiago   Seoul   Singapore   Sydney   Taipei   Toronto

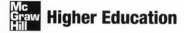

Higher Education

COMPUTERS IN THE MEDICAL OFFICE, FOURTH EDITION

Published by McGraw-Hill, a business unit of The McGraw-Hill Companies, Inc., 1221 Avenue of the Americas, New York, NY 10020. Copyright ©, 2005, 2001 by The McGraw-Hill Companies, Inc. All rights reserved. No part of this publication may be reproduced or distributed in any form or by any means, or stored in a database or retrieval system, without the prior written consent of The McGraw-Hill Companies, Inc., including, but not limited to, in any network or other electronic storage or transmission, or broadcast for distance learning.

Some ancillaries, including electronic and print components, may not be available to customers outside the United States.

This book is printed on recycled, acid-free paper containing 10% postconsumer waste.

2 3 4 5 6 7 8 9 0 QPD/QPD 0 9 8 7 6 5

ISBN 0-07-294856-6

Publisher: *David T. Culverwell*
Senior sponsoring editor: *Roxan Kinsey*
Developmental editor: *Patricia Forrest*
Editorial Coordinator: *Connie Kuhl*
Project manager: *Peggy S. Lucas*
Lead production supervisor: *Sandy Ludovissy*
Media project manager: *Sandra M. Schnee*
Media technology producer: *Janna Martin*
Senior coordinator of freelance design: *Michelle D. Whitaker*
Cover designer: *Studio Montage*
Cover images: Keyboard and Monitor: © *Photodisc, Signature Series Volume 21;* Diskette: *Art Explosion/Nova Development Corporation*
Supplement producer: *Brenda A. Ernzen*
Compositor: *Carlisle Communications, Ltd.*
Typeface: *11/13.5 Palatino*
Printer: *Quebecor World, Dubuque, IA*

Codeveloped by McGraw-Hill Higher Education and Chestnut Hill Enterprises, Inc.
chestnuthl@aol.com

The Student Data Disk, illustrations, instructions, and exercises in *Computers in the Medical Office* are compatible with the NDCMedisoft Advanced Patient Accounting for Windows software available at the time of publication. Adaptations may be necessary for use with subsequent versions of the software. Text changes will be made in reprints when possible.

All brand or product names are trademarks or registered trademarks of their respective companies.

CPT five-digit codes, nomenclature, and other data are copyright © 2003 American Medical Association. All rights reserved. No fee schedules, basic unit, relative values or related listings are included in CPT. Chestnut Hill Enterprises, Inc., and the AMA assume no liability for the data contained herein.

All names, situations, and anecdotes are fictitious. They do not represent any person, event, or medical record.

www.mhhe.com

Brief Contents

Contents

CHAPTER 4   ENTERING PATIENT INFORMATION   57

CHAPTER 5   WORKING WITH CASES   79

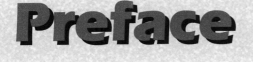

Preface

Demand for health care services is increasing, due to technological advances and to an aging population. Administrative duties in medical offices are also becoming more involved with technology. Computers are now used in almost all medical practices. Students who aim to find an administrative job in the health care industry will find that computer skills are often a prerequisite for employment.

This text/workbook, *Computers in the Medical Office*, prepares students for administrative tasks in health care practices. The text/workbook introduces and simulates situations using NDCMedisoft Advanced, a widely used medical administrative software. While progressing through NDCMedisoft's menus and windows, students learn to input patient information, schedule appointments, and enter transactions. In addition, they produce various lists and reports, and learn to create insurance claims. These invaluable skills are important in effective financial management of health care practices.

Although this text/workbook features NDCMedisoft Advanced, its concepts are general enough to cover most administrative software intended for health care providers. Students who complete *Computers in the Medical Office* should be able to use other medical administrative software with a minimum of training.

TEXT/WORKBOOK OVERVIEW

Computers in the Medical Office is divided into four parts. The first, "Introduction to Computers in the Medical Office," covers the general flow of information in a medical office and the role that computers play. HIPAA concepts, including the Privacy Rule, Security Rule, and Transaction and Code Sets Rule, are presented.

Part 2, "NDCMedisoft Advanced Training," teaches students how to start NDCMedisoft, input data, and use NDCMedisoft to bill patients, file claims, record data, print reports, and schedule appointments. The sequence takes the student through NDCMedisoft in a clear, concise manner. Each chapter includes a number of exercises that are to be done at the computer. These exercises give the student realistic experience using an administrative medical software program.

Part 3, "Applying Your Knowledge," completes the learning process by requiring the student to perform a series of tasks using NDCMedisoft. Each task is an application of the knowledge required in the medical office.

Part 4, a section of Source Documents, gives the student the data needed to complete the exercises. These forms, including patient information forms and encounter forms, are similar to those used in medical offices.

A glossary is included in the back of the book for reference.

COMPUTER SUPPLIES AND EQUIPMENT

The Student Data Disk that comes with the text/workbook is included in two formats: floppy disk and CD-ROM, and provides a base of case study information. Other equipment and supplies needed are as follows:

- PC with 400 MHz or greater processor speed
- 128 MB RAM
- 500MB available hard disk space (if saving data to hard disk)
- CD-ROM 2X or faster disk drive
- Windows 98, ME, NT, 2000, or XP operating system
- NDCMedisoft Advanced, Version 9 *(free to adopters)*
- Floppy disk drive
- Blank, formatted floppy disk for each student
- Printer

NDCMedisoft Advanced is free to schools adopting *Computers in the Medical Office*. Information on ordering and installing the software is located in the Instructor's Manual that accompanies the text/workbook.

CHAPTER STRUCTURE

At the beginning of each chapter, students are provided with a preview of what will be studied:

What You Need to Know   Describes the basic knowledge required in order to complete the chapter.

Objectives   Describes the primary areas of knowledge that can be acquired by studying the chapter and performing the exercises.

Key Terms   Presents an alphabetic list of important vocabulary terms found in the chapter. Key terms are printed in bold-faced type and defined when introduced in the text/workbook. Key term definitions also appear in the left margin of the page where they are first used.

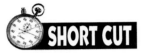

Throughout the instructional chapters, the narrative is supported by numerous figures and tables for reference. These instructional portions of the chapter include *Short Cut* and *Tip* features to enhance the learning experience (see icons in left margin). Computer exercises follow the portions of instructional material to reinforce what was just read.

Various types of testing are supplied in the *Chapter Review* at the end of each chapter in Parts 1 and 2. *Using Terminology* and *Checking Your Understanding* test the student's knowledge of the chapter's key terms and content. *Applying Knowledge* and *At the Computer* encourage the student to use critical thinking skills and apply practical knowledge using the computer.

SUPPLEMENTARY MATERIAL

An *Instructor's Manual* provides the instructor with answers to chapter exercises, answers to Chapter Review questions/exercises, teaching suggestions, SCANS and AAMA correlations, and information on ordering and installing NDCMedisoft Advanced Patient Accounting software. The CD also contains the ExamView Pro test generator program.

ABOUT THE AUTHOR

Susan M. Sanderson, senior technical writer for Chestnut Hill Enterprises, Inc., has developed successful products for McGraw-Hill for more than ten years. She has authored all Windows-based editions of *Computers in the Medical Office*. She has also written *Patient Billing, Capstone Billing Simulation,* and NDCMedisoft simulations for other medical office/insurance programs. Her most recent textbook program, *Introduction to Help Desk Concepts and Skills,* was published in 2003 by Osborne/McGraw-Hill. Susan has worked with instructors to site-test materials and has provided technical support to McGraw-Hill customers. Susan has experience in business training, instructional design, and computer-based presentations. She is a graduate of Drew University, with further study at Columbia University.

ACKNOWLEDGMENTS

For insightful reviews, criticisms, helpful suggestions, and information, we would like to acknowledge the following:

Dolly R. Horton, CMA
Mayland Community College

Char Swanson
Herzing College, Lakeland Division

Valeria D. Truitt
Craven Community College

Joanne D. Valerius, MPH, RHHA
College of St. Catherine, Minnesota

Sandra Masten, MS, RHIA
Florida Metropolitan University

Dawn M. Lyon, RN
Saint Clair County Communtiy College

Introduction to Computers in the Medical Office

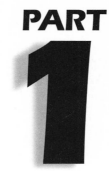

The Medical Office Billing Process and HIPAA

OBJECTIVES

When you finish this chapter, you will be able to:

◆ Describe the billing tasks that are regularly performed in medical offices, including scheduling appointments, gathering and recording patient information, recording diagnoses and procedures, filing insurance claims and billing patients, reviewing and recording payments, and balancing the accounts.

◆ Discuss the HIPAA Privacy Rule.

◆ Identify the major types of health plans.

◆ Discuss the process required to balance a medical office's accounts.

KEY TERMS

accounting cycle
accounts receivable (AR)
Acknowledgment of Receipt of
    Notice of Privacy Practices
capitation
coinsurance
copayment
diagnosis code
encounter form
explanation of benefits (EOB)
fee-for-service
health maintenance organization (HMO)
health plan

HIPAA (Health Insurance
    Portability and
    Accountability Act of 1996)
HIPAA Privacy Rule
managed care
patient information form
payer
policyholder
preferred provider organization (PPO)
premium
procedure code
remittance advice (RA)

THE BILLING CYCLE

From a business standpoint, the key to the financial health of a medical practice is billing and collecting fees for services. Without a steady flow of money coming in, payroll cannot be met, supplies cannot be ordered, and utility bills cannot be paid. To maintain a steady cash flow, specific billing tasks must be completed in a regular cycle and in a timely manner. These tasks include:

◆ Scheduling patients' appointments

◆ Gathering and recording patient information

◆ Recording procedures and services performed

◆ Filing insurance claims and billing patients

◆ Reviewing and recording payments

◆ Balancing the accounts

SCHEDULING APPOINTMENTS

The billing cycle begins when a patient requests an appointment. New appointments are usually requested by telephone; follow-up appointments are typically scheduled when the patient is at the front desk, having just seen the provider.

For a new patient, basic information (such as the patient's name and phone number) is recorded when the appointment is made. Information about the patient's insurance coverage is also usually gathered. Most patients have medical insurance that helps pay for medical services; some patients pay these costs themselves. To ensure that the provider receives payment for medical services, it is important for patients to understand the practice's payment policy.

RECORDING AND PROTECTING THE PRIVACY OF PATIENT INFORMATION

patient information form
form that includes a patient's personal, employment, and insurance data needed to complete an insurance claim.

Patients who are first visiting the practice are asked to complete two important forms: a patient information form and an Acknowledgment of Receipt of Notice of Privacy Practices.

The Patient Information Form

The **patient information form** contains the personal, employment, and medical insurance information needed to collect payment for the provider's services (see Figure 1-1 on page 5).

As illustrated in Figure 1-1, some patient information forms include other information, such as:

◆ Student status

◆ Patient allergies

◆ Referring provider

FAMILY CARE CENTER
285 Stephenson Boulevard
Stephenson, OH 60089-4000
614-555-0000

PATIENT INFORMATION FORM

Patient					

Last Name	First Name	MI	Sex __ M __ F	Date of Birth / /

Address	City	State	Zip

Home Ph # ( )	Marital Status	Student Status

SS#	Allergies:

Employment Status	Employer Name	Work Ph # ( )	Primary Insurance ID#

Employer Address	City	State	Zip

Referred By	Ph # of Referral ( )

Responsible Party (Complete this section if the person responsible for the bill is not the patient)

Last Name	First Name	MI	Sex __ M __ F	Date of Birth / /

Address	City	State	Zip	SS#

Relation to Patient __ Spouse __ Parent __ Other	Employer Name	Work Phone # ( )

Spouse, or Parent (if minor):	Home Phone # ( )

Insurance (If you have multiple coverage, supply information from both carriers)

Primary Carrier Name	Secondary Carrier Name
Name of the Insured (Name on ID Card)	Name of the Insured (Name on ID Card)
Patient's relationship to the insured __ Self __ Spouse __ Child	Patient's relationship to the insured __ Self __ Spouse __ Child
Insured ID #	Insured ID #
Group # or Company Name	Group # or Company Name
Insurance Address	Insurance Address
Phone #	Copay $	Phone #	Copay $

Other Information

Is patient's condition related to: __ Employment __ Auto Accident (if yes, state in which accident occurred: ___)	__ Other Accident
Date of Accident: / / Date of First Symptom of Illness: / /	

Authorization

I hereby authorize release of information necessary for my insurance company to process my claim. The above information is correct to the best of my knowledge. Signed: _____ Date: _____	I hereby authorize payment directly to FAMILY CARE CENTER insurance benefits otherwise payable to me. I understand that I am financially responsible for charges not paid in a timely manner by my insurance. Signed: _____ Date: _____

Figure 1-1 **Patient information form**

◆ Reason for visit

◆ Accident information, if appropriate

This form is filed in the patient's medical record and is updated when the patient reports a change, such as a new address or a change in medical insurance. Many offices ask patients to update these forms periodically to ensure that the information is current and accurate.

The patient information form also requires the patient's signature or a parent's or guardian's signature if the patient is a minor, is mentally incapacitated, or is incompetent. The signature authorizes the health plan or government program to send payments directly to the provider rather than to the patient.

The Acknowledgment of Receipt of Notice of Privacy Practices Form

HIPAA (Health Insurance Portability and Accountability Act of 1996) is a federal law governing many aspects of health care, such as electronic transmission standards and the security of health care records. As part of this act's Administrative Simplification provisions, the **HIPAA Privacy Rule** protects individually identifiable health information. Health information is information about a patient's past, present, or future physical and mental health and payment for health care. If this information is created or received by a health care provider electronically and if it can be used to identify the person, it is *protected health information* (PHI). Except for treatment, payment, and health care operations, the Privacy Rule limits the release of protected health information without the patient's consent.

Under the HIPAA Privacy Rule, medical practices must have a written Notice of Privacy Practices. This document describes the medical office's practices regarding the use and disclosure of PHI. It also establishes the office's privacy complaint procedures, explains that disclosure is limited to the minimum necessary information that is required, and discusses how consent for other types of information release is obtained.

Medical practices are required to display the Notice of Privacy Practices in a prominent place in the office. They also must give patients a form called the **Acknowledgment of Receipt of Notice of Privacy Practices,** illustrated in Figure 1-2. The office must make a good faith effort to obtain a patient's written acknowledgment of having received and read the Notice of Privacy Practices.

HIPAA (Health Insurance Portability and Accountability Act of 1996) federal government act that set forth guidelines for standardizing the electronic data interchange of administrative and financial transactions, exposing fraud and abuse in government programs, and protecting the security and privacy of health information.

HIPAA Privacy Rule regulations for protecting individually identifiable information about a patient's past, present, or future physical and mental health and payment for health care that is created or received by a health care provider.

Acknowledgment of Receipt of Notice of Privacy Practices under the HIPAA Privacy Rule, a form that new patients are requested to review and sign to be informed of the medical office's privacy practices.

Acknowledgment of Receipt of Privacy Practices Notice

PART A: The Patient.

Name: _____

Address: _____

Telephone: _____ E-mail: _____

Patient Number: _____ Social Security Number: _____

PART B: Acknowledgment of Receipt of Privacy Practices Notice.

I, _____ , acknowledge that I have received a Notice of Privacy Practices.

Signature: _____ Date: _____
If a personal representative signs this authorization on behalf of the individual, complete the following:

Personal Representative's Name: _____

Relationship to Individual: _____

PART C: Good Faith Effort to Obtain Acknowledgment of Receipt.

Describe your good faith effort to obtain the individual's signature on this form: _____

_____

_____

Describe the reason why the individual would not sign this form. _____

_____

_____

SIGNATURE.
I attest that the above information is correct.

Signature: _____ Date: _____

Print Name: _____ Title: _____
Include this acknowledgment of receipt in the individual's records.

Figure 1-2 **Acknowledgment of Receipt of Notice of Privacy Practices Form**

RECORDING DIAGNOSES AND PROCEDURES

When the patient sees the provider, the complaint(s) and symptom(s) are entered in the patient's medical record. The diagnosis, which is the physician's opinion of the nature of the patient's illness or injury, as well as the procedures, which are the services performed, are recorded. Prescribed medications are also listed.

When diagnoses and procedures are reported to health plans, code numbers are used in place of narrative description. An electrocardiogram is not reported as an electrocardiogram or an ECG, but as 93000. Coding is a way of translating a description of a condition or procedure into a shorter, standardized format. Standardization allows information to be shared among physicians, office personnel, health plans, and others without losing the precise meaning. Diagnosis and procedure codes are very precise. Health plans base much of their claim approval decisions on the information indicated by diagnosis and procedure codes. Thus, the medical office staff members who work with coding must have specialized knowledge.

diagnosis code *a standardized value that represents a patient's illness, signs, and symptoms.*

A patient's diagnosis is communicated to a health plan as a **diagnosis code,** a code found in the *International Classification of Diseases* (ICD). Diagnosis codes provide health plans with very specific information about the patient's illness(es), sign(s), and symptom(s). Errors in coding can delay the processing of claims and can result in reduced payment or denial of a claim.

procedure code *a code that identifies a medical service.*

Similarly, a **procedure code** is a standardized five-digit code that specifies which medical procedures and tests were performed. The most commonly used system of procedure codes is found in *Current Procedural Terminology,* Fourth Edition, also known as the CPT, or CPT-4. The CPT was developed by the American Medical Association (AMA) to provide a standardized system for describing diagnostic procedures, such as an office visit to examine a patient, and therapeutic procedures, such as surgery and immunizations.

encounter form *a list of the procedures and charges for a patient's visit.*

After entering diagnostic and procedural information in the patient's medical record, the physician completes an **encounter form,** also known as a superbill (see Figure 1-3). The encounter form lists procedures and codes relevant to the particular specialty of the medical office and may also include a list of typical diagnoses. It may provide a place for office visit charges and payments. The information on encounter forms should be checked on an annual basis to be sure that all diagnoses, procedures, and fees, if listed, are current.

FILING INSURANCE CLAIMS AND BILLING PATIENTS

During a typical day, dozens of patients visit the medical office. They have a variety of problems and needs, and they receive different services from the provider. When patients receive services from a medical practice, the costs are paid by the patients or by their medical insurance.

Many patients are covered by some type of insurance. Medical insurance represents an agreement between a person, known as the

ENCOUNTER FORM

DATE _____

PATIENT NAME _____

PROVIDER _____

CHART # _____

OFFICE VISITS - SYMPTOMATIC	
99201	OF--New Patient Minimal
99202	OF--New Patient Low
99203	OF--New Patient Detailed
99204	OF--New Patient Moderate
99205	OF--New Patient High
99211	OF--Established Patient Minimal
99212	OF--Established Patient Low
99213	OF--Established Patient Detailed
99214	OF--Established Patient Moderate
99215	OF--Established Patient High

PREVENTIVE VISITS	
NEW	
99381	Under 1 Year
99382	1 - 4 Years
99383	5 - 11 Years
99384	12 - 17 Years
99385	18 - 39 Years
99386	40 - 64 Years
99387	65 Years & Up
ESTABLISHED	
99391	Under 1 Year
99392	1 - 4 Years
99393	5 - 11 Years
99394	12 - 17 Years
99395	18 - 39 Years
99396	40 - 64 Years
99397	65 Years & Up

PROCEDURES	
12011	Simple suture--face--local anes.
29125	App. of short arm splint; static
29425	App. of short leg cast, walking
45378	Colonoscopy--diagnostic
45380	Colonoscopy--with biopsy
50390	Aspiration of renal cyst by needle
71010	Chest x-ray, single view, frontal

PROCEDURES	
71020	Chest x-ray, two views, frontal & lateral
71030	Chest x-ray, complete, four views
73070	Elbow x-ray, AP & lateral views
73090	Forearm x-ray, AP & lateral views
73100	Wrist x-ray, AP & lateral views
73510	Hip x-ray, complete, two views
73600	Ankle x-ray, AP & lateral views
80048	Basic metabolic panel
80061	Lipid panel
82270	Blood screening, occult; feces
82947	Glucose screening--quantitative
82951	Glucose tolerance test, three specimens
83718	HDL cholesterol
84478	Triglycerides test
85007	Manual differential WBC
85018	Hemoglobin
85025	Complete CBC w/auto diff WBC
85651	Erythrocyte sedimentation rate--non-auto
86585	Tuberculosis, tine test
87076	Culture, anerobic isolate
87077	Bacterial culture, aerobic isolate
87086	Urine culture and colony count
87430	Strep test
87880	Direct streptococcus screen
90471	Immunization administration
90703	Tetanus injection
90782	Injection
92516	Facial nerve function studies
93000	Electrocardiogram--ECG with interpretation
93015	Treadmill stress test, with physician...
96900	Ultraviolet light treatment
99070	Supplies and materials provided

FAMILY CARE CENTER

NOTES

REFERRING PHYSICIAN	UPIN

AUTHORIZATION #

DIAGNOSIS

PAYMENT AMOUNT

Figure 1-3 **Encounter Form**

policyholder a person who buys an insurance plan; the insured.

health plan a plan, program, or organization that provides health benefits.

premium the periodic amount of money the insured pays to a health plan for insurance coverage.

policyholder, and a **health plan.** A health plan is any plan, program, or organization that provides health benefits; it may be an insurance company, also called a carrier, a government program, or a managed care organization (MCO). The policyholder's payments to the health plan for insurance coverage are called **premiums.** In exchange for the premiums, the health plan agrees to pay for the insured's medical services according to the terms of the policy.

To receive payment, most medical practices must complete or produce documents for health plans and patients. One kind of document is an insurance claim. The claim forms of most health plans ask for the same basic information. For the most part, health care claims are created using medical billing programs and are sent electronically to health plans. In some cases, a paper claim is printed.

Charges that are not covered by a health plan are billed to the patient. Patients are sent bills that list all services performed, along with the associated charges for a particular visit. Most medical practices have a regular schedule, perhaps daily or weekly, for mailing claims to patients. For example, some practices bill half the patients on the fifteenth of the month and the other half on the thirtieth.

Overview of Medical Insurance

There are many sources of medical insurance in the United States. Most policyholders are covered by group policies, often through their employers. Some people have individual plans. Insurance coverage may be supplied by a private company, such as CIGNA, or by a government plan. CMS—Centers for Medicare and Medicaid Services—runs the Medicare and Medicaid programs. The most common government plans are:

- ◆ **Medicare** Medicare is a federal health plan that covers people aged sixty-five and over, people with disabilities, and dependent widows.

- ◆ **Medicaid** People with low incomes who cannot afford medical care are covered by Medicaid, which is cosponsored by federal and state governments. Qualifications and benefits vary by state.

- ◆ **TRICARE** TRICARE is a government program that covers medical expenses for dependents of active duty members of the uniformed services and for retired military personnel. Formerly known as CHAMPUS, it also covers dependents of military personnel who were killed while on active duty.

- ◆ **CHAMPVA** The Civilian Health and Medical Program of the Veterans Administration is for veterans with permanent service-related disabilities and their dependents. It also covers surviving spouses and dependent children of veterans who died from service-related disabilities.

◆ **Workers' Compensation** People with job-related illnesses or injuries are covered under workers' compensation insurance. Workers' compensation benefits vary according to state law.

Whether it is a private company or government program, the health plan is called a **payer.** The term *third-party payer* is also used because the primary relationship is between the provider and the patient, and the health plan is the third party.

Different types of medical insurance can be purchased. In a **fee-for-service** plan, which was the first type of plan to be widely used, policyholders are repaid for costs for health care obtained because of illnesses and accidents. The policy lists the medical services that are covered and the amounts that are paid. The benefit may be for all or part of the charges. For example, the policy may indicate that 80 percent of charges for surgery are covered and that the policyholder is responsible for paying the other 20 percent. The portion of charges that an insured person must pay is known as **coinsurance.**

The leading insurance system today is **managed care.** Most people who are insured through their employers are covered by some form of managed care. A managed care organization (MCO) controls both the financing and the delivery of health care to policyholders. The MCO reaches agreements with physicians and other health care providers that control fees.

In some managed care plans, providers are paid a fixed amount per month to provide necessary, contracted services to patients who are plan members. This fixed prepayment is referred to as **capitation.** The amount is based on several factors, including the number of plan members in the insured pool and their ages. The capitated rate per enrollee is paid to the provider even if the patient does not receive any medical services during the time period covered by the payment. Similarly, the provider receives the same capitated rate if a patient is treated more than once during the time period. In other plans, negotiated per-service fees are paid. These fees are lower than the provider's regular rates for the services.

The most common type of managed care health plan is a **preferred provider organization (PPO).** A PPO is a network of providers under contract to an MCO to perform services for plan members at discounted fees. Usually, members may choose to receive care from doctors or providers outside the network, but they pay a higher cost.

Another common type of managed care system is a **health maintenance organization (HMO).** In an HMO, patients pay fixed rates at regular intervals, such as monthly, that cover whatever services they need for that period. In some HMOs, patients also pay a **copayment**—a small fixed fee, such as $10—at the time of the office visit. Usually, patients in an HMO must choose from a specific group of health care providers. If they seek services from a provider who is not in the health plan, the MCO does not pay for the care.

Processing Claims

For a health plan to pay a claim, certain information about the patient must be shared. The health plan needs to know the procedures the provider performed while the patient was in the office. The date of the visit and the location of the visit must be indicated. The health plan also requires basic information about the provider who is treating the patient, including the provider's name and/or the provider's identification number. There may be a group number and an individual identification number for a provider who is part of a group practice.

The information needed to create a claim is found on the patient information form and the encounter form. After the claims are created, they are submitted electronically by transferring information from a computer in the provider's office to a computer in the payer's office. In some situations, a paper claim may be prepared.

When the claim is received by the payer, it is reviewed and processed. If the patient's insurance is a fee-for-service plan, the payer compares the fees to the schedule of benefits in the patient's policy and determines the amount of benefit to be paid. If the patient's insurance is a PPO, the insurance company pays a contracted fee to the provider, and the patient pays the copayment directly to the provider.

REVIEWING AND RECORDING PAYMENTS

remittance advice (RA) an explanation of benefits transmitted electronically by a payer to a provider.

explanation of benefits (EOB) paper document from a payer that shows how the amount of a benefit was determined.

After the amount of the benefit is determined, the payer issues a payment. At the same time, it issues a **remittance advice (RA)** or **explanation of benefits (EOB).** Usually, an RA is sent electronically to the provider; the patient receives a paper EOB. An RA or EOB indicates what was paid and how the amount was determined. The payer sends the payment to the provider or to the policyholder to whom it is owed.

When the RA arrives at the provider's office, it is reviewed for accuracy. If an error is found, a request for a review of the claim must be filed with the payer. When a paper check is enclosed or an electronic payment is made, the amount of the payment is recorded. Depending on the rules of the health plan, the patient may be billed for an outstanding balance. In other circumstances, an account adjustment is made.

BALANCING THE ACCOUNTS

accounting cycle the flow of financial transactions in a business.

accounts receivable (AR) monies that are flowing into a business.

The **accounting cycle** is the flow of financial transactions in a business—from making a sale to collecting payment for the goods or services delivered. In a medical practice, this is the cycle from seeing and treating the patient to receiving payments for services provided.

Accounting software can be used to track **accounts receivable (AR)**—monies that are coming into the practice—and to produce financial reports. Reports are usually created at the end of each day and at the end of the month, quarter, and year.

The report generated at the end of each day lists all charges, payments, and adjustments entered during that day. To balance out a day, transactions listed on encounter forms (charges and payments) and totals from deposit tickets are compared against the computer-generated end-of-day report. A monthly report summarizes the financial activity of the entire month. This report lists charges, payments, and adjustments and the total accounts receivable for the month. It is possible to balance out the month by totaling the daily charges, payments, and adjustments, and comparing the totals to the amounts listed on the monthly report.

It is good practice to periodically print reports that list the outstanding balances owed to the practice by health plans or patients. There are also reports that provide current information on the status of patient and insurance billing. Regular review of these reports can alert the billing staff to accounts that require action to collect the amount due. In addition to these reports, most accounting programs provide other useful report tools that offer a clear picture of the practice's financial health at any point in time. Timely printing of reports also helps the office staff meet claim filing deadlines and collect unpaid insurance payments.

CHAPTER REVIEW

USING TERMINOLOGY

Match the terms on the left with the definitions on the right.

__u__ 1. accounting cycle

__m__ 2. accounts receivable (AR)

__n__ 3. Acknowledgment of Receipt of Notice of Privacy Practices

__K__ 4. capitation

__q__ 5. coinsurance

__h__ 6. copayment

__S__ 7. diagnosis code

__D__ 8. encounter form

__A__ 9. explanation of benefits (EOB)

__j__ 10. fee-for-service

__O__ 11. health maintenance organization (HMO)

__V__ 12. health plan

__E__ 13. HIPAA (Health Insurance Portability and Accountability Act of 1996)

__C__ 14. HIPAA Privacy Rule

__L__ 15. managed care

__B__ 16. patient information form

__F__ 17. payer

a. A paper document from a health plan that lists the amount of a benefit and explains how it was determined.

b. A document that contains personal, employment, and medical insurance information about a patient.

c. Federal government act that set guidelines for standardizing the electronic data interchange of administrative and financial transactions, exposing fraud and abuse in government programs, and protecting the security and privacy of health information.

d. A form listing procedures relevant to the specialty of a medical office, used to record the procedures.

e. Regulations for protecting individually identifiable information about patients.

f. Private or government organization that insures or pays for health care.

g. An electronic document from a health plan that lists the amount of a benefit and explains how it was determined.

h. A small fixed fee paid by the patient at the time of an office visit.

i. An individual who has contracted with a health plan for coverage.

j. Payments made to a health plan by a policyholder for coverage.

k. A fixed amount that is paid to a provider in advance to provide medically necessary services to patients.

l. A type of insurance in which the carrier is responsible for the financing and delivery of health care.

m. A term used to describe money coming in to a business.

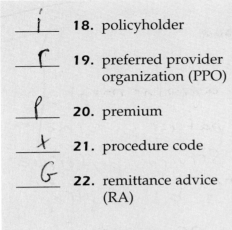

_i_ 18. policyholder

_r_ 19. preferred provider organization (PPO)

_p_ 20. premium

_t_ 21. procedure code

_G_ 22. remittance advice (RA)

n. Under the HIPAA Privacy Rule, a form that new patients must read and sign to be informed of the medical office's privacy practices.

o. A type of managed care system in which the plan pays fixed rates at regular intervals.

p. An insurance plan in which policyholders are reimbursed for health care costs.

q. Under an insurance plan, the portion or percentage of the charges that the patient is responsible for paying.

r. A network of health care providers who agree to provide services to plan members at a discounted fee.

s. A value that stands for a patient's illness, signs, or symptoms.

t. A number that represents medical procedures that were performed.

u. The flow of financial transactions in a business.

v. A plan, program, or organization that provides health benefits.

CHECKING YOUR UNDERSTANDING

Write "T" or "F" in the blank to indicate whether you think the statement is true or false.

_T_ 23. Many patient information forms contain a place for the patient to sign to authorize the patient's health plan to send payments directly to a provider.

_F_ 24. CPT-4 codes have eight digits.

_F_ 25. "Coinsurance" refers to a small fixed fee that must be paid by the patient at the time of an office visit.

_T_ 26. The HIPAA Privacy Rule protects patients' private information.

Answer the question below in the space provided.

27. List the six basic categories of billing tasks in a medical office.

Scheduling patients' appointments

Gathering + recording patient information

Recording procedures + services performed

Filing insurance ~~forms~~ claims + billing pts

Reviewing + recording payments

Balancing the account

Choose the best answer.

_b_ **28.** A patient information form contains information such as name, address, employer, and:
 a. procedure code
 b. insurance coverage
 c. charges for procedures performed

_C_ **29.** A health maintenance organization (HMO) is one example of:
 a. a fee-for-service health plan
 b. a government plan
 c. a managed care health plan

_C_ **30.** In a managed care health plan, a _____ is usually collected from the patient at the office visit.
 a. deductible
 b. patient statement
 c. copayment

_C_ **31.** The most commonly used system of medical procedure codes is found in the:
 a. CPT
 b. ICD
 c. CMS-1500

_C_ **32.** Information about a patient's medical procedures that is needed to create an insurance claim is found on the:
 a. remittance advice
 b. Acknowledgment of Receipt of Notice of Privacy Practices
 c. encounter form

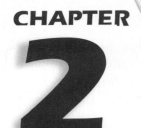

CHAPTER 2

Medical Billing Programs

OBJECTIVES

When you finish this chapter, you will be able to:

◆ Discuss the role of information technology in medical offices.

◆ Describe the purpose of the HIPAA Security Rule.

◆ Explain how the HIPAA Transaction and Code Sets Standards relate to insurance claims.

◆ Discuss the use of computer programs in medical office scheduling and billing.

KEY TERMS

audit/edit report
business associate
clearinghouse
database
edit
electronic data interchange (EDI)
electronic funds transfer (EFT)
electronic medical record (EMR)

HIPAA Security Rule
HIPAA Transaction and Code Sets Standards
information technology (IT)
walkout statement
X12-837 Health Care Claim (837P)

INFORMATION TECHNOLOGY IN MEDICAL OFFICES

information technology (IT) development, management, and support of computer-based hardware and software systems.

Medical office assistants use **information technology (IT)**—computer hardware and software information systems—to handle administrative tasks electronically in almost all physician practices. For example, most offices use medical billing programs. The computer user enters information about the practice's providers, patients, health plans, procedure codes, diagnosis codes, charges, and payments in the program's **databases,** which are collections of related facts. The computer program can then be used to schedule appointments, verify insurance eligibility, produce insurance claims, create financial reports, accept electronic payments, and perform other tasks.

database a collection of related facts.

electronic medical record (EMR) electronic collection and management of health data.

Information technology is also used for storing, accessing, and sharing health information electronically. Many physician practices have invested in **electronic medical record (EMR)** systems to record clinical data. These systems involve creating and storing physicians' reports of examinations, surgical procedures, tests, and X-rays electronically. Hospitals, which have enormous amounts of patient data, collect and manage health data and information electronically. Professionals in the health information management (HIM) field handle both administrative and clinical hospital systems.

ADVANTAGES OF COMPUTER USE

In the past, most of the administrative and financial work done in medical offices involved printed information. Appointments were recorded in scheduling books; insurance claims were printed on paper forms; and physicians' schedules were often filled in by hand in appointment books. Clinical reports, too, such as the patients' medical records and test results, were filed on paper. This work is faster and easier with computers, so information technology applications are increasingly important in medical offices, and computer literacy is a basic requirement for employment in an administrative position.

In physician practices, there are a number of advantages to performing tasks with a computer instead of on paper:

◆ Information is stored in electronic files that can be used by more than one person at a time. The office's computers can be linked in a network, which allows them to share files in the central database. Without a computer database, it is difficult for someone to update a document if another person is working on it.

◆ Information is easy to find. Instead of looking in different file cabinets and folders, patient information can quickly be retrieved and displayed on the computer screen.

◆ Less storage space is needed, since data are stored on computer media, not on paper.

- Computer databases are more efficient than manual filing systems, so they save enormous amounts of time. For example, when medical records are stored electronically, a staff member does not have to pull patient charts at the start of each day and file them at the end of the day. Instead, physicians can quickly access and update records as they see patients, using computer equipment in examining rooms.

- Computer use also reduces errors. Information is entered once, proofed, and then used over and over again. For example, the patient's address and insurance policy number are entered once and accessed when needed to create claims, bills, or correspondence.

Medical billing programs, especially, greatly streamline the important process of creating and following up on health care claims sent to payers and bills sent to patients. Here are examples:

- In a large medical practice with a group of providers and thousands of patients, the phone rings, and a patient would like to know the amount owed on an account. With a computerized billing program, the medical office assistant enters the first few letters of the patient's last name, and the patient's account data appear on the monitor. The outstanding balance is communicated to the patient.

- The wrong diagnosis code has been entered on an insurance claim, and the claim has been rejected by the payer. To resubmit the claim without the use of a computer would require completing the entire form again by hand. Using a computerized billing program, the error is corrected and a new claim sent, making payment more rapid and improving cash flow.

A NOTE OF CAUTION: WHAT COMPUTERS CANNOT DO

While computers do increase efficiency and reduce errors, they are no more accurate than the individual entering the data. If the person makes an error while entering data, the information the computer produces will be incorrect. Computers are precise and unforgiving. While the human brain knows that "flu" is short for influenza, the computer does not know this, and it regards them as two distinct conditions. If a computer user accidentally enters a name as "ORourke" instead of "O'Rourke," a person might know what is meant; the computer does not. It would probably respond with a message such as "No such patient exists in the database."

Many human errors occur during data entry, such as pressing the wrong key on the keyboard. Other errors are due to a lack of computer literacy—not knowing how to use a program to accomplish the tasks. For this reason, knowledge of the use of computer programs and proper training in data-entry techniques so that errors are caught are essential for medical office personnel who handle administrative work.

HIPAA AND SECURITY OF INFORMATION

More and more, patient data are transmitted electronically. For example, the results of blood work completed by an outside lab can be sent to the physician's office via computer. An EMR program is capable of receiving this electronic information and storing it in the appropriate patient record. Once clinical information is entered into the computer, it can be transmitted to another computer with just a few commands. This can be especially helpful in emergency situations. For example, suppose a patient who had coronary bypass surgery eight weeks ago is admitted to the hospital complaining of chest pain. The computer at the physician's office can transmit clinical information on the patient's condition to a computer at the hospital in seconds. Results of prior tests and lab work, such as electrocardiograms, could be sent, as well as a list of medications currently taken by the patient. In a case where time is critical, the computer can be a lifesaving device.

Storing patient records on the computer raises the issue of computer security and the confidentiality of patient records. The HIPAA Privacy Rule (see page 6) governs the practice's privacy procedures to protect patients' health information. Similarly, the **HIPAA Security Rule** outlines the administrative, technical, and physical safeguards required to prevent unauthorized access to protected health care information. The security standards help safeguard confidential health information.

As one security measure, many medical offices assign passwords to individuals who have access to computer files, thereby limiting access to data stored on the computer. Access is granted on an as-needed basis. For example, the individual responsible for scheduling may not be able to access medical records or billing data. On the other hand, the physicians and several others (such as the practice manager) most likely have access to all databases.

As additional security, computer programs keep track of data entry and create an audit trail—a way to trace who has accessed information and when. When new information is entered or existing information is changed, a log is created to record the time and date of the entry as well as the name of the computer operator. This log is stored and may be reviewed by the practice manager on a regular basis to detect irregularities. In addition, if an error has been made, the log makes it possible to determine who made the error and when it was entered.

HIPAA Security Rule regulations outlining the minimum administrative, technical, and physical safeguards required to prevent unauthorized access to protected health care information.

HIPAA AND ELECTRONIC EXCHANGE OF INFORMATION

electronic data interchange (EDI) the exchange of routine business transactions from one computer to another using publicly available communications protocols.

HIPAA Transaction and Code Sets Standards regulations requiring electronic transactions such as claim transmission to use standardized formats.

Just as clinical records are increasingly exchanged electronically, so are the financial transactions on the business side of the health care industry. Electronic transmission—called **electronic data interchange (EDI)**—involves sending data from computer to computer. Many different EDI systems have been used in health care, causing a confusing array of software programs to decipher messages. To improve the efficiency of health care electronic transactions, the **HIPAA Transaction and Code Sets Standards** have been implemented. These standards describe a particular electronic format that providers and payers must use to send and receive health care transactions. They also establish standard medical code sets, such as ICD and CPT-4, for use in health care transactions.

The electronic formats are based on EDI standards called ASC X12, after the initials of the national committee that developed them, and a number has been assigned to each standard transaction. The HIPAA standards cover the following key electronic transactions between medical offices and payers and that contain patient-identifiable, health-related administrative information:

◆ X12-270/271 Health Care Eligibility Benefit Inquiry and Response
Questions and answers about whether patients' health plans cover planned treatments and procedures

◆ X12-837 Health Care Claim or Encounter
Data about the billing provider who requests payment, the patient, and the diagnoses and procedures that a provider sends to a payer

◆ X12-276/277 Health Care Claim Status Request and Response
Questions and answers between providers—such as medical offices and hospitals—and payers about claims that are due to be paid

◆ X12-278 Health Care Services Review—Request for Review and Response
Questions and answers between patients, or providers on their behalf, and managed care organizations for approval to see medical specialists

◆ X12-835 Claims Payment and Remittance Advice
The payment and RA that is sent from the payer to the provider; the payment may be via **electronic funds transfer (EFT)** from the payer directly to the provider's bank, similar to an ATM transaction

electronic funds transfer (EFT) a system that transfers money electronically.

USING MEDICAL BILLING PROGRAMS

Medical billing programs are used to keep track of accounts receivable, or payments coming in from patients and health plans, and accounts payable, or amounts owed to suppliers and staff. Keeping accurate financial records is critical to a practice's survival. Accurate records are needed to meet financial obligations and for tax reporting purposes. And, as in any business, accurate financial reports let management know whether the medical office is profitable.

Medical offices use various accounting systems to keep track of their finances, but they are all similar. Initially, the program is prepared for use by entering basic facts about the practice. Often a computer consultant or an accountant helps set up the records about the practice. Then the provider database is entered, including descriptions of each physician's office hours and facts about referring physicians and lab services. Finally, the insurance carrier (health plan) database is entered. It contains information about the health plans that most patients use. Each database is linked, or related, to each of the others by having at least one fact in common.

A medical billing system automatically generates completed claims by drawing needed information from its databases of information. NDCMedisoft, the computerized medical billing program used in *Computers in the Medical Office*, is an example of a computer program used in medical offices.

APPOINTMENTS

Medical billing programs often contain computerized scheduling programs to keep track of patient appointments. (Chapter 8 of this text/workbook covers this task in depth.) If the person requesting an appointment is an established patient of the practice, the scheduler searches for an available time slot that is suitable for the patient, and enters the appointment. Figure 2-1 shows an example of a computerized appointment schedule.

Using a scheduling program, the scheduler can easily cancel or reschedule appointments. Computers are also used to print daily lists of appointments for the providers in the practice. They store information about time reserved for hospital rounds, surgeries, seminars, lunches, and time out of the office. In addition, patient recall appointment notices can be generated on a timely basis.

One of the major advantages of computerized scheduling is the ability to easily find scheduled appointments in the system. For example, when a patient calls to ask when her or his next appointment is scheduled, the medical office assistant enters the patient's name in a search box, and the computer program locates the appointment.

Family Care Center

Rudner, John   **Monday, April 9, 2007**

Time	Name	Phone	Length	Notes
Monday, April 09, 2007				
8:00a	Staff Meeting		60	
1:15p	Gardiner, John	(614)726-9898	45	
2:30p	Bell, Herbert	(614)030-1111	60	
3:30p	Fitzwilliams, John	(614)002-1111	30	
4:00p	Patterson, Leila	(614)666-0099	15	
4:15p	Klein, Randall	(614)022-2693	30	

Figure 2-1 *Sample NDCMedisoft Appointment List for a Provider*

Computer scheduling also simplifies the entry of repeated appointments. Rather than needing to look through an appointment book for acceptable dates and times, the medical office assistant can have the computer program perform the search and display available dates and times.

CLAIMS AND BILLS

Billing in medical offices is based on two basic types of information:

♦ **Patient Data** Personal information about the patient, as well as information on the patient's medical insurance coverage, is entered in the program's patient database.

♦ **Transaction Data** Transaction information is taken from the encounter form and keyed into the computer program. It includes the date of the visit, diagnosis and procedures codes, lab work, prescribed medications, and payments.

Claims—the 837P

When all transaction information has been entered and checked, the medical billing program is instructed to create a claim. The program organizes the necessary databases and selects the data from each database as needed to produce a complete claim.

X12-837 Health Care Claim (837P) *HIPAA-standard format for electronic transmission of a professional claim from a provider to a health plan.*

In most physician practices, the claim is the HIPAA-standard **X12-837 Health Care Claim,** or **837P.** This claim is called the professional claim because it is used to bill for a physician's services. A hospital's claim is called an institutional claim, and there are also HIPAA dental claims and drug claims. Some small medical offices are exempt from the HIPAA requirement to send electronic claims. These practices use the CMS-1500 paper claim, which has most of the same information as the 837P Health Care Claim.

Claims may be transmitted directly between the provider's computer system and the payer's computer system, or the Internet may be used for communications between providers and health plans.

Clearinghouses

clearinghouse a service company that receives electronic or paper claims from the provider, checks and prepares them for processing, and transmits them in HIPAA-compliant format to the correct carriers.

To produce HIPAA-standard electronic claims, a medical office may choose to employ a clearinghouse instead of preparing its own claims. A **clearinghouse** is a service bureau that collects electronic insurance claims from medical practices and forwards the claims to the appropriate health plans (see Figure 2-2). Clearinghouses translate claim data to fit the HIPAA standard.

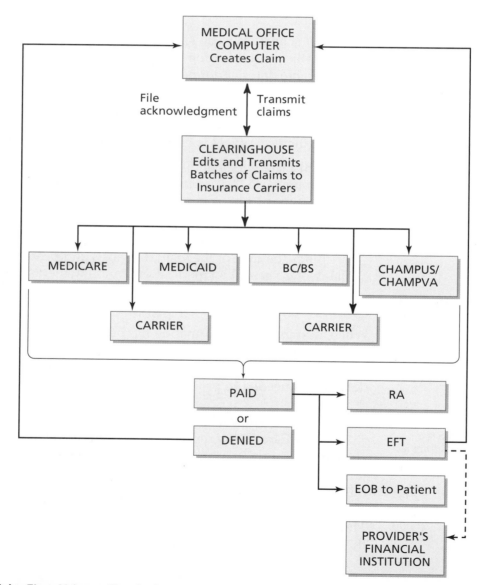

Figure 2-2 **Claim Flow Using a Clearinghouse**

When a clearinghouse receives a claim, it performs a computer **edit**, meaning that it checks to see that all necessary information is included. The edit checks obvious facts, such as whether the charges and procedure codes are appropriate for the gender of the patient and whether the patient's date of birth is not later than the date of service. For example, a pregnancy-related charge for a male patient would fail the edit process.

An **audit/edit report** is used to communicate problems that need to be corrected to the medical office (see Figure 2-3). Ensuring "clean" claims before transmission to payers greatly reduces the number of claim rejections and speeds payment.

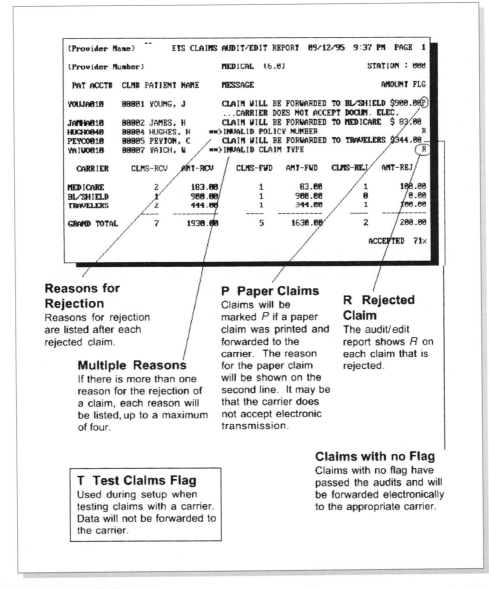

Reasons for Rejection
Reasons for rejection are listed after each rejected claim.

Multiple Reasons
If there is more than one reason for the rejection of a claim, each reason will be listed, up to a maximum of four.

P Paper Claims
Claims will be marked *P* if a paper claim was printed and forwarded to the carrier. The reason for the paper claim will be shown on the second line. It may be that the carrier does not accept electronic transmission.

R Rejected Claim
The audit/edit report shows *R* on each claim that is rejected.

T Test Claims Flag
Used during setup when testing claims with a carrier. Data will not be forwarded to the carrier.

Claims with no Flag
Claims with no flag have passed the audits and will be forwarded electronically to the appropriate carrier.

Figure 2-3 *Sample Audit/Edit Report*

Billing Services

Some practices also hire medical billing services to prepare claims. When billing services or other outside professional services such as an accounting firm are used, the pratice is required by HIPAA to have a contract with such **business associates.** The contract has procedures that the business associate must follow to ensure their compliance with HIPAA rules on privacy, security, and transactions.

business associate an organization providing services to a health care provider that involve processing protected health information, such as an accounting firm or billing service.

PAYMENTS

walkout statement a document listing charges and payments that is given to a patient after an office visit.

If the patient has made a payment after a visit, the amount is entered in the medical billing program, and a **walkout statement,** which lists the charges and the amount paid by the patient, is printed for the patient (see Figure 2-4).

Payers' payments are usually in the form of a single check that covers a number of claims (see Figure 2-5). The remittance advice (RA) that arrives with the payment gives details about each payment, such as:

♦ Provider identifier

♦ Total provider payment amount

♦ Total coinsurance amount

♦ Total contractual adjustment amount

These payments must be correctly entered in the medical billing program. This process may be done by hand, as the medical office assistant examines each payment's details and matches payments with claims. Some practices use a software program called *autoposting,* which is a part of the medical billing program. These programs access the electronic data in the HIPAA claim payment remittance advice and automatically post the payments to the system.

Family Care Center
285 Stephenson Boulevard
Stephenson, OH 60089
(614)555-0000

Page: 1

9/6/2007

Patient:	Susan Arlen 310 Oneida Lane Stephenson, OH 60089	**Instructions:** Complete the patient information portion of your insurance claim form. Attach this bill, signed and dated, and all other bills pertaining to the claim. If you have a deductible policy, hold your claim forms until you have met your deductible. Mail directly to your insurance carrier.
Chart #:	ARLENSU0	
Case #:	24	

Date	Description	Procedure	Modify	Dx 1	Dx 2	Dx 3	Dx 4	Units	Charge
9/6/2007	OF--established patient, focused	99212		466.0				1	46.00
9/6/2007	East Ohio PPO Copayment	EAPCOPAY						1	-25.00
9/6/2007	East Ohio PPO Copayment	EAPCOPAY		466.0				1	25.00

Figure 2-4 **Walkout Statement**

Payer A 123 Main Street Anywhere, USA		5678
	Date: Today's date	
Pay to the Order of: Your Business Name		$ 4,567.82
Four thousand five hundred sixty seven and 82/100 -		
First Bank of Anywhere 345 Main Street Anywhere, USA		
For	Official Signature of Payer A	

Summary Information (= the "check" information) Total Paid = $4,567.82		
Details of Claim #1	adjustments	Amount paid
Details of Claim #2	adjustments	Amount paid
Details of Claim #3	adjustments	Amount paid
Details of Claim #4	adjustments	Amount paid

Figure 2-5 **Sample Payment**

CHAPTER REVIEW

USING TERMINOLOGY

Match the terms on the left with the definitions on the right.

_F_   **1.** audit/edit report

_D_   **2.** business associate

_J_   **3.** clearinghouse

_L_   **4.** database

_B_   **5.** edit

_K_   **6.** electronic data interchange (EDI)

_E_   **7.** electronic funds transfer (EFT)

_I_   **8.** electronic medical records (EMR)

_M_   **9.** HIPAA Security Rule

_J_   **10.** HIPAA Transaction and Code Sets Standards

_G_   **11.** information technology (IT)

_H_   **12.** walkout statement

_A_   **13.** X12-837 Health Care Claim (837P)

a. A claim used by physicians' offices to bill for services.

b. The process of checking a claim to see that all required information is included.

c. Computer hardware and software systems.

d. An organization that provides services (such as claims processing or billing services) to a health care provider.

e. The movement of money via electronic systems.

f. A clearinghouse report that lists errors in a claim.

g. Regulations that require electronic transactions to use standardized formats.

h. A document listing charges and payments that is given to a patient after an office visit.

i. The electronic collection and management of health information.

j. An organization that receives claims from a provider, checks and prepares them for processing, and transmits them to insurance carriers in HIPAA-compliant format.

k. The transfer of business transactions from one computer to another using communications protocols.

l. A collection of related information.

m. Regulations outlining the minimum safeguards required to prevent unauthorized access to health care information.

CHECKING YOUR UNDERSTANDING

Write "T" or "F" in the blank to indicate whether you think the statement is true or false.

_____T_____ **14.** The HIPAA Transaction and Code Sets Standards specify standard medical code sets, such as ICD-9-CM and CPT-4.

_____F_____ **15.** Computer programs may use audit trails to help ensure the privacy and confidentiality of patient health care information.

_____F_____ **16.** All medical offices, regardless of size, must use the HIPAA-standard X12-837 claim.

_____T_____ **17.** The HIPAA standards require a practice that uses a clearinghouse to have a contract that states the procedures that must be followed to ensure HIPAA compliance.

_____T_____ **18.** Computerized databases are more efficient than manual filing systems.

Answer the question below in the space provided.

19. List five advantages of using computers in a medical practice.

It's more organized meaning less storage space is needed.
Info is easier to find info.
Files can be used by more than one person at a time
Computer use reduces errors
It save an enormous amount of time.

Choose the best answer.

_____A_____ **20.** The HIPAA Security Rule specifies the _____, technical, and physical safeguards required to prevent unauthorized access to health care information.
a. administrative
b. clinical
c. legal

_B_ **21.** Electronic medical records are used to record data such as physicians' reports of examinations, surgical procedures, tests results, and:
   a. billing codes
   b. X-rays
   c. insurance claims

_C_ **22.** Many medical offices assign _____ to individuals who have access to computer data, as a security measure.
   a. identification numbers
   b. private offices
   c. passwords

_A_ **23.** The HIPAA-standard electronic format for the exchange of payment and remittance advice is the:
   a. X12-835
   b. X12-278
   c. X12-271

_C_ **24.** _____ reports are designed to provide payers with "clean" claims, thus reducing the number of claim rejections due to missing or incorrect data.
   a. clearinghouse
   b. electronic data interchange
   c. audit/edit

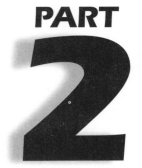

NDCMedisoft Advanced Training

PART 2

Introduction to NDCMedisoft

WHAT YOU NEED TO KNOW

To use this chapter, you need to know how to:

◆ Start your computer and Microsoft Windows (98 or later version).

◆ Use the keyboard and mouse.

OBJECTIVES

When you finish this chapter, you will be able to:

◆ Start NDCMedisoft.

◆ Use the Student Data Disk.

◆ Move around the NDCMedisoft menus.

◆ Use the NDCMedisoft toolbar.

◆ Enter, edit, and delete data in NDCMedisoft.

◆ Save and back up NDCMedisoft data.

◆ Use NDCMedisoft's Help features.

◆ Make a backup copy of the database files while exiting NDCMedisoft.

◆ Exit NDCMedisoft.

KEY TERMS

backup data
knowledge base
MMDDCCYY format

WHAT IS NDCMEDISOFT?

NDCMedisoft is a patient accounting software program. Information on patients, providers, insurance carriers, and patient and insurance billing is stored and processed by the system. NDCMedisoft is widely used by medical practices throughout the United States. It is typically used to accomplish the following daily work in a medical practice:

◆ Enter information on new patients, and change information on established patients as needed

◆ Enter transactions, such as charges, to patients' accounts

◆ Record payments and adjustments from patients and insurance companies

◆ Print walkout statements and remainder statements for patients

◆ Submit insurance claims to payers

◆ Print standard reports

◆ Create custom reports

◆ Schedule appointments

Many of the general working concepts used in operating NDCMedisoft are similar to those in other software programs. Thus, you should be able to transfer many skills taught in this book to other patient accounting programs.

HOW NDCMEDISOFT DATA ARE ORGANIZED AND STORED

Information entered into NDCMedisoft is stored in databases. As defined in Chapter 2, a database is a collection of related pieces of information.

NDCMEDISOFT DATABASES

NDCMedisoft stores these major types of data:

◆ **Provider Data** The provider database has information about the physician(s) as well as the practice, such as its name and address, phone number, and tax and medical identifier numbers.

◆ **Patient Data** Each patient information form is stored in the patient database. The patient's unique chart number and personal information—name and address, phone number, birth date, Social Security number, gender, marital status, and employer—are examples of information stored in this database.

◆ **Insurance Carriers** The insurance carrier database contains information on each carrier's EDI requirements for claims, often referred to as electronic claim submission.

- **Diagnosis Codes** The diagnosis code database contains the *International Classification of Diseases,* Ninth Revision, *Clinical Modification* (ICD) codes that indicate the reasons service is provided. The codes entered in this database are those most frequently used by the practice. The practice's encounter form or superbill often serves as a source document when the NDCMedisoft system is first set up.

- **Procedure Codes** The procedure code database contains the data needed to create charges. The *Current Procedural Terminology* (CPT) codes most often used by the practice are selected for this database. The practice's encounter form is often a good source document for the codes. Other claim data elements, such as place of service (POS) and the charge for each procedure, are also stored in the procedure code database.

- **Transactions** The transaction database stores information about each patient's visits, diagnoses, and procedures, as well as received and outstanding payments. Transactions in the form of charges, payments, and adjustments are also stored in the transaction database.

Within NDCMedisoft, each database is linked, or related, to each of the others by having at least one fact in common. For example, information entered in the patient database is shared with the transaction database, linking the two. Information is entered only once; NDCMedisoft selects the data from each database as needed.

THE STUDENT DATA DISK

Before a medical office begins using NDCMedisoft, basic information about the practice and its patients must be entered in the computer. For the exercises you will complete in this book, the preliminary work has been done for you. The NDCMedisoft database for these exercises is located on the Student Data Disk located inside the back cover.

MAKING A COPY OF THE STUDENT DATA DISK

Before you begin using the Student Data Disk, you need to make a working copy of it, following the instructions below. When you are finished making the disk copy, store the original Student Data Disk in a safe place. You may need to use it to make another copy if the working disk is accidentally damaged or lost.

Note: These instructions assume the use of a floppy disk. If you are using an alternate media for saving your work, ask your instructor for help.

Complete the following steps to make a copy of the Student Data Disk.

Note: These instructions assume that Microsoft Windows 98 or a later version is installed on your computer.

1. Turn on the computer and monitor.

2. After the Windows desktop is displayed, insert the Student Data Disk in the 3 1/2" floppy drive (drive A).

3. Double-click the My Computer icon on the desktop. (In some versions of Windows, open the Start menu to display the My Computer icon.) The My Computer window is displayed.

4. Click the icon labeled 3 1/2 Floppy (A:).

5. On the File menu, select Copy Disk. The Copy Disk dialog box is displayed.

6. Make sure the Copy From and Copy To windows both have 3 1/2 Floppy (A:) highlighted or displayed.

7. Click the Start button. The computer begins reading the files on the source disk. You can monitor the computer's progress by viewing the bar above the words "Reading source disk."

8. When the system prompts you to insert the disk you want to copy to (the destination disk), eject the Student Data Disk from the drive.

9. Insert a blank disk in the floppy drive, and click the OK button. The files are copied to the destination disk. Again, you can monitor the progress by looking at the bar above the words "Writing to destination disk."

10. When the copy is completed, the message "Copy completed successfully" is displayed. Eject the disk from the drive, and label it "Working Copy FCC8."

11. Close the Copy Disk dialog box by clicking the Close button.

12. Close the My Computer dialog box by clicking the Close button (in this case, the X in the upper-right corner).

STARTING NDCMEDISOFT AND RESTORING THE BACKUP FILE

The following instructions take you through the steps of starting the NDCMedisoft program the first time the program is used with this text. These steps start the program, create a new directory and data set name for the Family Care Center files, and restore the backup file to the new directory.

1. While holding down the F7 key, click Start, Programs, NDCMedisoft, and NDCMedisoft Advanced Patient Accounting to start NDCMedisoft. When the Find NDCMedisoft Database dialog box appears, release the F7 key. (The F7 key bypasses any starting directions that may have been left in the program by a previous user.) This dialog box asks you to enter the NDCMedisoft data directory.

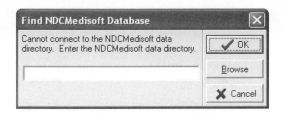

2. Click inside the white data entry box to make it active. Then key **C:\MediData** in the space provided (where C is the letter that represents the hard drive you will be using). The dialog box should now look like this:

3. Click the OK button. An Information dialog box appears with the following message, "This is not an existing root data directory. Do you want to create a new one?"

4. Click Yes. *Note:* If a Warning Box appears with information about registering the program, click the Register Later button. The Create Data dialog box is displayed.

5. Click the Create a New Set of Data button. The Create a New Set of Data dialog box appears. In the upper box, key *Family Care Center.* In the lower box, key *FCC8.* The dialog box should now look like this:

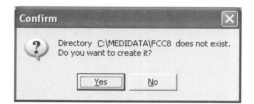

6. Click the Create button. A Confirm dialog box is displayed.

7. Click the Yes button. The Practice Information dialog box appears. In the Practice Name box, key *Family Care Center.* The remaining boxes can remain blank. The dialog box should now look like this:

8. Click the Save button. The main window of the NDCMedisoft program is displayed. Your screen should look like this:

9. Insert the working copy of the Student Data Disk in the floppy drive. (This is usually the A: drive; if your computer uses a different letter to represent the floppy drive, please substitute that letter for "A:" whenever it appears in these instructions.)

10. Open the File menu and locate the Restore Data option.

11. Click Restore Data. A Warning dialog box is displayed.

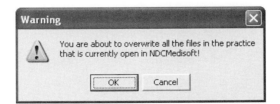

12. Click the OK button. The Restore dialog box is displayed. In the top box, key *A:\FCC8.mbk* if it is not already displayed. The dialog box should now look like this:

```
┌─────────────────────────────────────────────────┐
│ Restore                                      [X]  │
├─────────────────────────────────────────────────┤
│  Backup File Path and Name                        │
│  ┌──────────────────────────────────┐  ┌──────┐  │
│  │ A:\FCC8.mbk                      │  │ Find │  │
│  └──────────────────────────────────┘  └──────┘  │
│  Existing Backup Files                            │
│  ┌──────────────────────────────────────────────┐│
│  │ FCC8.mbk                                      ││
│  │                                               ││
│  │                                               ││
│  │                                               ││
│  └──────────────────────────────────────────────┘│
│                                                   │
│  Password:                                        │
│  ┌──────────────────────────────────────────────┐│
│  │                                               ││
│  └──────────────────────────────────────────────┘│
│                                                   │
│  Destination Path              ┌──────────────┐   │
│  ┌──────────────────────────┐  │ Start Restore│   │
│  │ C:\Medidata\FCC8\        │  └──────────────┘   │
│  └──────────────────────────┘                     │
│  Backup Progress               ┌──────────────┐   │
│  ┌──────────────────────────┐  │ [X]  Close   │   │
│  │         0%               │  └──────────────┘   │
│  └──────────────────────────┘                     │
│  File Progress                 ┌──────────────┐   │
│  ┌──────────────────────────┐  │      Help    │   │
│  │         0%               │  └──────────────┘   │
│  └──────────────────────────┘                     │
│  ┌──────────────────────────────────────────────┐│
│  └──────────────────────────────────────────────┘│
└─────────────────────────────────────────────────┘
```

13. Click the Start Restore button. A Confirm dialog box is displayed.

```
┌─────────────────────────────────────┐
│ Confirm                        [X]   │
├─────────────────────────────────────┤
│  (?)  About to restore file A:\FCC8.mbk │
│                                      │
│      ┌──────┐   ┌────────┐           │
│      │  OK  │   │ Cancel │           │
│      └──────┘   └────────┘           │
└─────────────────────────────────────┘
```

14. Click the OK button. After the program restores the database to the hard drive, an Information dialog box is displayed, indicating that the restore is complete. Click OK.

```
┌──────────────────────────────┐
│ Information          [X]      │
├──────────────────────────────┤
│  (i)  Restore complete.       │
│                               │
│        ┌──────┐               │
│        │  OK  │               │
│        └──────┘               │
└──────────────────────────────┘
```

15. You are returned to the main NDCMedisoft window. To open the newly restored data, open the File menu and locate the Open Practice option.

16. Click Open Practice. The Open Practice dialog box is displayed, with the Family Care Center practice name listed.

Open Practice

Family Care Center	✓ OK
	✗ Cancel
	New
	Delete
	Add Tutorial
	Help

17. To open the Family Care Center database files, click the OK button.

18. The database is now ready for use. (*Hint:* If the main NDCMedisoft window does not fill the screen, click the Maximize button to expand it.)

19. To verify that the data has been restored from the Student Data Disk, click Practice Information on the File menu. The Practice Information dialog box should now look like this:

Practice Information

Practice | Billing Service

Practice Name: Family Care Center
Street: 285 Stephenson Boulevard

City: Stephenson   State: OH
Zip Code: 60089

Phone: (614)555-0000   Extension:
Fax Phone: (614)555-0001
Type: Medical
Federal Tax ID: 033987562

Extra 1:
Extra 2:

Save
Cancel
Help

20. Close the Practice Information dialog box.

21. For now, keep the NDCMedisoft program open, as it is required to complete the remaining exercises in the chapter.

THE NDCMEDISOFT MENU BAR

NDCMedisoft offers choices of actions through a series of menus. Commands are issued by clicking an option on the menu bar or by clicking a shortcut button on the toolbar. The menu bar lists the names of the menus in NDCMedisoft: File, Edit, Activities, Lists, Reports, Tools, Window, Help, and Services (see Figure 3-1). Beneath each menu name is a pull-down menu with one or more options.

File Menu   The File menu is used to enter information about the medical office practice when first setting up NDCMedisoft. It is also used to back up data, restore data, set program security options, and change the program date (see Figure 3-2).

Edit Menu   The Edit menu contains the basic commands needed to move, change, and delete information (see Figure 3-3). These commands are Cut, Copy, Paste, and Delete.

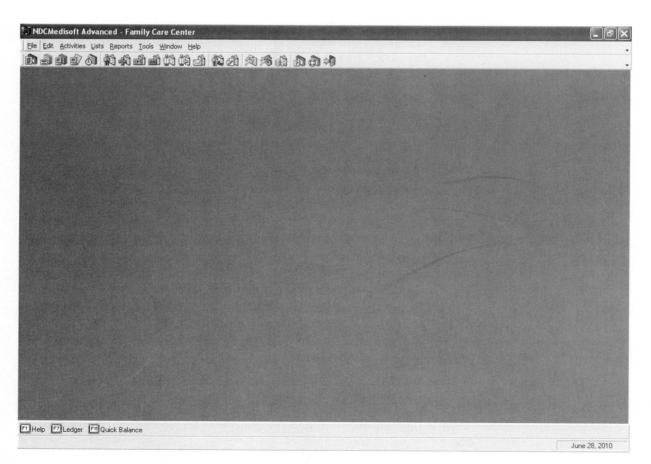

Figure 3-1 **Main NDCMedisoft Window**

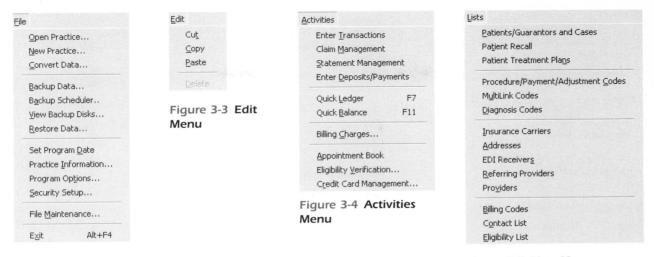

Figure 3-3 **Edit Menu**

Figure 3-4 **Activities Menu**

Figure 3-2 **File Menu**

Figure 3-5 **Lists Menu**

Activities Menu Most medical office data collected on a day-to-day basis are entered through options on the Activities menu (see Figure 3-4). This menu is used to enter financial transactions, create insurance claims, manage patient statements, view summaries of patient account information, calculate billing charges, and to access Office Hours, NDCMedisoft's built-in appointment scheduler. Transactions include charges, payments, and adjustments.

Lists Menu Information on new patients, such as name, address, and employer, is entered through the Lists menu (see Figure 3-5). If an established patient's information needs to be changed, it is updated through this menu. The Lists menu also provides access to lists of codes, insurance carriers, and providers. These lists may be updated and printed when necessary.

Reports Menu The Reports menu is used to print reports about patients' accounts and the practice (see Figure 3-6 on page 44). NDCMedisoft comes with a number of standard report formats, such as day sheets, aging reports, and patient ledgers. Practices may create their own report formats using the Design Custom Reports and Bills option.

Tools Menu The built-in calculator is accessed through the Tools menu. Other options on the Tools menu can be used to view the contents of a file as well as a profile of the computer system (see Figure 3-7 on page 44).

Window Menu Using the Window menu, it is possible to switch back and forth between several open windows (see Figure 3-8 on page 44). The Window menu also has an option to close all windows.

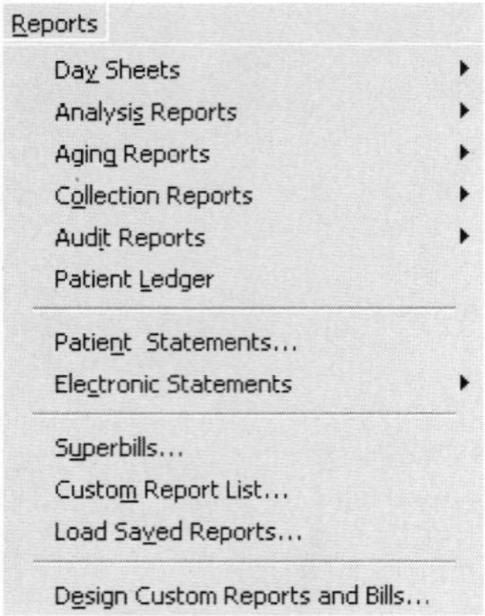

Reports

Day Sheets ▶
Analysis Reports ▶
Aging Reports ▶
Collection Reports ▶
Audit Reports ▶
Patient Ledger
_____
Patient Statements...
Electronic Statements ▶
_____
Superbills...
Custom Report List...
Load Saved Reports...
_____
Design Custom Reports and Bills...

Figure 3-6 **Reports Menu**

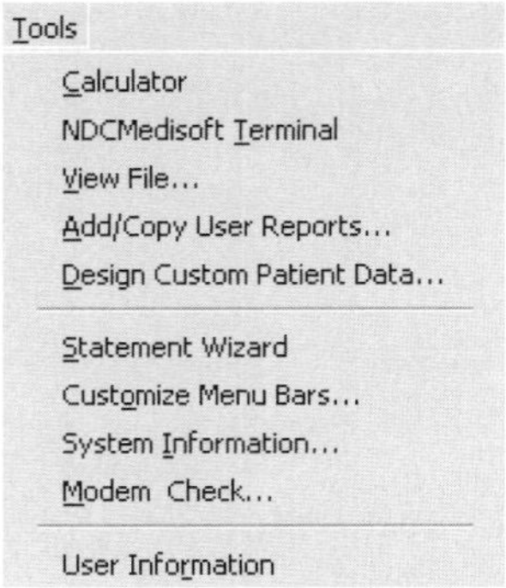

Tools

Calculator
NDCMedisoft Terminal
View File...
Add/Copy User Reports...
Design Custom Patient Data...
_____
Statement Wizard
Customize Menu Bars...
System Information...
Modem Check...
_____
User Information

Figure 3-7 **Tools Menu**

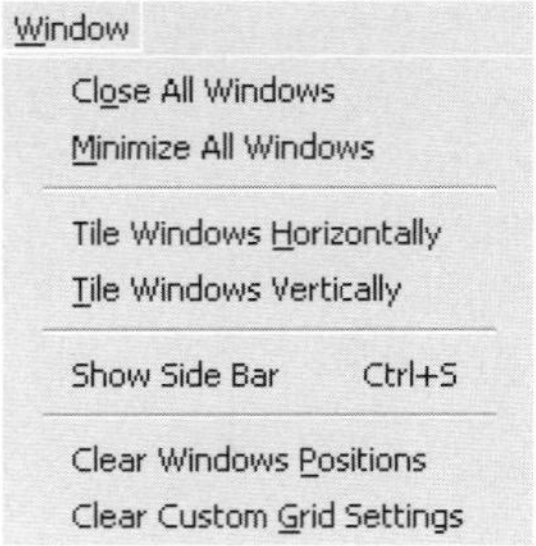

Window

Close All Windows
Minimize All Windows
_____
Tile Windows Horizontally
Tile Windows Vertically
_____
Show Side Bar   Ctrl+S
_____
Clear Windows Positions
Clear Custom Grid Settings

Figure 3-8 **Window Menu**

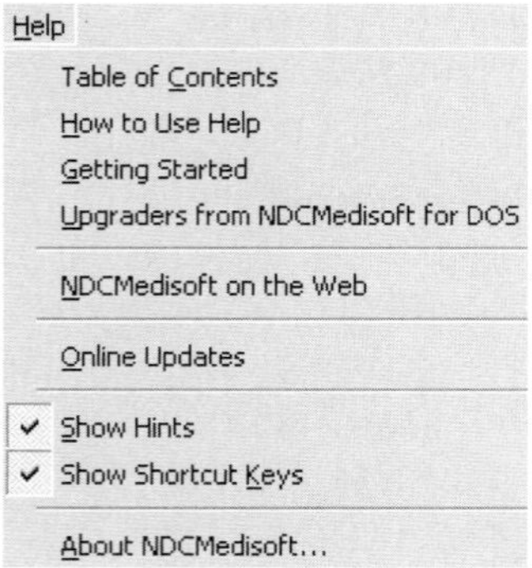

Help

Table of Contents
How to Use Help
Getting Started
Upgraders from NDCMedisoft for DOS
_____
NDCMedisoft on the Web
_____
Online Updates
_____
✓ Show Hints
✓ Show Shortcut Keys
_____
About NDCMedisoft...

Figure 3-9 **Help Menu**

Help Menu   The Help menu, shown in Figure 3-9, is used to access NDCMedisoft's built-in Help feature and also provides a link to NDCMedisoft support on the World Wide Web.

Exercise 3-1

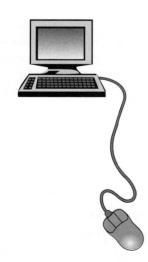

Practice using the NDCMedisoft menus.

1. **Start NDCMedisoft, if it is not already running.**

2. **Click the Lists menu on the menu bar.**

3. **Click Patients/Guarantors and Cases. The Patient List dialog box is displayed.**

4. **Click the Close button at the bottom of the dialog box.**

5. **Click the Activities menu.**

6. **Click Enter Transactions. The Transaction Entry dialog box appears.**

7. **Click the Close button.**

THE NDCMEDISOFT TOOLBAR

Located below the menu bar, the toolbar contains a series of buttons with icons that represent the most common activities performed in NDCMedisoft. These buttons are shortcuts for frequently used menu commands. The toolbar displays twenty buttons (see Figure 3-10 on page 46 and Table 3-1).

Table 3-1   NDCMedisoft Toolbar Buttons

Button	Button Name	Opens	Activity
	Transaction Entry	Transaction Entry dialog box	Enter, edit, or delete transactions
	Credit Card Management	Credit Card Management dialog box	Process credit card payments
	Claim Management	Claim Management dialog box	Create and transmit insurance claims
	Statement Management	Statement Management dialog box	Create statements
	Appointment Book	Office Hours	Schedule appointments
	Patient List	Patient List dialog box	Enter patient information
	Insurance Carrier List	Insurance Carrier List dialog box	Enter insurance carriers
	Procedure Code List	Procedure/Payment/Adjustment List dialog box	Enter procedure codes
	Diagnosis Code List	Diagnosis Code List dialog box	Enter diagnosis codes
	Provider List	Provider List dialog box	Enter providers
	Referring Provider List	Referring Provider List dialog box	Enter referring providers
	Address List	Address List dialog box	Enter addresses
	Patient Recall Entry	Patient Recall Entry dialog box	Enter Patient Recall data
	Custom Report List	Open Report dialog box	Open a custom report
	Quick Ledger	Quick Ledger dialog box	View a patient's ledger
	Quick Balance	Quick Balance dialog box	View a patient's balance
	Enter Deposits and Apply Payments	Deposit List dialog box	Enter deposits and payments
	Show/Hide Hints	Show or Hide Hints	Turn the Hints feature on and off
	Help	NDCMedisoft Help	Access NDCMedisoft's built-in help feature
	Exit Program	Exit Program	Exit the NDCMedisoft program

Figure 3-10 **NDCMedisoft Toolbar**

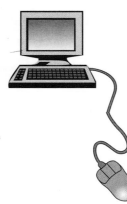

Exercise 3-2

Practice using buttons on the toolbar.

1. **Click the Provider List button. The Provider List dialog box opens.**

2. **Close the dialog box.**

3. **Click the Procedure Code List button. The Procedure/Payment/Adjustment List dialog box is displayed.**

4. **Close the dialog box.**

ENTERING AND EDITING DATA

All data, whether patients' addresses or charges for procedures, are entered into NDCMedisoft through the menus on the menu bar or through the buttons on the toolbar. Selecting an option from the menus or toolbar brings up a dialog box. The Tab key is used to move between text boxes within a dialog box. In some dialog boxes, information is entered by keying data into a text box. For example, a patient's name would be keyed directly into a text box. At other times selections are made from a list of choices already present. For example, when entering the name of the provider a patient is seeing, the provider is selected from a drop-down list of providers already in the system.

DATES   NDCMedisoft is a date-sensitive program. When transactions are entered in the program, the dates must be accurate, or the data will be of little value to the practice. Many times, date-sensitive information is not entered into NDCMedisoft on the same day that the event or transaction occurred. For example, Friday afternoon's office visits may not be entered into the program until Monday. If the NDCMedisoft Program Date is not changed to Friday's date before entering the data, all the information entered on Monday will be stored as Monday's transactions. For this reason, it is important to know how to change the NDCMedisoft Program Date.

For most of the exercises in this book, you will need to change the NDCMedisoft Program Date to the date specified at the beginning of the exercise. The following steps are used to change the NDCMedisoft Program Date:

July, 2010
Sun Mon Tue Wed Thu Fri Sat
1 2 3
4 5 6 7 8 9 10
11 12 13 14 15 16 17
18 19 20 21 22 23 24
25 26 27 28 29 30 31
Today: 7/12/2010

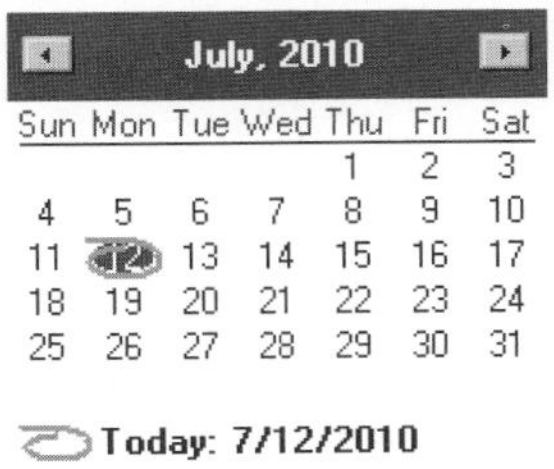

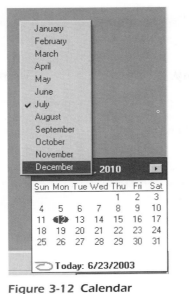

Figure 3-11 NDCMedisoft Pop-Up Calendar

January
February
March
April
May
June
July
August
September
October
November
December
, 2010
Sun Mon Tue Wed Thu Fri Sat
1 2 3
4 5 6 7 8 9 10
11 12 13 14 15 16 17
18 19 20 21 22 23 24
25 26 27 28 29 30 31
Today: 6/23/2003

Figure 3-12 Calendar Month Pop-Up List

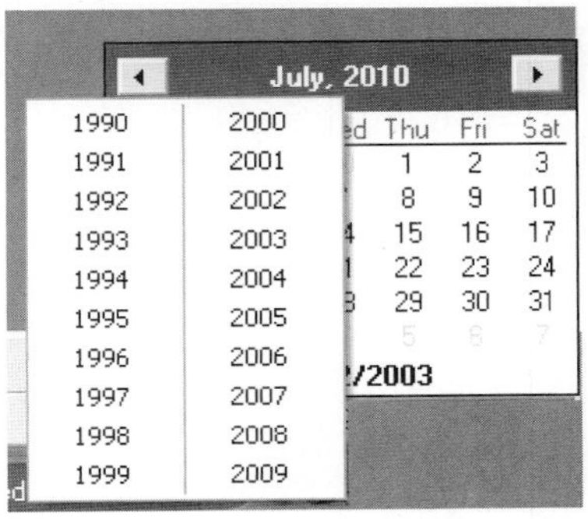
July, 2010
1990 2000
1991 2001
1992 2002
1993 2003
1994 2004
1995 2005
1996 2006
1997 2007
1998 2008
1999 2009
Thu Fri Sat

Figure 3-13 Calendar Year Pop-Up List

1. Click Set Program Date on the File menu. A pop-up calendar is displayed (see Figure 3-11).
2. To change the month, click the name of the current month, and a pop-up list of months appears (see Figure 3-12). Click the desired month on the pop-up list.
3. To change the year, follow the same procedure. Click the current year, and select the desired year from the pop-up list (see Figure 3-13). Note that only 1990 through 2009 are listed. To change the calendar to 2010, click 2009, and then click the right arrow button to advance one month at a time until 2010 is reached.
4. Select the desired day of the month by clicking on that date in the calendar. The calendar closes, and the desired date is displayed on the status bar.

MMDDCCYY format a specific way in which dates must be keyed, in which "MM" stands for the month, "DD" stands for the day, "CC" represents century, and "YY" stands for the year.

In most NDCMedisoft dialog boxes, dates are entered in the MMDDCCYY format. The **MMDDCCYY** format is a specific way in which dates must be keyed. "MM" stands for the month, "DD" stands for the day, "CC" represents century, and "YY" stands for the year. Each day, month, century, and year entry must contain two digits, and no punctuation can be used. For example, February 1, 2010, would be keyed as "02012010."

Note that if a future date is entered, NDCMedisoft displays a Confirm dialog box (see Figure 3-14 on page 48). When this box appears throughout the exercises in this book, click No.

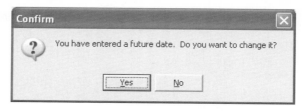

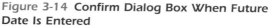

Figure 3-14 **Confirm Dialog Box When Future Date Is Entered**

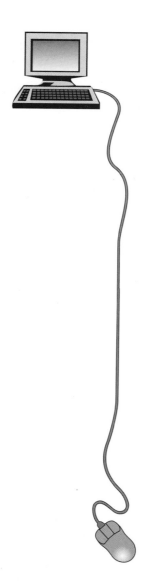

Exercise 3-3

Practice entering information and correcting errors.

1. Click the Activities menu.

2. Click Enter Transactions.

3. Click the triangle button in the Chart box. The Chart drop-down list is opened (see Figure 3-15).

4. To select James Smith, key the first two letters of his chart number (SMITHJA∅): **SM.** Notice that when "SM" is keyed, the system goes to the entry for the first patient whose chart number begins with "SM," in this case James Smith.

5. Press the Tab key.

6. To edit a transaction, click in the field that needs to be changed. Click in the Procedure field. Notice that the entry in the field becomes highlighted.

7. Click again in the Procedure field. A pop-up list of procedure codes is displayed.

8. Select a new code from the list by clicking on it. Scroll down the pop-up list of codes and click 99396. Notice that the new code is displayed in the Procedure field, but the entry in the Amount field has not changed. This does not happen until the Tab key is pressed. Press the Tab key now, and watch the entry in the Amount field change.

9. Press the Tab key repeatedly, and watch as the cursor moves from box to box.

10. Exit the Transaction Entry dialog box by clicking the Close button or by clicking the close icon in the top right corner of the dialog box. An Information box is displayed, asking whether the changes should be saved (see Figure 3-16). In this case, click the No button. The changes are not saved and the Transaction Entry window closes.

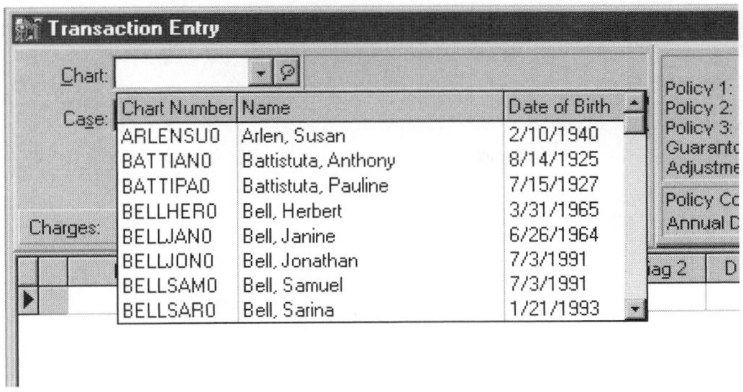

Figure 3-15 **Transaction Entry Chart Drop-Down List**

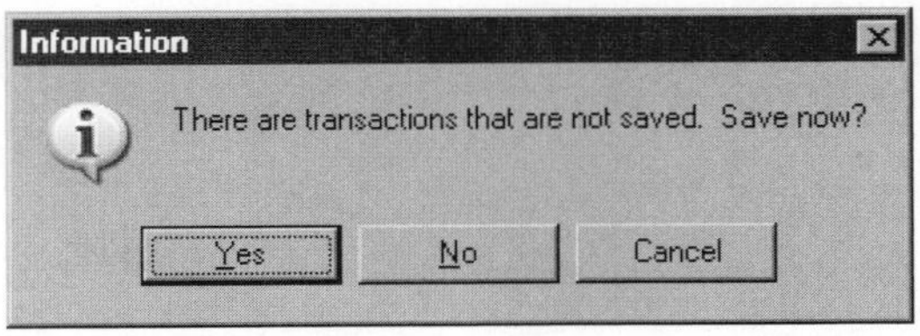

Figure 3-16 **Transaction Entry Save Warning Dialog Box**

SAVING AND DELETING DATA

Information entered into NDCMedisoft is saved by clicking the Save button that appears in most dialog boxes. In some NDCMedisoft dialog boxes, there are buttons for deleting data. For example, to delete an insurance carrier, the entry for the carrier is clicked in the Insurance Carrier List dialog box. Then the Delete button is clicked. NDCMedisoft will ask for a confirmation before deleting the data. In other dialog boxes, such as the Patient/Guarantor dialog box, there is no button for deleting data. In this situation, select the text that is to be deleted, and click the right mouse button. A shortcut menu is displayed that contains an option to delete the entry.

USING NDCMEDISOFT HELP

NDCMedisoft offers users three different types of help.

Hints   As the cursor moves over certain fields, hints appears on the status bar at the bottom of the screen. For example, in Figure 3-17, on page 50, the status bar displays a hint about editing the selected record.

Built-in   For more detailed help, NDCMedisoft has an extensive help feature built into the program itself, which is accessed through the Help menu.

Online   The Help menu also provides access to NDCMedisoft help available on the NDCMedisoft corporate Web site, http://www.ndcmedisoft.com. The Web site contains a searchable **knowledge base,** which is a collection of up-to-date technical information about NDCMedisoft products.

knowledge base a collection of up-to-date technical information.

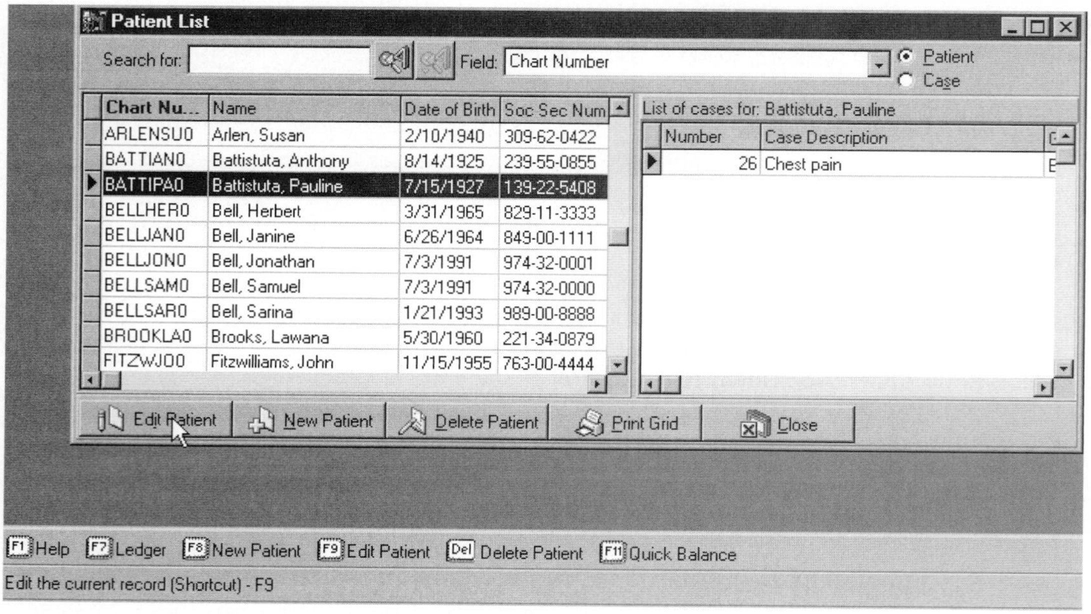

Figure 3-17 Hint Displayed on Status Bar

Exercise 3-4

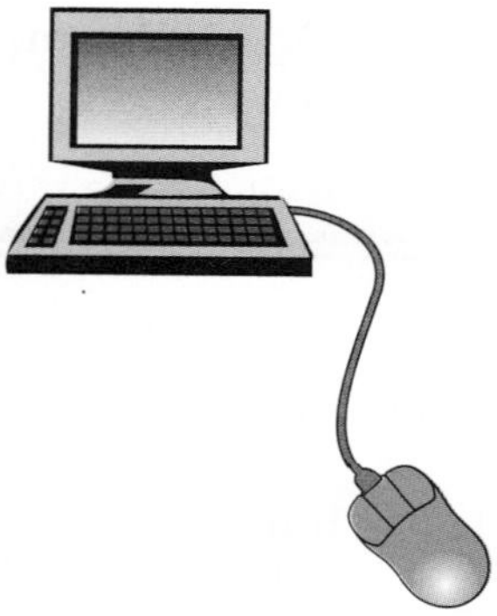

Practice using NDCMedisoft's built-in help feature.

1. Click the Help menu.

2. Click Table of Contents. NDCMedisoft displays a list of topics for which help is available.

3. Locate Diagnosis Entry in the left column. Click on Diagnosis Entry. Information on entering diagnosis codes is displayed on the right side of the window.

4. Click the Close button in the upper right corner to close the Help window.

Exercise 3-5

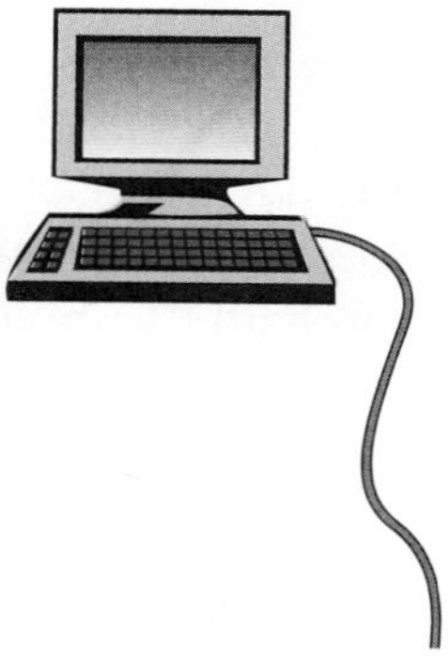

Practice using NDCMedisoft's online help.

1. Access the Internet. Click NDCMedisoft on the Web > Knowledge Base on the Help menu (see Figure 3-18). The knowledge base area of the Web site is displayed.

2. Select Medisoft Patient Accounting on the drop-down list that appears.

3. Enter Transaction Entry.

4. Click the Search button. A list of articles related to transaction entry appears.

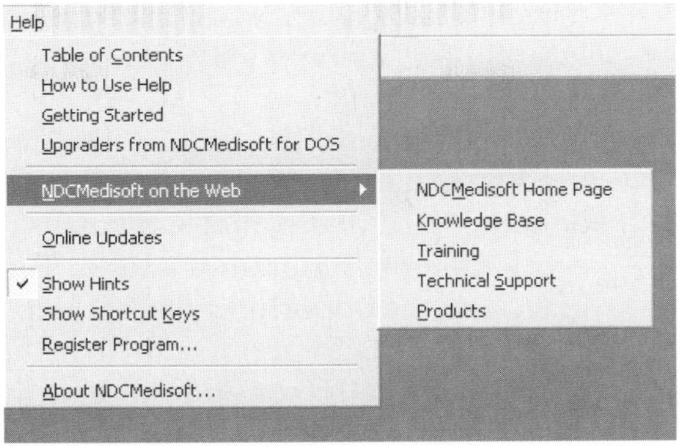

Figure 3-18 **NDCMedisoft on the Web Submenu**

5. **Select an article to read, and click on the title. The article appears.**

6. **Terminate your Internet connection, if appropriate.**

EXITING NDCMEDISOFT

NDCMedisoft is exited by clicking Exit on the File menu or by clicking the Exit button on the toolbar. To avoid the inconvenience of exiting NDCMedisoft when the computer is needed for a different program, and then restarting it, NDCMedisoft can be made temporarily inactive by using the Minimize button, the first of the three small buttons displayed in the upper-right corner of the window. NDCMedisoft can be reactivated at any time by clicking the NDCMedisoft button on the Windows taskbar.

MAKING A BACKUP FILE WHILE EXITING NDCMEDISOFT

backup data a copy of data files made at a specific point in time that can be used to restore data to the system.

Data are periodically saved on removable media, such as CDs or floppy disks, through a process known as backing up. **Backup data** is an extra copy of data files made at a specific time that can be used to restore data in the event they are accidentally lost or destroyed. Backups are performed on a regular schedule, determined by the practice. Many practices back up data at the end of each day.

In an instructional environment, files are also backed up regularly to store each student's work securely and separately. If you are a student working in a computer lab, it is important to make a backup copy of your work after you complete the exercises in each chapter. This ensures that you can restore your work during the next session and be sure of using your own data, even if another student uses the computer during the interim or if, for any reason, the data on the hard drive have been changed or corrupted. Backup files may be saved to a variety of media (floppy disk, CD, hard drive, network drive). Check with your instructor to determine the appropriate location for saving your backup files.

In NDCMedisoft, the Backup Data option on the File menu can be used to make a backup copy of the active database at any time. By default, NDCMedisoft also displays a Backup Reminder dialog box every time the program is exited. The Backup Reminder dialog box gives you the opportunity to back up your work every time you exit NDCMedisoft. To perform the backup, the Back Up Data Now button is clicked. To continue to exit the program without making a backup, the Exit Program button is clicked. The following exercise provides practice.

Exercise 3-6

Practice backing up your work when exiting NDCMedisoft. *Note:* This exercise assumes files are being backed up to a floppy drive (A:). If this is not the case, substitute the appropriate drive letter for the location of your backup file.

1. To exit NDCMedisoft, click Exit on the File menu, or click the Exit button on the toolbar.

2. The Backup Reminder dialog box appears, displaying three options: Back Up Data Now, Exit Program, or Cancel (see Figure 3-19). To begin the backup, make sure your working copy of the Student Data Disk is inserted in Drive A:. Then click Back Up Data Now.

3. The Backup dialog box is displayed (see Figure 3-20). Depending on the last time the dialog box was accessed, the Destination File Path and Name box may already contain the entry A:\FCC8.mbk. If the box is blank, or if it contains something other than this, key *A:\FCC8.mbk* in the Destination File Path and Name box.

Backup Reminder

Your data should be kept safe. A backup of your data should be made on a different disk or tape. A backup is a copy of your data files that can be used if your working data files are lost or damaged. IF YOUR DATA BECOMES DAMAGED, YOUR ONLY RECOURSE IS TO RESTORE YOUR DATA FROM A BACKUP THAT YOU HAVE MADE.

A backup of your data should be made on a DAILY basis, using a different diskette (or tape) for each day of the week.

PLEASE, BACK UP YOUR DATA!

[Back Up Data Now]   [Exit Program]   [Cancel]

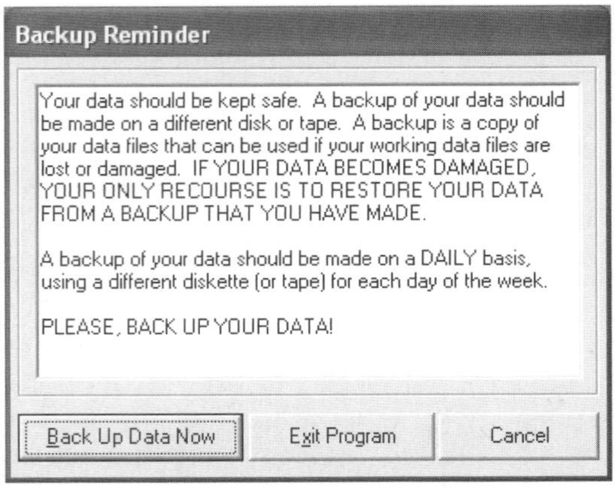

Figure 3-19 Backup Reminder Dialog Box

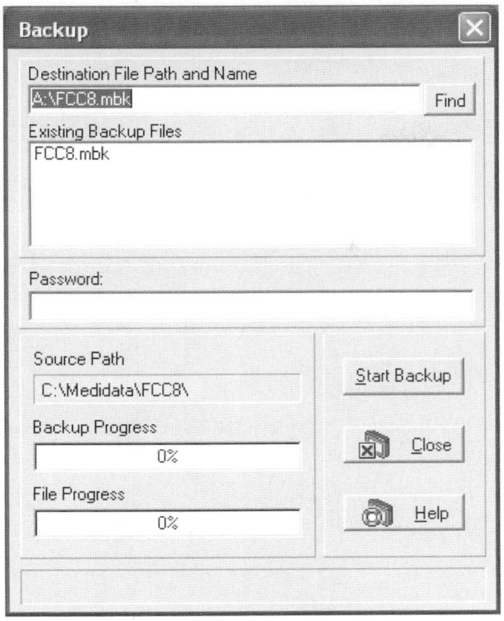

Figure 3-20 Backup Dialog Box

4. **NDCMedisoft automatically displays the location of the data-base files to be backed up in the Source Path box in the lower half of the dialog box. Click the Start Backup button.**

5. **The program backs up the latest database files to the disk in Drive A:, and displays an Information dialog box indicating that the backup is complete. Click OK to continue.**

6. **The Backup dialog box disappears, and the NDCMedisoft program closes.**

RESTORING THE BACKUP FILE

When a new NDCMedisoft session begins, the following steps can be used to restore the backup file if required. If you share a computer in an instructional environment, it is recommended that you perform a restore before each new session to be sure you are working with your own data. *Note:* These instructions assume files are being backed up to a floppy drive (A:). If this is not the case, substitute the appropriate drive letter for your backup file.

To restore A:\FCC8.mbk to C:\Medidata\FCC8:

1. Start NDCMedisoft.

2. Check the program's title bar at the top of the screen to make sure the Family Care Center data set is the active data set. (If it is not, use the Open Practice option on the File menu to select it.)

3. Insert your working copy of the Student Data Disk in Drive A:.

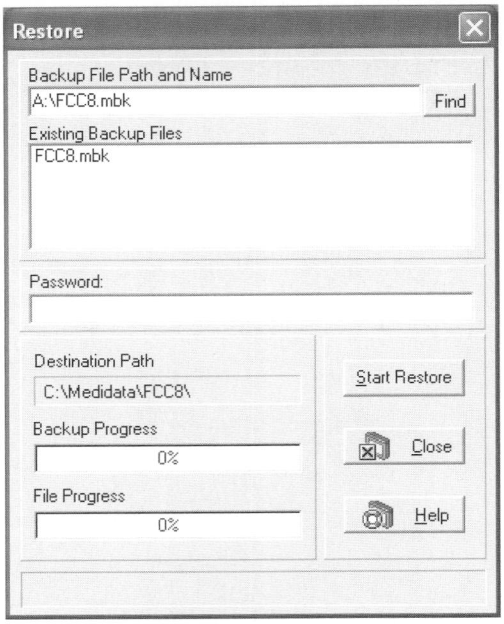

Figure 3-21 Restore Dialog Box

4. Open the File menu and click Restore Data.

5. When the Warning box appears, click OK.

6. The Restore dialog box appears (see Figure 3-21). In the Backup File Path and Name box at the top of the dialog box (if the following name is not already displayed), key *A:\FCC8.mbk*.

7. The Destination Path at the bottom of the box should already say C:\Medidata\FCC8\. Do not change this.

8. Click the Start Restore button.

9. When the Confirm box appears, click OK.

10. After the files are restored, an Information dialog box appears, indicating the restore is complete. Click OK to continue.

11. The Restore dialog box disappears. You are ready to begin the next session.

USING TERMINOLOGY

Match the terms on the left with the definitions on the right.

___C___ 1. backup data

___A___ 2. knowledge base

___B___ 3. MMDDCCYY format

a. A searchable collection of up-to-date technical information.

b. A way in which dates must be keyed.

c. A copy of data files made at a specific point in time that can be used to restore data to the system.

CHECKING YOUR UNDERSTANDING

Answer the questions below in the space provided.

4. Describe two ways of issuing a command in NDCMedisoft.

_____

_____

5. What are two ways data are entered in a box?

1) through the menubar

2) through the button on the toolbar

6. What three types of NDCMedisoft help are available?

Hints, Builtin and online

_____

7. Which menu provides access to Office Hours, NDCMedisoft's scheduling feature?

_____

_____

8. What is the purpose of the buttons on the toolbar?

_____

_____

9. What is the format for entering dates in NDCMedisoft?

_____

_____

10. Describe two ways of exiting NDCMedisoft.

_____

_____

APPLYING KNOWLEDGE

11. Use NDCMedisoft's built-in Help to look up information on the following topics:

   • How to enter diagnosis codes

   • How to print procedure code lists

AT THE COMPUTER

Answer the following questions at the computer.

12. How many options are there in the Reports menu?

13. What is the first choice on the Lists menu?

14. List the options on the Activities menu.

15. Set the NDCMedisoft Program Date to December 1, 2010, and then exit NDCMedisoft.

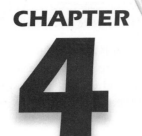

CHAPTER 4

Entering Patient Information

WHAT YOU NEED TO KNOW

To use this chapter, you need to know how to:
◆ Start NDCMedisoft.
◆ Move around the NDCMedisoft menus.
◆ Use the NDCMedisoft toolbar.
◆ Enter and edit data in NDCMedisoft.
◆ Exit NDCMedisoft.

OBJECTIVES

When you finish this chapter, you will be able to:
◆ Use the NDCMedisoft Search feature.
◆ Assign a chart number for a new patient.
◆ Enter personal and employer information for a new patient.
◆ Locate and change information for an established patient.

KEY TERMS

chart number
guarantor

HOW PATIENT INFORMATION IS ORGANIZED IN NDCMEDISOFT

Figure 4-1 Patient List Shortcut Button

Patient information is accessed through the Patient List dialog box. The Patient List dialog box is displayed when Patients/Guarantors and Cases is clicked on the Lists menu or when the corresponding shortcut button is clicked on the toolbar (see Figure 4-1).

The Patient List dialog box (see Figure 4-2) is divided into two primary sections. The left side of the window displays information about patients, and the right side of the window contains information about cases. Cases are covered in Chapter 5. At the top right side of the Patient List dialog box are two radio buttons: Patient and Case. When the Patient radio button is clicked, the left side of the window becomes active. Correspondingly, when the Case radio button is clicked, the right side of the window becomes active. The command buttons at the bottom of the dialog box vary, depending on which side of the window is active. When the Patient window is active, the command buttons at the bottom of the screen include Edit Patient, New Patient, Delete Patient, Print Grid, and Close.

The Patient window contains the following data: Chart Number, Name, Date of Birth, Social Security Number, Patient ID #2, Patient Type, Phone 1, Provider, Last Name, Billing Code, and Patient Indicator. There is not enough room in the Patient window to display all this information, so only a portion is visible at one time. The additional patient information can be viewed by using the scroll bar, maximizing the dialog box, or by resizing the Patient area of the dialog box (see Figure 4-3).

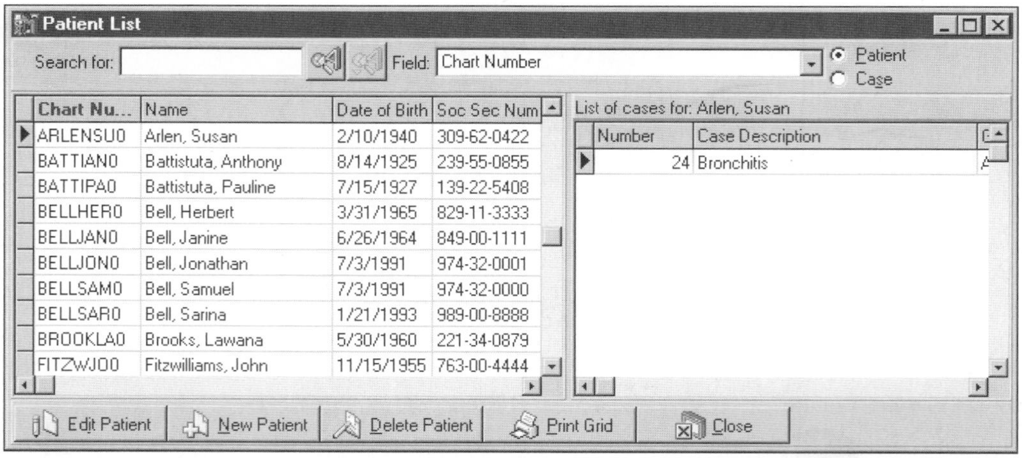

Figure 4-2 Patient List Dialog Box

Chart Nu...	Name	Date of Birth	Soc Sec Num	Patient ID #2	Patient Type	Phone 1	Provider	Last Name	Billing Code	Patient Indicator
ARLENSU0	Arlen, Susan	2/10/1940	309-62-0422		Patient	(614)315-2233	5	Arlen		
BATTIAN0	Battistuta, Anthony	8/14/1925	239-55-0855		Patient	(614)500-3619	4	Battistuta		
BATTIPA0	Battistuta, Pauline	7/15/1927	139-22-5408		Patient	(614)500-3619	4	Battistuta		
BELLHER0	Bell, Herbert	3/31/1965	829-11-3333		Patient	(614)030-1111	2	Bell		
BELLJAN0	Bell, Janine	6/26/1964	849-00-1111		Patient	(614)030-1111	3	Bell		
BELLJON0	Bell, Jonathan	7/3/1991	974-32-0001		Patient	(614)030-1111	2	Bell		
BELLSAM0	Bell, Samuel	7/3/1991	974-32-0000		Patient	(614)030-1111	2	Bell		
BELLSAR0	Bell, Sarina	1/21/1993	989-00-8888		Patient	(614)030-1111	3	Bell		
BROOKLA0	Brooks, Lawana	5/30/1960	221-34-0879		Patient	(614)027-4242	4	Brooks		
FITZWJO0	Fitzwilliams, John	11/15/1955	763-00-4444		Patient	(614)002-1111	2	Fitzwilliams		

Figure 4-3 Expanded Patient Window

ENTERING NEW PATIENT INFORMATION

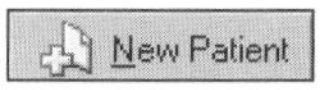

Figure 4-4 New Patient Button

Information on a new patient is entered in NDCMedisoft by clicking the New Patient button at the bottom of the Patient List dialog box (see Figure 4-4). This action opens the Patient/Guarantor dialog box (see Figure 4-5). The Patient/Guarantor dialog box contains two tabs: the Name, Address tab and the Other Information tab.

NAME, ADDRESS TAB

The Name, Address tab is where basic patient information is entered.

Chart Number

chart number *a unique number that identifies a patient.*

The **chart number** is a unique number that identifies a patient. In NDCMedisoft, a chart number links all the information about a patient that is stored in the different databases, such as name,

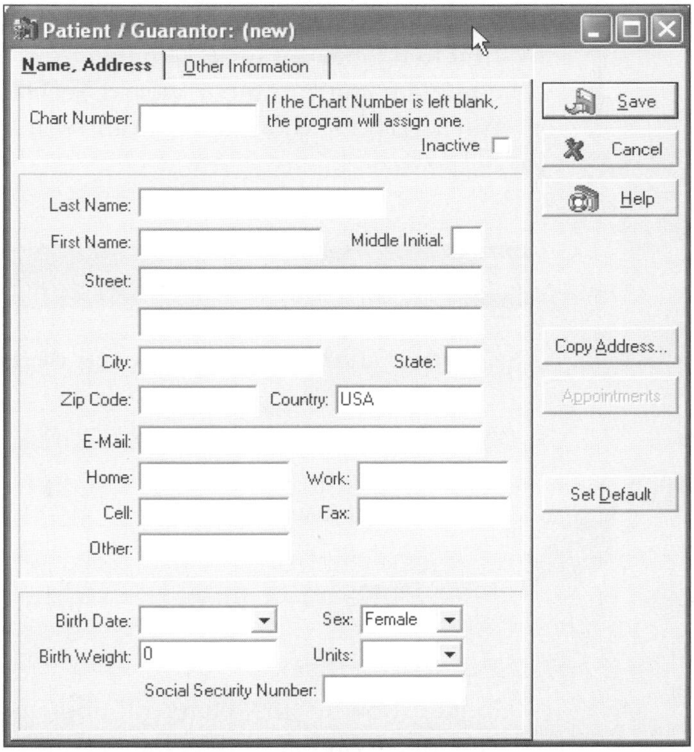

Figure 4-5 Patient/Guarantor Dialog Box with Name, Address Tab Active

address, charges, and insurance claims. Each patient is assigned an eight-character chart number. If the chart number box for a patient is left blank, the system will assign a chart number.

Medical practices may use different methods for assigning chart numbers, although these general guidelines must be followed:

◆ No special characters, such as hyphens, periods, or spaces, are allowed.

◆ No two chart numbers can be the same.

For the purposes of this book, the following method will be used for assigning chart numbers:

◆ The first five characters of the chart number are the first five letters of a patient's last name. If the patient's last name is less than five characters, add the beginning letters of the patient's first name.

◆ The next two characters are usually the first two letters of a patient's first name. (If the first two letters of the first name were used to complete the first five letters, the next two letters of the patient's first name are used.)

◆ The last character is always a zero, displayed in this book with the symbol "∅."

For example, the chart number for John Fitzwilliams would begin with the first five letters of his last name (FITZW), followed by the first two letters of his first name (JO), followed by a zero (∅). John's complete chart number would be FITZWJO∅. Following the same rules, John's daughter Sarah would have a chart number of FITZWSA∅.

Exercise 4-1

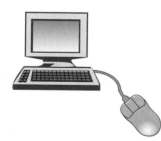

Create a chart number for each of these patients.

Albert Wong _____

Jessica Sypkowski _____

John James _____

Personal Data

In addition to the chart number, personal information about a patient is entered in the Name, Address tab.

Name, Address, and Phone Numbers   NDCMedisoft provides fields for name and address, as well as a number of fields for contact methods. There are boxes for e-mail address, home phone, work phone, cell phone, fax, and other. Phone and fax numbers must be entered without parentheses or hyphens. NDCMedisoft automatically adds these.

Birth Date   The patient's birth date is entered in the Birth Date box using the MMDDCCYY format.

Sex   This drop-down list contains choices for the patient's gender, male or female.

Birth Weight   If the patient is a newborn, the birth weight is entered in this field.

Units   This field indicates whether the birth weight is listed in pounds or grams.

Social Security Number   The nine-digit Social Security number is entered without hyphens; NDCMedisoft automatically adds hyphens.

OTHER INFORMATION TAB   The Other Information tab within the Patient/Guarantor dialog box contains facts about a patient's employment and other miscellaneous information (see Figure 4-6).

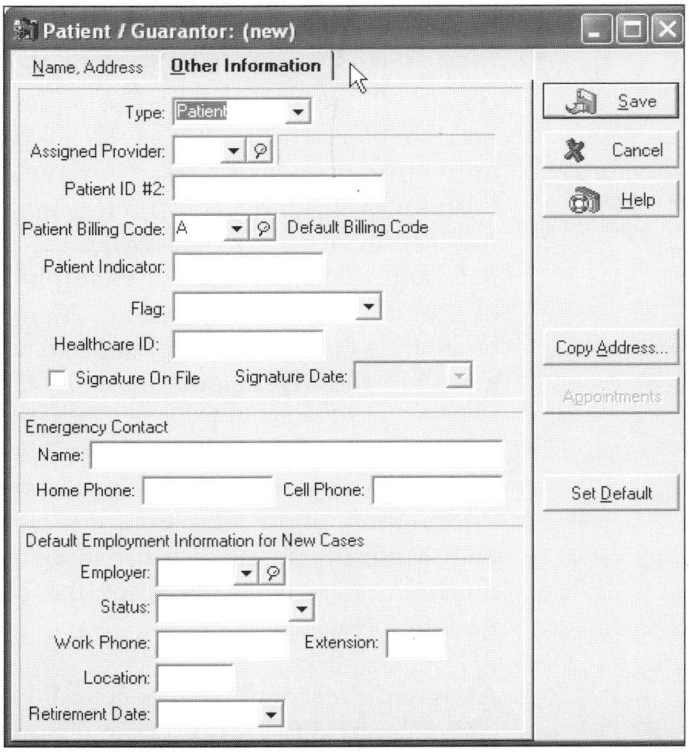

Figure 4-6 **Other Information Tab**

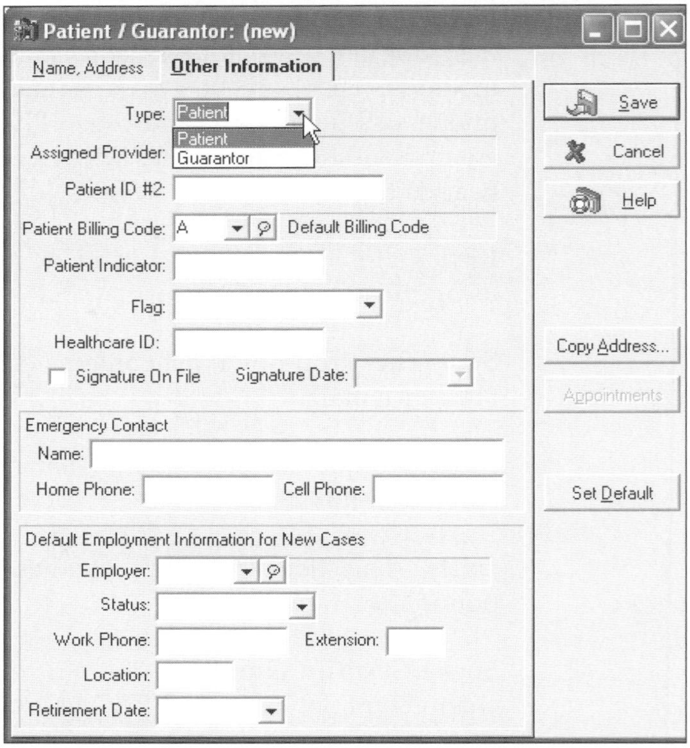

Figure 4-7 **Other Information Tab with Type Drop-Down List Displayed**

Type   The Type drop-down list is used to designate whether, for billing purposes, an individual is a patient or guarantor (see Figure 4-7).

In the NDCMedisoft Patient/Guarantor dialog box, individuals are classified into two categories: patient and guarantor. "Patient" is used to refer to individuals who are patients of the practice, whether or not they are also the insurance policyholders. The term **guarantor** (also known as the *insured*) refers to the person who is the holder of the insurance policy that covers the patient. The guarantor may or may not be the patient. For example, a parent may not be a patient of the practice, but the parent's insurance policy may provide coverage for a child who is a patient. In this case, the child is the patient, and the parent is the guarantor.

guarantor *an individual who is not a patient of the practice, but who is the insurance policyholder for a patient of the practice.*

Information about the patient is always entered in NDCMedisoft in the Name, Address tab. When the patient is not the policyholder, information about the guarantor must also be entered in the NDCMedisoft database for insurance claims to be processed. This information is collected from the patient information or patient update form.

Assigned Provider   The Assigned Provider drop-down list contains codes assigned to the doctors in the practice (see Figure 4-8). The code for the specific doctor who provides care to this patient is selected.

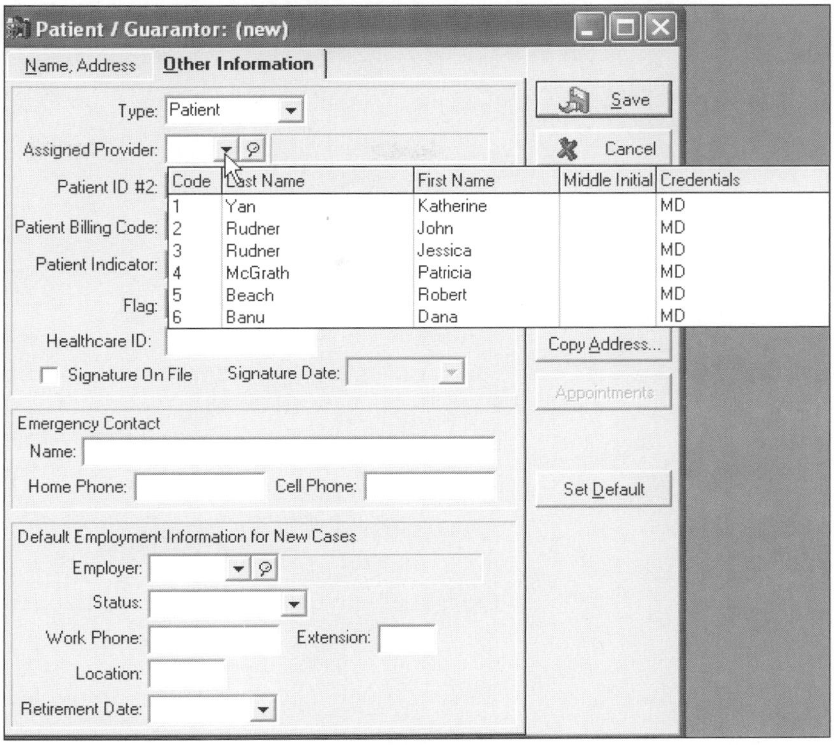

Figure 4-8 Other Information Tab with Assigned Provider Drop-Down List Displayed

Patient ID #2   The Patient ID #2 box is used by some medical practices as a second identification system in addition to chart numbers.

Patient Billing Code   The Patient Billing Code is an optional field used to categorize patients according to the billing codes that the practice has set up in NDCMedisoft. For example, Billing Code A might be for patients with insurance coverage and B for cash patients. Some practices use billing codes to classify patients according to a billing cycle—patients with Billing Code A are billed on the first of the month and those with Code B on the fifteenth of the month. The Patient Billing Code field is not used in the exercises in this book.

Patient Indicator   The Patient Indicator is an optional field that practices can use to classify types of patients, such as workers' compensation patients or cash patients.

Flag   The flag field can be used to group patients in categories set up by the practice.

Healthcare ID   The Healthcare ID is not used at present; it is included for future implementation of the HIPAA legislation.

Signature on File   A check mark in the Signature on File check box means that the patient's signature is on file for the purpose of submitting insurance claims. This box must be completed. If it is not, insurance carriers will not accept and process insurance claims.

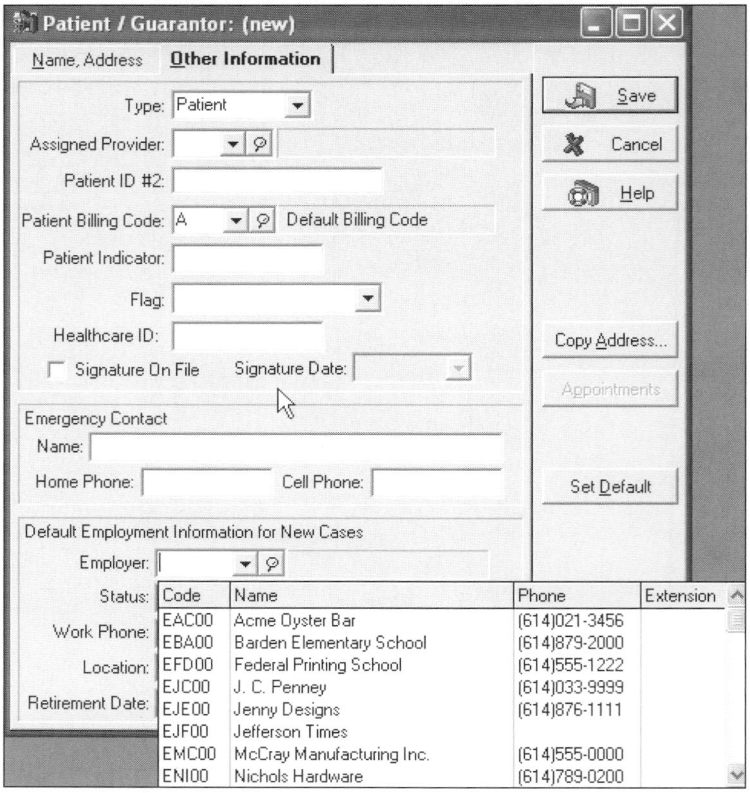

Figure 4-9 **Other Information Tab with Employer Drop-Down List Displayed**

Signature Date   The date keyed in the Signature Date box is the date the patient signed the insurance release form.

Emergency Contact   Information about how to contact someone in case of a patient emergency is entered in these fields.

Employer   The code for the patient's employer is selected from the drop-down list of employers that are in the database (see Figure 4-9). If the patient's employer is not in the database, this information must be entered before the code can be selected. (This process is described later in the chapter.)

Status   The Status drop-down list displays the following choices for the patient's employment status: Not employed, Full time, Part time, Retired, and Unknown (see Figure 4-10).

Work Phone and Extension   Work phone numbers should be entered without parentheses and hyphens.

Location   Some companies have multiple locations. If the patient supplies information on the specific company location, it is entered in this box.

Retirement Date   The Retirement Date box is filled in only if the patient is already retired. Retirement dates should be entered in the MMDDCCYY format.

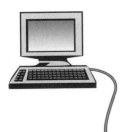

Figure 4-10 **Other Information Tab with Status Drop-Down List Displayed**

When all fields in the Name, Address tab and the Other Information tab have been filled in, entries should be checked for accuracy. If any information needs to be changed, it can easily be corrected. Once the information has been checked and necessary corrections made, data are saved by clicking the Save button.

SHORT CUT The Copy Address button in the Patient/Guarantor dialog box saves time when entering patients with the same address, such as family members. Clicking on the Copy Address button provides a way to copy demographic information from a patient already in the database.

Exercise 4-2

Using Source Document 1 (located in Part 4 of this book), complete the Patient/Guarantor dialog box for Hiro Tanaka, a new patient of Dr. Yan's.

1. Hold down the F7 key and start NDCMedisoft. Enter the location of the NDCMedisoft data in the Find NDCMedisoft Directory box and click OK. (If you are unsure what to enter, ask your instructor.) When the Open practice dialog box appears, verify that Family Care Center is highlighted and click OK.

2. On the Lists menu, click Patients/Guarantors and Cases, or click the corresponding shortcut button on the toolbar.

3. Scroll down the list of patients to make sure Hiro Tanaka is not already in the patient database.

4. Click the New Patient button.

5. Create a chart number for this patient. Click the Chart Number box, and enter the chart number.

6. Click the Last Name box, and fill in the patient information. Fill in the rest of the boxes (for which you have data) on the Name, Address tab, pressing the Tab key to move from box to box.

7. Click the Other Information tab, and fill in the appropriate boxes. Be sure to select an Assigned Provider (Dr. Yan is Tanaka's assigned provider); if you don't, subsequent exercises in this chapter will not work.

8. Make no entries in the following boxes: Patient ID #2, Patient Indicator, Flag, Healthcare ID, and Emergency Contact. Accept the default entry in the Patient Billing Code box. Click the Signature on File box and enter *10/04/2010* as the Signature Date. A Confirm box appears, stating that you have entered a future date and asking whether you want to change it. Click No. A Warning box is displayed, stating that the date entered is in the future. Click OK.

9. Since Tanaka's employer is not in the database, leave the employer boxes blank for now.

10. Check your entries for accuracy, and make corrections if necessary.

11. Click the Save button to save the data on Tanaka.

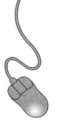

12. Verify that Tanaka has been added to the list in the Patient List dialog box.

13. Close the Patient List dialog box.

Adding an Employer to the Address List

If the patient's employer does not appear on the Employer drop-down list in the Other Information tab, it must be entered using the Address feature. Addresses are entered by clicking the Addresses command on the Lists menu, which displays the Address List dialog box (see Figure 4-11).

Clicking the New button at the bottom of the Address List dialog box displays the Address dialog box (see Figure 4-12).

The Address dialog box contains the following boxes:

Code   The code for an employer should begin with the letter "E," to indicate that this is an employer. Codes can be a combination of

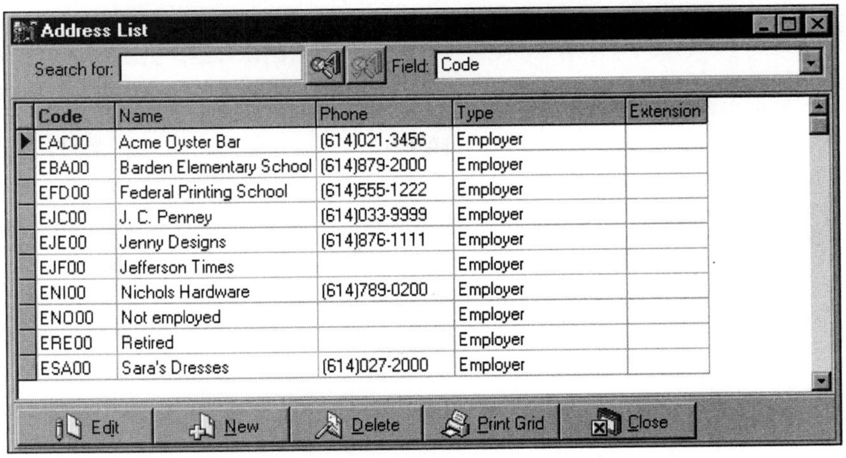

Figure 4-11 **The Address List Dialog Box**

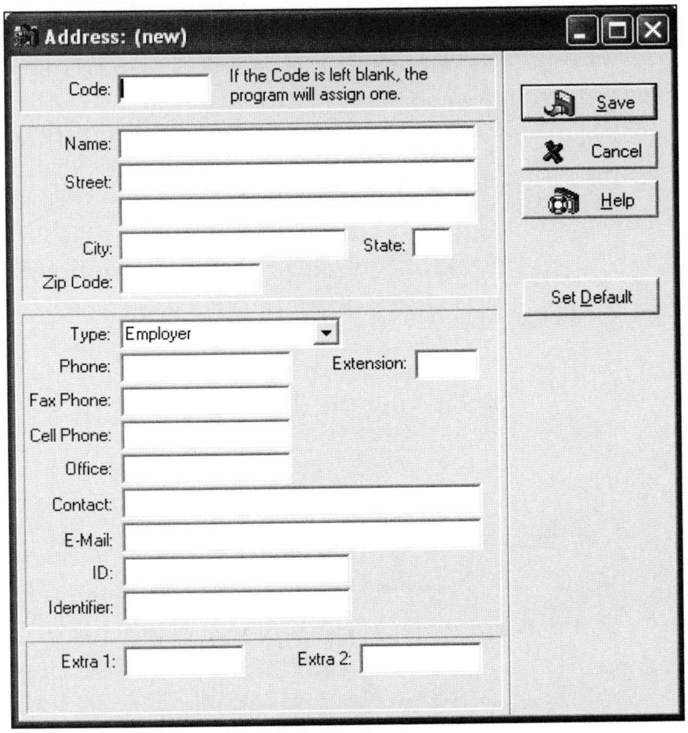

Figure 4-12 **Address Dialog Box**

letters and numbers, up to a maximum of five characters. If a code is not assigned, the system will assign one.

Name and Address The employer's name is entered in the Name box. This field allows up to thirty characters. The employer's street, city, state (two characters only), and ZIP code are entered in the boxes provided.

Type   The Type drop-down list displays a list of kinds of address-es: Attorney, Employer, Facility, Laboratory, Miscellaneous, and Referral Source. For example, when an employer's address is being entered, "Employer" would be selected.

Phone, Extension, Fax Phone, Cell Phone   In the Phone box, the employer's phone number is entered, without parentheses or hyphens. If there is an extension, it is entered in the Extension box. If there is a cell phone, it is entered in the Cell Phone box. The employer's fax number is entered in the Fax Phone box.

Contact   The Contact box is used to enter the name of an individual at the place of employment. If there is no contact person, the box is left blank.

E-mail   This box provides a field for the employer's e-mail address.

ID   If there is an identification number for the employer, it is entered in the ID box.

Identifier   The Employer Identification Number (EIN) Identifier issued by the Internal Revenue Service is entered in this field.

Extra 1, Extra 2   The Extra 1 and Extra 2 boxes are available to keep track of any additional information that needs to be recorded and stored for future reference.

When all information on the employer has been entered, it is saved by clicking the Save button.

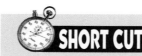 **SHORT CUT**   Throughout NDCMedisoft, the F8 function key serves as a shortcut for entering data. For example, clicking once in the Employer box on the Other Information tab and then pressing function key F8 brings up the Address dialog box, in which a new employer can be entered. The F8 key shortcut enables users to enter data in another part of the NDCMedisoft program without leaving the current dialog box. Once the F8 key is pressed, the dialog box used to enter new addresses is opened, with the Patient/Guarantor dialog box still open in the background (see Figure 4-13).

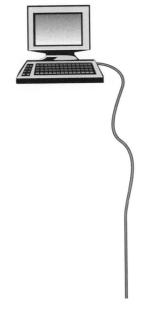

Figure 4-13 Address Dialog Box with Patient/Guarantor Dialog Box Visible in Background

Exercise 4-3

Practice entering information about an employer.

1. Click Addresses on the Lists menu. The Address List dialog box is displayed.

2. Click the New button at the bottom of the dialog box. The Address dialog box is displayed.

3. In the Code box, key *EMCØØ* for McCray Manufacturing, Inc. ("E" for employer, followed by the first two letters of the employer's name, followed by two zeros.) Press the Tab key.

4. Key *McCray Manufacturing Inc.* in the Name box. Press the Tab key.

5. In the Street box, key *1311 Kings Highway.* Press the Tab key twice.

6. Key *Stephenson* in the City box. Press the Tab key.

7. Key *OH* in the State box. Press the Tab key.

8. Key *60089* in the Zip Code box. Press the Tab key.

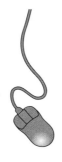

9. Verify that "Employer" is displayed in the Type box. If it is not, click Employer in the drop-down list and press the Tab key.

10. Key *6145555000* in the Phone box. Press the Tab key.

11. Leave the remaining boxes blank.

12. Click the Save button to store the information you have entered.

13. Click the Close button to exit the Address List dialog box.

SEARCHING FOR PATIENT INFORMATION

A patient who comes to a medical practice for the first time fills out a patient information form. The information on this form needs to be entered into the NDCMedisoft patient/guarantor database before any insurance claims can be submitted. However, before information on a patient is entered into the system, it is important to search the database to be certain that the patient information has not already been entered into the program.

NDCMedisoft provides two options for conducting searches: Search For and Field boxes, and Locate.

SEARCH FOR AND FIELD OPTION

The Search For and Field boxes at the top of many dialog boxes provide a quick way to search for information in NDCMedisoft (see Figure 4-14).

The Search For box contains the text that is to be searched. The entry in the Field box controls how the list is sorted. Figure 4-15 displays the Field options in the Patient List dialog box.

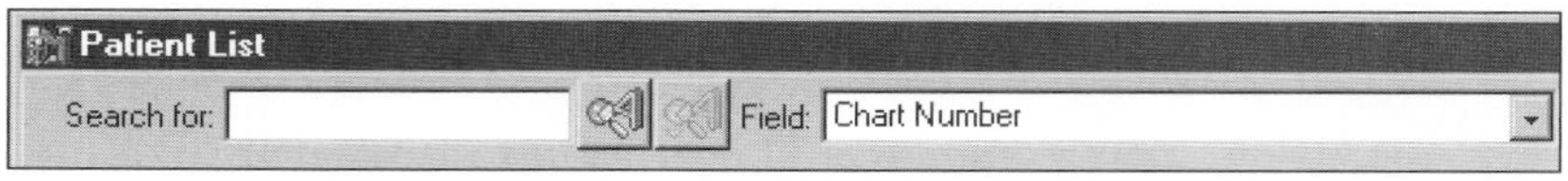

Figure 4-14 **Search For and Field Boxes**

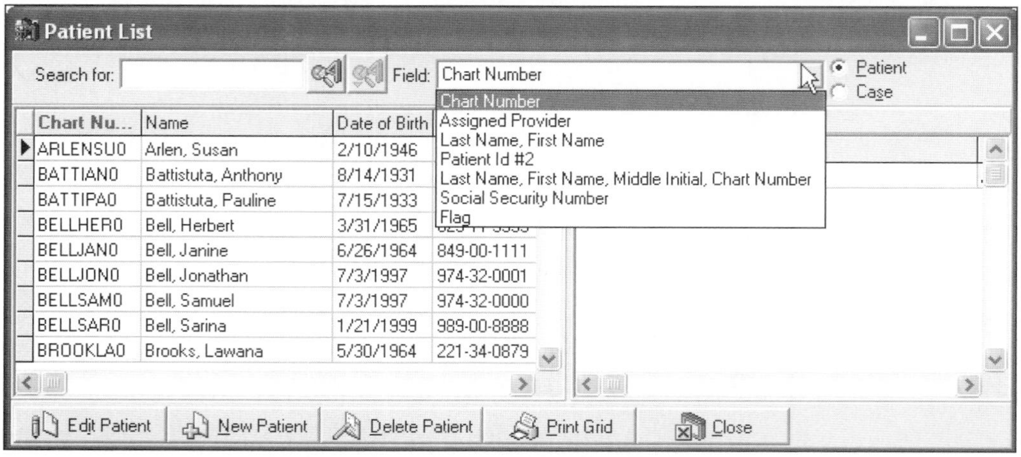

Figure 4-15 **Field Options in the Patient List Dialog Box**

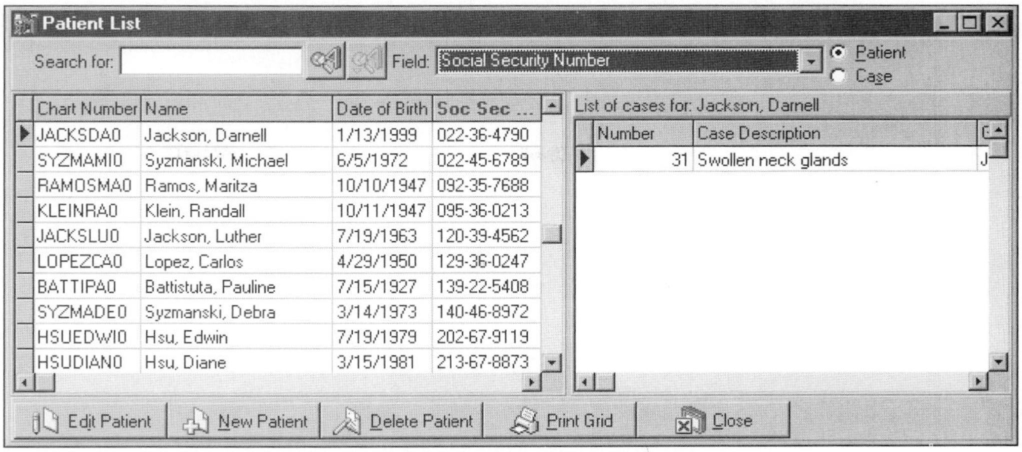

Figure 4-16 List Window Sorted by Social Security Number

When a selection is made in the Field box, the information is resorted by the selected criteria. For example, if Social Security Number is selected in the Field box, the entries in the List window are listed in numerical order by Social Security Number, from lowest to highest (see Figure 4-16).

The Search For and Field feature is used in the following NDCMedisoft dialog boxes: Patient List, Insurance Carrier List, Procedure/Payment/Adjustment List, Diagnosis List, Address List, Provider List, and Referring Provider List. The Claim Management/Statement Management, and Deposit List dialog boxes contain similar features called Search and Sort By. Table 4-1 displays the Field box options for each of these NDCMedisoft dialog boxes.

After an entry is made in the Field box, the search criterion is entered in the Search For field. As each letter or number is entered, the list automatically filters out records that do not match. For example, if the Field box is set to Last Name, First Name in the Patient List dialog box, and "S" is entered in the Search For field, the program

Table 4-1   Field Options for NDCMedisoft Searches

List Window	Field Options
Patient List	Chart Number; Assigned Provider; Last Name, First Name; Patient Id #2; Last Name, First Name, Middle Initial, Chart Number; Social Security Number; Flag
Insurance Carrier List	Code, Name, Iod
Procedure/Payment/Adjustment List	Code 1, Description, Type
Diagnosis List	Code 1, Description
Address List	Code, Name, Type
Provider List	Code; Last Name, First Name
Referring Provider List	Code; Last Name, First Name
Claim Management	Batch 1, 2, or 3; Carrier 1, 2, or 3; Chart Number; Claim Number; Date Created; or EMC Receiver 1, 2, or 3
Statement Management	Batch Number, Chart Number, Date Created, Initial Billing Date, Last Billing Date, Statement Number
Deposit List	Amount, Date-Description, Date-Payor, Description, Insurance Code, Patient Chart, Payor

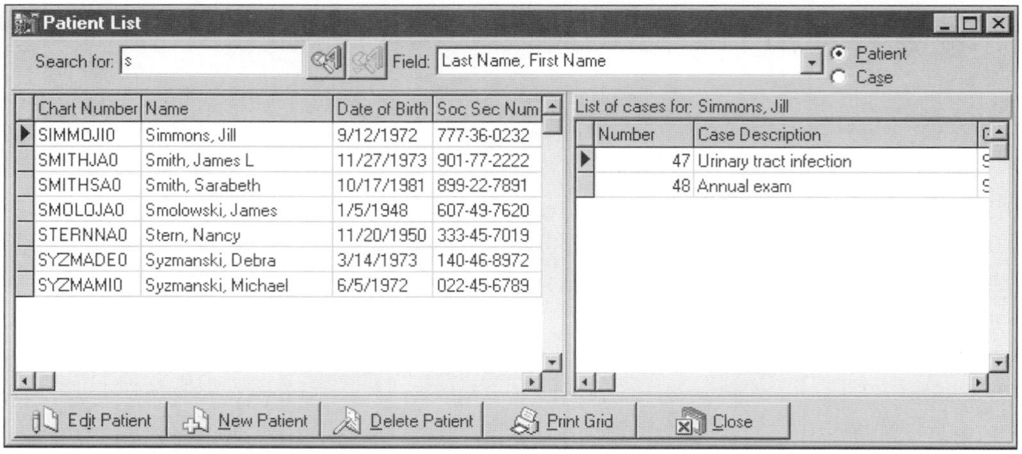

Patient List

Chart Number	Name	Date of Birth	Soc Sec Num
SIMMOJI0	Simmons, Jill	9/12/1972	777-36-0232
SMITHJA0	Smith, James L	11/27/1973	901-77-2222
SMITHSA0	Smith, Sarabeth	10/17/1981	899-22-7891
SMOLOJA0	Smolowski, James	1/5/1948	607-49-7620
STERNNA0	Stern, Nancy	11/20/1950	333-45-7019
SYZMADE0	Syzmanski, Debra	3/14/1973	140-46-8972
SYZMAMI0	Syzmanski, Michael	6/5/1972	022-45-6789

Search for: s   Field: Last Name, First Name   ● Patient ○ Case

List of cases for: Simmons, Jill

Number	Case Description
47	Urinary tract infection
48	Annual exam

Edit Patient   New Patient   Delete Patient   Print Grid   Close

Figure 4-17 Patient List Dialog Box with Search Set for Last Name Beginning with "S"

eliminates all data from the list except patients whose last names begin with S (see Figure 4-17).

To restore the Patient list to its default setting (all patients listed), delete the entry in the Search for box.

Exercise 4-4

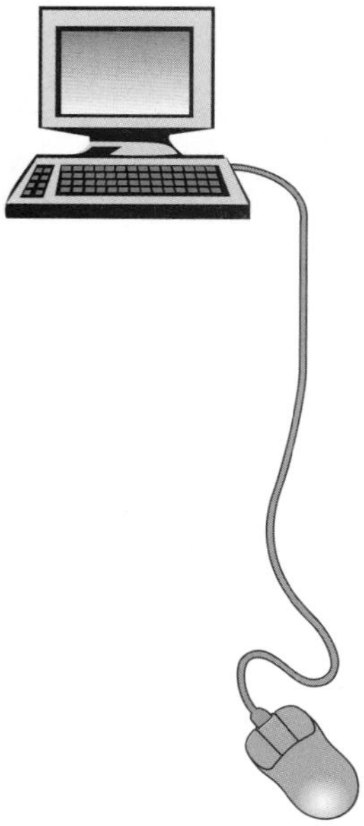

Use the Search feature to locate information on James Smolowski.

1. **On the Lists menu, click Patients/Guarantors and Cases or click the corresponding shortcut button. The Patient List dialog box is displayed, and the cursor is blinking in the Search For box. Confirm that the entry in the Field box is Last Name, First Name. If it is not, change it to Last Name, First Name.**

2. **Enter the first letter of the patient's last name. Notice that when you keyed "S," the list window filtered the data so that only those patients whose last names begin with "S" are listed. Now enter the second letter of his last name, "m." The list now displays only those patients whose last names begin with the letters "Sm." Now enter the third letter, "o." Smolowski is the only patient whose name begins with the letters "Smo," so he is the only patient listed.**

3. **To restore the Patient window so that all patients are listed, delete the letters entered in the Search For box.**

4. **Click the Close button to exit the Patient List dialog box.**

LOCATE BUTTONS OPTION Another option for finding information in NDCMedisoft is the use of the Locate buttons (see Figure 4-18).

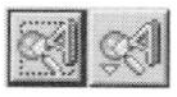

Figure 4-18 Locate Buttons

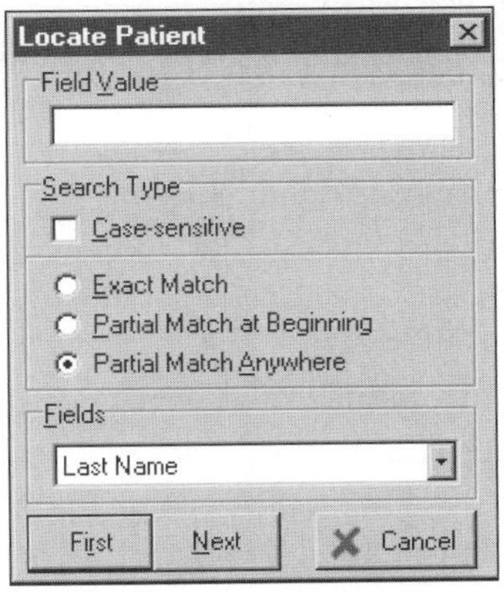

![Locate Patient dialog box showing Field Value text box, Search Type with Case-sensitive checkbox, Exact Match, Partial Match at Beginning, Partial Match Anywhere radio buttons, Fields drop-down with Last Name, and First, Next, Cancel buttons]

Figure 4-19 Locate Patient dialog Box

When a Locate button is clicked, the Locate dialog box is displayed. The Fields drop-down list contains options for filtering data (see Figure 4-19).

Field Value

The information entered in the Field Value box at the top of the window can be part of a name, birth date, payment date or amount, or assigned provider. Any combination of numbers and letters can be used.

Search Type

Case-Sensitive Use to make the search sensitive to uppercase and lowercase letters.

Exact Match Use when the entry in the Field Value box is exactly as entered in the program.

Partial Match at Beginning Use when unsure of the correct spelling or entry at the end of the word.

Partial Match Anywhere Use when unsure of the correct spelling or entry.

Fields

The Fields box provides a drop-down list from which to choose the field that contains the information that is being matched. For example, if searching for a patient by last name, select the Last Name field. The available fields are determined by the type of information you are working with. For example, if you are looking for a particular Chart Number, you have nineteen fields from which to choose as the basis of your search. Searching for cases gives access to up to ninety-one fields.

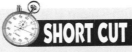 **SHORT CUT** To make searching easier, right-click a column heading in a window that contains several columns. From the shortcut menu that appears, select Locate or press Ctrl + L. This opens a Locate window that defaults the Fields selection to the column you selected.

Once the criteria are selected, clicking the First button starts a search for the first match to the criteria. If a match is found, the Locate window is closed and the search result is highlighted in the Search window. If a match is not found, a message is displayed.

Clicking the Next button begins a search for the next match, and so on.

When the program reaches the end of the list, a message is displayed indicating that the search is complete.

EDITING INFORMATION ON AN ESTABLISHED PATIENT

From time to time, established patients notify the practice that they have moved, changed jobs or insurance carriers, or changed other information. When this happens, information needs to be updated in NDCMedisoft's patient/guarantor database.

The process of changing information on an established patient is similar to that of entering information for a new patient. The Patients/Guarantors and Cases command is selected from the Lists menu. A search is usually performed to locate the chart number of the patient whose record needs to be updated. Clicking the edit button displays the Patient/Guarantor dialog box, where changes can be made. Clicking the Save button stores the changes.

Exercise 4-5

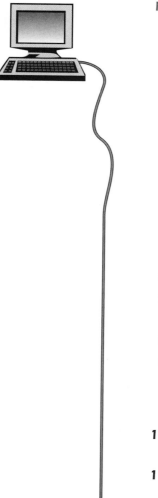

Practice searching for and editing information on Hiro Tanaka.

1. Open the Patient List dialog box. Confirm that the Field box entry is Last Name, First Name.

2. Search for Hiro Tanaka by keying the first few letters of her last name in the Search For box. Notice that as soon as the "T" is entered, all patients except Tanaka disappear from the Patient List window, because Tanaka is the only patient whose last name begins with "T."

3. Click the Edit Patient button.

4. Click the Other Information tab.

5. Click the triangle button in the Employer box. Click McCray Manufacturing Inc. on the drop-down list. Notice that the program automatically enters the phone number in the Work Phone box.

6. Select Full time from the Status drop-down list.

7. Click the Save button to store the information you have entered.

8. Close the Patient List dialog box.

9. Create a backup of your work and exit NDCMedisoft by selecting Exit on the File menu. The Backup Reminder dialog box is displayed. If you are backing up to a floppy disk, make sure your working copy of FCC8 is in the floppy drive.

10. Click the Back Up Data Now button. The Backup dialog box appears.

11. Enter the file path and file name in the Destination File Path and Name box or click the Find button and browse to the desired location. The file name should be FCC8-4.mbk (the

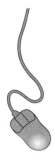

database name followed by the chapter number). The file path will vary depending on your computer and whether you are saving data to a floppy disk or to a network drive. Ask your instructor for the file path.

12. Click the Start Backup button. NDCMedisoft creates a backup file. When it is complete, an Information box is displayed, indicating that the backup is complete. Click OK. The Backup dialog box closes and the program is shut down.

CHAPTER REVIEW

USING TERMINOLOGY

Define the terms in the space provided.

1. chart number

   _____

   _____

2. guarantor

   _____

   _____

CHECKING YOUR UNDERSTANDING

Answer the questions below in the space provided.

3. To search for Paul Ramos, can you key either "Paul" or "Ramos"? Explain.

   _____

   _____

4. Create a chart number for a patient named William Burroughs.

   _____

   _____

5. Sam Wu has no insurance of his own but is covered by his wife's insurance policy. How would you indicate this in the Patient/Guarantor dialog box?

   _____

   _____

6. Which tab in the Patient/Guarantor dialog box is used to store information on a patient's assigned provider?

   _____

   _____

7. How would you enter the Social Security number 123-45-6789?

_____

_____

APPLYING KNOWLEDGE

Answer the following question in the space provided.

8. Jane Taylor-Burke comes to the office. She thinks she saw Dr. Yan a few years ago for a flu shot, but she is not sure. You need to decide whether to enter Ms. Taylor-Burke as a new patient in the NDCMedisoft database. What should you do?

_____

_____

AT THE COMPUTER

Answer the following questions at the computer.

9. How many patients in the database have the last name of Smith?

10. List the name of the patient who is found when you search for the letters "JO."

11. What is Li Y. Wong's chart number?

12. In the Patient List dialog box, search for information on Leila Patterson. What steps did you take to find the information?

CHAPTER 5

Working with Cases

WHAT IS A CASE?

A **case** is a grouping of transactions for visits to a physician's office organized around a condition. When a patient comes for treatment, a case is created.

Cases are set up to contain the transactions that relate to a particular condition. For example, all treatments and procedures for bronchial asthma would be stored in a case called "bronchial asthma." Services performed and charges for those services are entered in the system and linked to the bronchial asthma case.

WHEN TO SET UP A NEW CASE

A new case should be set up each time a patient comes to see the physician for a new condition or when there is a change in the provider or insurance carrier. For example, suppose a patient has been seeing a physician regularly for treatment of bronchial asthma. All the transactions for this treatment would be contained in one case. Then suppose the patient has an accident and comes in for treatment of a sprained ankle. The sprained ankle is a new condition. A new case would be set up in NDCMedisoft for the sprained ankle treatments.

When a patient changes insurance carriers, a new case should be set up, even if the same condition is being treated under the new carrier. This makes it easier to submit insurance claims to the appropriate carrier. Transactions that took place while the previous policy was in effect must be submitted under that policy. Transactions that occur after the change in policies must be submitted to the new carrier. By opening a new case, transactions for the two insurance carriers can be kept separate. The information needed to submit claims to the previous carrier is still intact, while information for claims under the new policy is current.

A patient may require more than one case per office visit if treatment is provided for two or more unrelated conditions. For example, a patient who visits the physician complaining of migraine headaches may also ask for an influenza vaccination. Since the two conditions are unrelated, two cases would need to be created: one for the migraine headaches, and one for the vaccination. In contrast, a patient who is treated for shortness of breath and chest pain during exertion would require one case, provided the physician determines that the two complaints are related to the same diagnosis.

It is common for patients to have more than one case open at any one time. In the example mentioned earlier, the patient's bronchial asthma case and sprained ankle case would be open at the same time. While the patient is being treated for the ankle injury, the bronchial asthma treatment is continuing. Some cases are for chron-

![Patient List dialog box screenshot showing a list of patients and cases. Top bar reads "Patient List". Search for field, Field: Last Name, First Name, with Patient and Case radio buttons (Case selected). The patient list includes columns Chart Number, Name, Date of Birth, Soc Sec Num with entries ARLENSU0 Arlen, Susan 2/10/1940 309-62-0422; BATTIAN0 Battistuta, Anthony 8/14/1925 239-55-0855; BATTIPA0 Battistuta, Pauline 7/15/1927 139-22-5408; BELLHER0 Bell, Herbert 3/31/1965 829-11-3333; BELLJAN0 Bell, Janine 6/26/1964 849-00-1111; BELLJON0 Bell, Jonathan 7/3/1991 974-32-0001; BELLSAM0 Bell, Samuel 7/3/1991 974-32-0000; BELLSAR0 Bell, Sarina 1/21/1993 989-00-8888; BROOKLA0 Brooks, Lawana 5/30/1960 221-34-0879. The right panel reads "List of cases for: Arlen, Susan" with columns Number and Case Description showing 24 Bronchitis. Bottom buttons: Edit Case, New Case, Delete Case, Copy Case, Print Grid, Close.]

Figure 5-1 **Patient List Dialog Box with Case Radio Button Clicked**

ic conditions and remain open a long time. Other cases, such as for treatment of influenza, may be of short duration. Cases are closed when the patient is no longer being treated for the condition, when the insurance policy in a case is no longer in effect, or when the patient leaves the practice.

CASE COMMAND BUTTONS

In NDCMedisoft, cases are created, edited, and deleted from within the Patient List dialog box. The Patient List dialog box is accessed by choosing Patients/Guarantors and Cases from the Lists menu. When the Case radio button in the Patient List dialog box is clicked, the following command buttons appear at the bottom of the Patient List dialog box: Edit Case, New Case, Delete Case, Copy Case, Print Grid, and Close (see Figure 5-1).

Edit Case

The Edit Case button is used to add, delete, or change information in an existing case. When the Edit Case button is clicked, the Case dialog box is displayed. Case information to be updated is contained in nine different tabs. For example, if a patient changes insurance carriers, information needs to be updated in the Policy 1, 2, or 3 tab. The only item in the Case dialog box that cannot be changed is the Case Number. All other boxes are edited by moving the cursor to the box and making the change, whether this involves rekeying, selecting and deselecting a check box, or clicking a different option on a drop-down list.

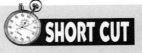 **SHORT CUT** Cases can also be opened for editing by double-clicking on the case number/ description in the Case window within the Patient List dialog box.

New Case

The New Case button creates a new case.

Delete Case

The Delete Case button deletes a case from the system if the case has no open transactions. Open transactions are charges that have not been fully paid by the insurance carrier or the policyholder. The Delete Case button should be used with caution; once deleted, information cannot be retrieved. Cases should be deleted only when it is definite that the patient's records will never be needed again. Medical offices usually have policies about when a patient's records are deleted. In most instances, it is more appropriate to close a case than to delete it. Cases are closed by clicking the Case Closed box in the Personal tab of the Case dialog box.

Cases are deleted in the Patient List dialog box. With the Case radio button clicked, the specific case to be deleted is selected by clicking the line that displays the case number and description. The case is then deleted by clicking the Delete Case button at the bottom of the dialog box. The system will ask, "Are you sure you want to delete this case?" Clicking the Yes button deletes the case from the system.

Copy Case

The Copy Case button copies all the information from an existing case into a new case. This feature is useful when creating a new case for a patient who already has a case in the system. Rather than reenter the information in all nine tabs, the information in the existing case is copied into a new case. Then the information that needs to be changed can be edited to reflect the new case. Sometimes the new case requires few changes; other times data must be changed in all the tabs of the Case folder. For this reason, when copying a case it is important to check each tab to make sure the copied information is accurate for the new case. The information that remains the same from the previous case can be left as is.

Print Grid

The Print Grid button is used to select or deselect columns of information in the Patient List dialog box.

Close

The Close button closes the Patient List dialog box.

SAVING CASES

After the information in all nine tabs has been checked for accuracy and edited as necessary, the case must be saved. Data recorded in the Case dialog box are stored by clicking the Save button on the right side of the Case dialog box. Clicking the Cancel button exits the Case dialog box without saving the newly entered information. The boxes that had new data entered will clear, and the screen will redisplay the Patient List dialog box.

ENTERING CASE INFORMATION

Clicking the New Case button or the Edit Case button brings up the Case dialog box (see Figure 5-2). Information about a patient is entered in nine different tabs in the Case dialog box:

- ◆ Personal
- ◆ Account
- ◆ Diagnosis
- ◆ Condition
- ◆ Miscellaneous
- ◆ Policy 1
- ◆ Policy 2
- ◆ Policy 3
- ◆ Medicaid and Tricare

chart a folder that contains all records pertaining to a patient.

The information required to complete the nine tabs comes from documents found in a patient's chart. The **chart** is a folder that contains all records pertaining to a patient. The patient information

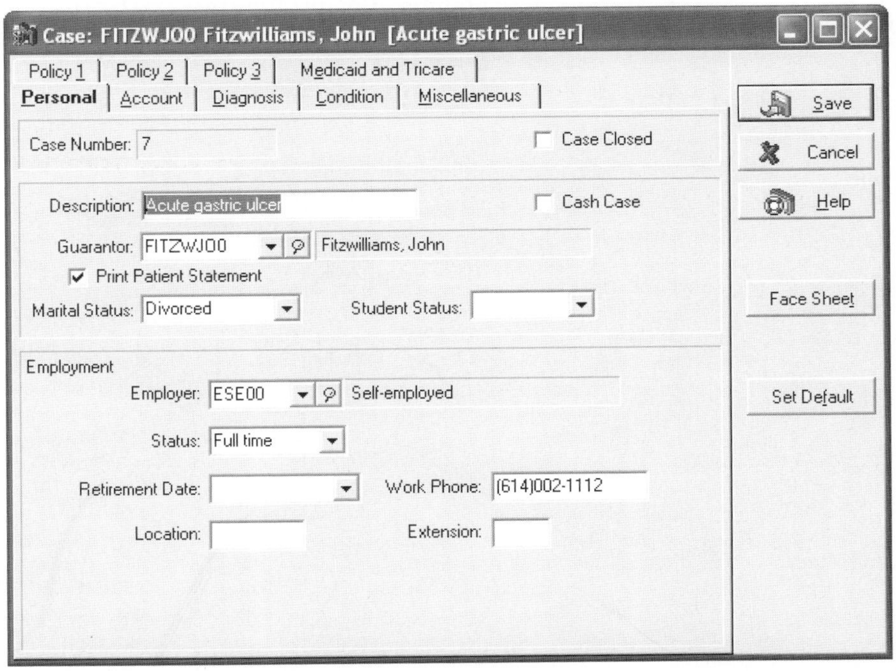

Figure 5-2 Case Dialog Box

form supplies basic information such as name and address as well as information about insurance coverage, allergies, whether the condition is related to an accident, and the referral source. The **record of treatment and progress** contains the physician's notes about a patient's condition and diagnosis. The encounter form is a list of services performed and charges for these procedures.

record of treatment and progress a physician's notes about a patient's condition and diagnosis.

PERSONAL TAB

The Personal tab contains basic information about a patient and his or her employment (see Figure 5-3).

Case Number The case number is a sequential number assigned by NDCMedisoft. To avoid confusion, case numbers are unique; no two patients ever have the same case number.

Case Closed A case is marked as closed by placing a check mark in the Case Closed box. At times it is appropriate to close a case. Closing a case indicates that no more data will be entered into the case. When is it appropriate to close a case? Policies vary from practice to practice, but generally cases are closed when a patient changes insurance carriers, has recovered completely from a condition (such as the flu), or is no longer a patient at the practice.

Description Information entered in the Description box indicates a patient's complaint, or reason for seeing a physician. For example, if a patient comes to see a physician for an annual physical examination, the Description box would read "annual physical." Other examples of entries are sore throat, stomach pains, dog bite, and accident at work. A patient's complaint can be found in his or her chart.

Cash Case If the Cash Case box is checked, the patient is paying cash and has no insurance coverage.

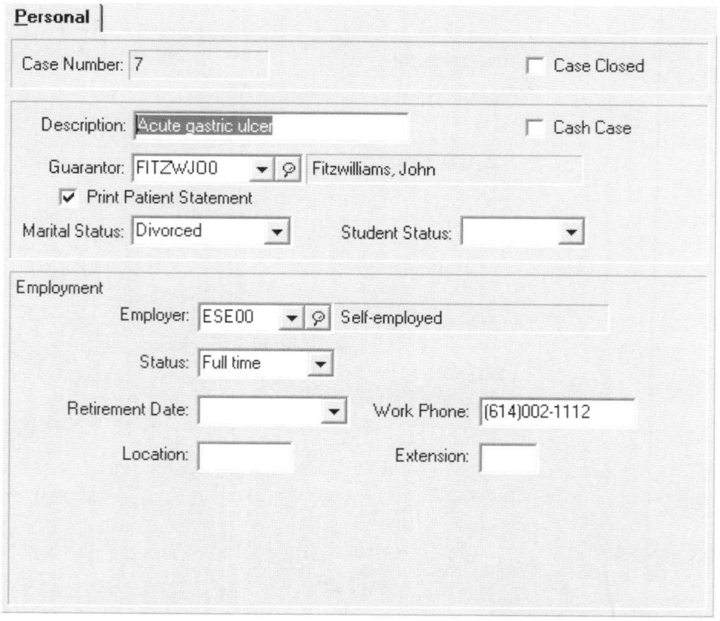

Figure 5-3 **Personal Tab**

Guarantor   The Guarantor box lists the name of the person responsible for paying the bill. The drop-down list contains the chart numbers and names of all potential guarantors in the database.

Print Patient Statement   If this box is checked, a statement for the patient is automatically printed when statements for the practice are printed.

Marital Status   The drop-down list provides the following choices to indicate a patient's marital status: Divorced, Legally separated, Married, Single, Unknown, or Widowed.

Student Status   The Student Status drop-down list is used to indicate whether a patient is a full-time student, a part-time student, or a non-student. If a patient's status is not known, the box should be left blank.

Employer   The Employer box contains the default employer information that has been entered in the Patient/Guarantor dialog box. If it is necessary to change the employer, the default can be overridden by clicking another employer code on the drop-down list.

Status   The Status box lists a patient's employment status as recorded in the Patient/Guarantor dialog box. To change the selection that appears in the Status box, another selection is clicked on the drop-down list. The options are Full-time, Not employed, Part-time, Retired, and Unknown.

Retirement Date   The Retirement Date box should be filled in only when a patient is already retired. There are two ways of entering the retirement date. The date can be entered in the Retirement Date box, or it can be selected from the calendar that appears when the Pop-Up Calendar button at the right of the box is clicked.

Location   If a patient has supplied a specific work location, such as "5th Avenue Branch," it is entered in the Location box.

Work Phone   The Work Phone box contains a patient's work phone number.

Extension   The Extension box lists a patient's work phone extension.

Exercise 5-1

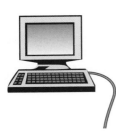

Create a new case for patient Hiro Tanaka, and enter information in the Personal tab. The information needed to complete this exercise is found on Source Document 1.

> Note: Steps 1 through 3 are required at the beginning of each chapter. These steps start NDCMedisoft, set the path to the correct data location, and restore the data saved at the end of the last work session.

Date: October 4, 2010

1. Hold down the F7 key and start NDCMedisoft. Enter the location of the NDCMedisoft data in the Find NDCMedisoft Directory box and click OK. (If you are unsure what to enter, ask your instructor.) When the Open practice dialog box appears, verify that Family Care Center is highlighted and click OK.

2. Restore the data from your last work session by selecting Restore Data on the File menu. When a Warning box appears, click OK. Enter the file path and file name in the File Destination Path and Name, or click the Find button and browse to the desired location. The file name should be FCC8-4.mbk (the database name followed by the chapter number that you last worked on). The file path will vary depending on your computer and network setup. Ask your instructor for the file path, and enter it here.

3. Click the Start Restore button. When a Confirm dialog box appears, click OK. NDCMedisoft restores the data. When it is complete, an Information box is displayed, indicating that the restore is complete. Click OK. The Restore box closes, and the main NDCMedisoft window is displayed.

4. Change the NDCMedisoft Program Date to the date listed above, October 4, 2010.

5. On the Lists menu, click Patients/Guarantors and Cases. The Patient List dialog box is displayed.

6. Search for Hiro Tanaka by keying *T* in the Search For box. The arrow should point to the entry line for Hiro Tanaka.

7. Click the Case radio button to activate the case portion of the Patient List dialog box.

8. Click the New Case button. The dialog box labeled "Case: TANAKHI∅ Tanaka, Hiro (new)" is displayed. The Personal tab is the current active tab. Notice that some information is already filled in.

9. Enter Tanaka's reason for seeing the doctor in the Description box.

10. Choose the correct entry for Tanaka's marital status from the drop-down list in the Marital Status box. The Student Status box can be left blank.

11. Notice that the information on Tanaka's employment is already filled in. The system copies the information entered in the Patient/Guarantor dialog box to the case file for you.

12. Check your entries for accuracy.

13. Click the Save button to save the case information you just entered. The Patient List dialog box redisplays. Notice that the case you just created is listed in the area of the dialog box labeled "List of cases for: Tanaka, Hiro."

14. Do not close the Patient List dialog box.

ACCOUNT TAB

The Account tab includes information on a patient's assigned provider, referring provider, and referral source, as well as other information that may be used in some medical practices but not others (see Figure 5-4).

Assigned Provider   The Assigned Provider box is automatically filled in with the code number and name of the assigned provider listed in the Patient/Guarantor dialog box. The drop-down list provides a complete list of providers in the practice. If necessary, the Assigned Provider selection can be changed by clicking another provider on the list.

referring provider *a physician who recommends that a patient see a specific other physician.*

Referring Provider   A **referring provider** is a physician who recommends that a patient see a specific other physician. The Referring Provider box contains the name of the physician who referred the patient to the practice. The referring provider's name and code are selected from the drop-down list. If the referring provider is not listed on the drop-down list, he or she will need to be added to the Referring Provider list, which is found on the Lists menu. It is not necessary to close the Case dialog box to add a referring provider to the database. When Referring Providers is clicked on the Lists menu, the Referring Provider List dialog box opens in front of the other dialog boxes displayed on the screen. Instructions for adding a referring provider to the database are covered later in this chapter.

Supervising Provider   Whenever the provider rendering services is being supervised by a physician, the supervising physician's information must be included on the claim.

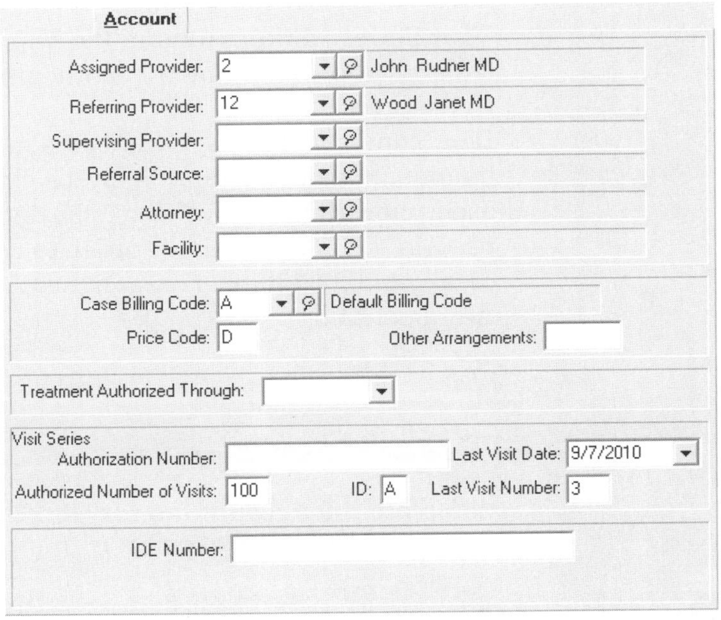

Figure 5-4 **Account Tab**

Referral Source   If known, the source of a patient's referral is selected from the drop-down list of choices.

Attorney   The Attorney box is used for accident cases. If a patient has an attorney, the name of the attorney should be selected from the drop-down list. If the attorney is not listed, he or she will need to be added to the system by clicking Addresses on the Lists menu and entering information about the attorney.

Facility   The Facility box lists the place where a patient is receiving treatment. A facility is selected from the drop-down list. When necessary, facilities can be added to the database by clicking Addresses on the Lists menu and entering the necessary information.

Case Billing Code   The Case Billing Code box is a one- or two-character box used by some practices to classify and sort patients by insurance carrier, diagnosis, billing cycle, or other kinds of information.

Price Code   The Price Code box determines which set of fees is used when entering transactions for this case. The Price Code fees are entered and stored in the Amounts tab of the Procedure/Payment/Adjustment dialog box, accessed through the Lists menu.

Other Arrangements   If a special arrangement is made for billing, it is indicated in the Other Arrangements box.

Treatment Authorized Through   A date can be entered in this box if the insurance carrier has authorized treatment only through a certain date.

Visit Series   Information in the Visit Series section of the Account tab is used primarily by psychotherapy practices and chiropractors.

IDE Number   The IDE Number is required when there is an investigational device exemption on the claim. An investigational device exemption (IDE) allows a newly developed medical device to be used in a clinical study in order to collect safety and effectiveness data. An IDE Number is assigned by the FDA (Food and Drug Administration).

Exercise 5-2

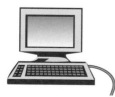

Complete the Account tab for Hiro Tanaka. The information needed to complete this exercise is found on Source Document 1.

Date: October 4, 2010

1. Confirm that Hiro Tanaka is still listed in the Patient List dialog box and that the Case radio button is selected.

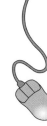

2. Click the Edit Case button to add information to Tanaka's case file. The Case dialog is displayed, with the Personal tab active.

3. Make the Account tab active. The word "Account" should now be displayed in boldface type, and the boxes on the Account tab should be visible.

4. Notice that the Assigned Provider box is already filled in with the name of Tanaka's assigned provider, Katherine Yan. The system copies this information from data stored in the Patient/Guarantor dialog box.

5. Click the name of Tanaka's referring provider on the Referring Provider drop-down list. Press Tab.

6. Notice that the entry in the Price Code box is "A." Since "A" is the list of price codes for Tanaka's insurance carrier, OhioCare HMO, you do not need to change the entry in this box.

7. Check your work for accuracy.

8. Save the changes. The Patient List dialog box is redisplayed.

9. Do not close the Patient List dialog box.

Adding a Referring Provider to the Database

If a referring provider is not listed in the Referring Provider drop-down list in the Account tab, he or she will need to be added to the database. To add a referring provider, click Referring Providers on the Lists menu. The Referring Provider List dialog box is then displayed (see Figure 5-5).

Clicking the New button brings up the Referring Provider dialog box, which is where information on a new referring provider is entered (see Figure 5-6 on page 90). The Referring Provider dialog box contains two tabs: Address and Default Pins.

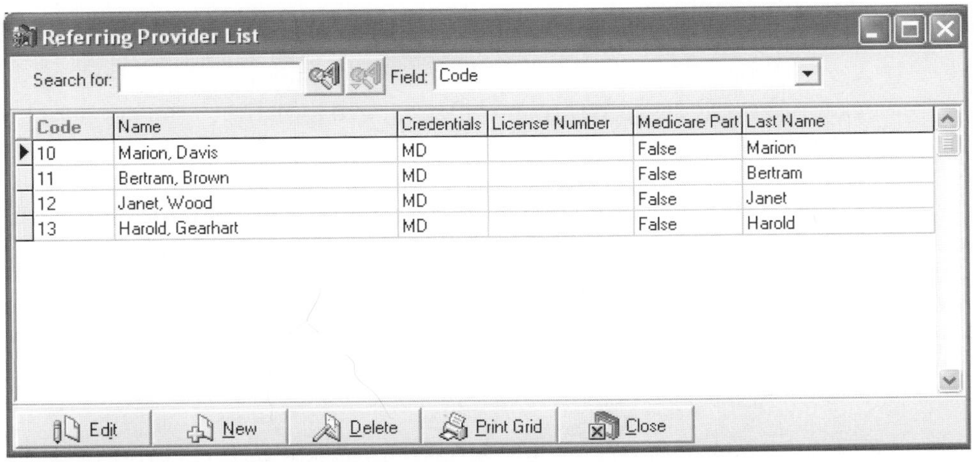

Referring Provider List

Search for: [ ] Field: Code [▼]

Code	Name	Credentials	License Number	Medicare Part	Last Name
▶ 10	Marion, Davis	MD		False	Marion
11	Bertram, Brown	MD		False	Bertram
12	Janet, Wood	MD		False	Janet
13	Harold, Gearhart	MD		False	Harold

Edit | New | Delete | Print Grid | Close

Figure 5-5 **Referring Provider List Dialog Box**

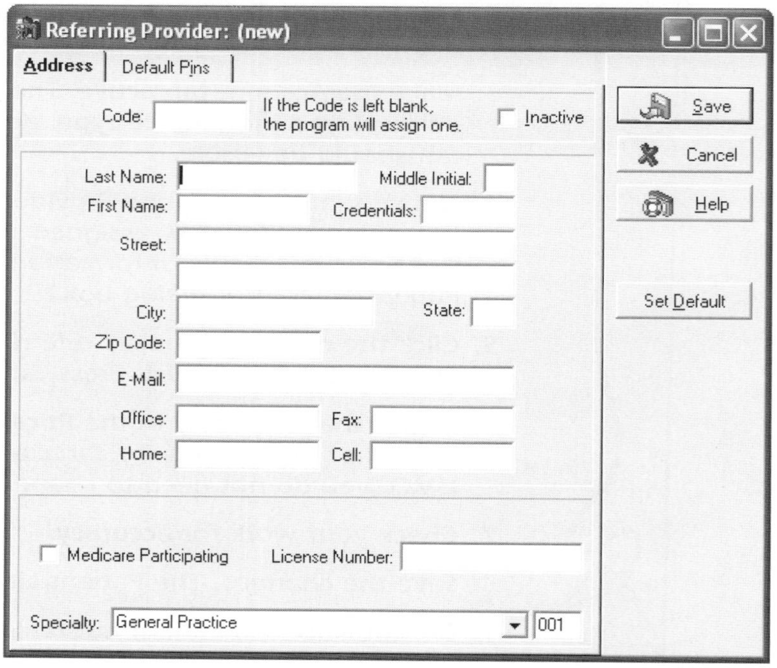

Figure 5-6 **Referring Provider Dialog Box**

ADDRESS TAB   The Address tab includes a provider's name, address, license number, specialty, and Medicare participation status (see Figure 5-6).

Code   The Code box contains a unique identification code assigned to a referring provider. It can be up to five characters long. If a code is not entered in the Code box, the system will assign one.

Inactive   The Inactive box is checked if a referring provider has not provided the practice with referrals for a specified period of time.

Name, Address, Email, and Phone Numbers   The Last Name, Middle Initial, First Name, Street, City, State, Zip Code, E-mail, Office, Home, Fax, and Cell boxes list basic information about a referring provider.

Credentials   The Credentials box lists a referring provider's professional credentials, such as MD, DO, PhD, or RN. This box can be up to three characters long.

Medicare Participating   If a referring provider is a participating Medicare provider, the Medicare Participating box is checked.

License Number   A referring provider's license number is listed in the License Number box.

Specialty   A referring provider's specialty is selected from the corresponding drop-down list. Specialty codes are assigned under HIPAA legislation to facilitate electronic billing.

DEFAULT PINS TAB The Default Pins tab contains identification numbers assigned to a referring provider (see Figure 5-7).

SSN/Federal Tax ID The SSN/Federal Tax ID box contains a provider's Social Security number or Federal Tax Identification number. The corresponding radio button should first be clicked to indicate whether the number to be entered is a Social Security number or a Federal Tax ID.

PINs In the boxes listed, a referring provider's PINs (provider identification numbers) are entered for each insurance type: Medicare, Medicaid, Tricare, Blue Cross/Shield, Commercial, PPO, and HMO.

UPIN The provider's Unique Physician Identifier Number (UPIN) is entered in the UPIN box. The UPIN code will eventually be replaced by the National Provider Identifier (NPI).

Extra 1, Extra 2 These boxes can be used to enter any additional information about the referring provider.

EDI ID The EDI ID box contains the identification number assigned to a physician by the EDI clearinghouse.

National Identifier The National Identifier field contains a provider's National Provider Identifier (NPI), which is a unique identification number assigned to health care providers, and used by all health plans.

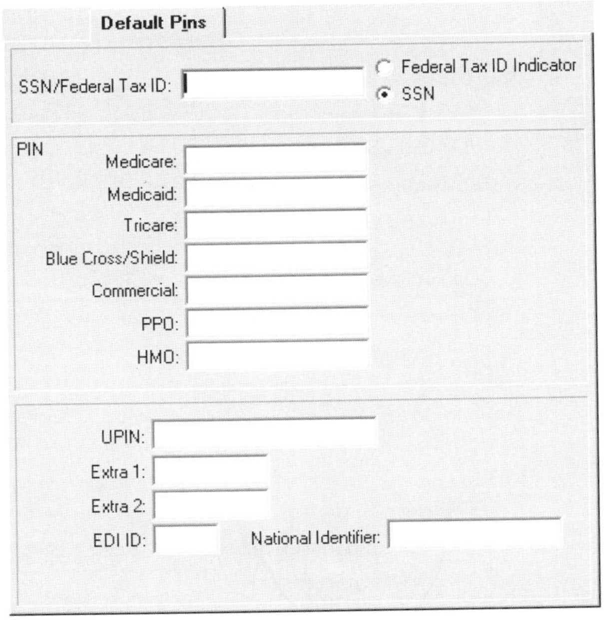

Figure 5-7 **Default Pins Tab**

When all the information about the referring provider has been entered and checked for accuracy, it is saved by clicking the Save button in the Referring Provider dialog box.

DIAGNOSIS TAB   The Diagnosis tab contains a patient's diagnosis, information about allergies, and electronic claim (EDI) notes (see Figure 5-8).

Default Diagnosis 1, 2, 3, and 4   A patient's diagnosis is selected from the drop-down list of diagnoses. If a patient has more than one diagnosis, the primary diagnosis is entered as Default Diagnosis 1. Up to four diagnoses can be entered for each case. If there are more than four diagnoses, a new case must be opened.

Allergies and Notes   If a patient has allergies or other special conditions that need to be recorded, they are entered in the Allergies and Notes box.

EDI Notes   If a patient's claims require special handling when submitted electronically, notes about the procedure, such as an explanation about the charges for supplies, are listed in this box.

EDI Report   The Report Type Code is a two-character code that indicates the title or contents of a document, report, or supporting item sent with electronic claims. The Report Transmission Code is a two-character code that defines the timing, transmission method, or format by which reports are sent with electronic claims. The value entered in the Attachment Control Number field is a unique reference number up to seven digits long.

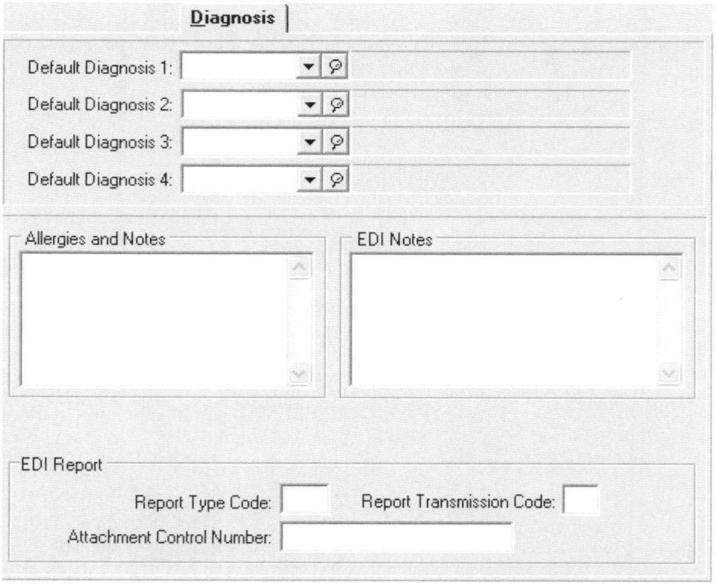

Figure 5-8 **Diagnosis Tab**

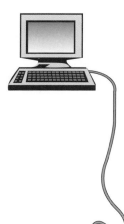

Exercise 5-3

Complete the Diagnosis tab for Hiro Tanaka. The information needed to complete this exercise is found on Source Documents 1 and 2.

Date: October 4, 2010

1. **Edit the case for Hiro Tanaka.**

2. **Make the Diagnosis tab active.**

3. **From the list of choices in the drop-down list, select Tanaka's diagnosis.**

4. **In the Allergies and Notes box, enter information on Tanaka's allergies.**

5. **Check your work for accuracy.**

6. **Save the changes. The Patient List dialog box is redisplayed.**

7. **Do not close the Patient List dialog box.**

CONDITION TAB   The Condition tab stores data about a patient's illness, accident, disability, and hospitalization (see Figure 5-9). This information is used by insurance carriers to process claims.

Injury/Illness/LMP Date   The date of a patient's injury, illness, or last menstrual period (LMP) is entered in the Injury/Illness/LMP Date box. (For an illness, the date when the symptoms first appeared is entered.)

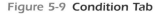

Figure 5-9 **Condition Tab**

Illness Indicator   The Illness Indicator box specifies whether a patient's condition is an illness, a last menstrual period, in the case of a pregnancy, or an injury.

First Consultation Date   The date of a patient's first visit for a particular condition is entered in the First Consultation Date box. The actual date can be entered, or the pop-up calendar can be activated and dates selected.

Date Similar Symptoms   If a patient has had similar symptoms in the past, enter the date of those symptoms in the Date Similar Symptoms box.

Same/Similar Symptoms   A check mark in the Same/Similar Symptoms box indicates that a patient has had the same or similar symptoms in the past.

Employment Related   If the Employment Related box is checked, it means that the illness or accident is in some way related to a patient's employment.

Emergency   If a patient sees the provider on an emergency visit, a check mark is entered in the Emergency box.

Accident—Related To   The Accident—Related To box indicates whether a patient's condition is related to an accident. The drop-down list offers three choices: Auto if an automobile accident is involved; No, if it is not accident-related; and Yes, if it is accident-related but not to an auto accident. If a patient's condition is accident-related, the State and Nature Of boxes should also be completed.

Accident—State   The abbreviation for the state in which the accident occurred is entered in this box.

Accident—Nature Of   This box provides additional information about the type of accident. The following choices can be selected from the drop-down list: Injured at home, Injured at school, Injured during recreation, Motorcycle injury, Work injury/Non-collision, and Work injury/Self employed.

Last X-ray Date   The date of the last X-rays for the current condition are entered in this box.

Death/Status   The Death/Status box indicates a patient's condition according to the Karnofsky Performance Status Scale. There are eleven options: Able to carry on normal activity, Cares for self, Dead, Disabled, Moribund (a terminal condition near death), Normal, Normal activity with effort, Requires considerable assistance, Requires occasional assistance, Severely disabled, and Very sick. If this information is not provided by the physician, the box should be left blank.

Dates—Unable to Work If a patient is unable to work, the dates of the absence from work are listed in these boxes.

Dates—Total Disability If a patient is totally disabled, the dates of the total disability are entered in these boxes.

Dates—Partial Disability If a patient is partially disabled, the dates of the partial disability are listed in these boxes.

Dates—Hospitalization If a patient is hospitalized, the dates of the hospitalization are entered in these boxes.

Workers' Compensation—Return to Work Indicator If a patient has been out of work on workers' compensation, the patient's return to work status is selected from the drop-down list of choices: Conditional, Limited, or Normal. If the status is Conditional or Limited, the Percent of Disability box should also be completed.

Workers' Compensation—Percent of Disability This box indicates a patient's percent of disability upon returning to work.

Last Worked Date The last day the patient worked is listed in this box.

Pregnant This box is checked if a woman is pregnant.

Estimated Date of Birth If the patient is pregnant, enter the date the baby is due.

Date Assumed Care This field is used when providers share postoperative care. Enter the date the provider assumed care for this patient.

Date Relinquished Care This field is used when providers share post-operative care. Enter the date the provider relinquished care of the patient.

Exercise 5-4

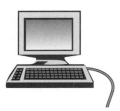

Complete the Condition tab for Hiro Tanaka. The information needed to complete this exercise is found on Source Documents 1 and 3.

Date: October 4, 2010

1. **Edit the case for Hiro Tanaka.**

2. **Make the Condition tab active.**

3. Enter the date of the injury in the Injury/Illness/LMP Date box.

4. Leave the Illness Indicator box blank.

5. In the First Consultation Date box, enter the date Tanaka first saw Dr. Yan for this condition. Press Tab. The program displays a Confirm message stating that the date entered is in the future, and asking whether you want to change it. Click No.

6. Since this visit resulted from a non-work-related accident, leave the Date Similar Symptoms box, the Same/Similar Symptoms box, and the Employment Related box blank.

7. Since this was an emergency visit, place a check mark in the Emergency box by clicking it.

8. Choose Auto in the Accident—Related To box.

9. In the Accident—State box, enter the two-letter abbreviation for the state in which the accident occurred.

10. Tanaka was injured while driving home from a softball game. Complete the Accident—Nature Of box regarding the type of accident with Injured during Recreation.

11. Enter the dates Tanaka was unable to work in the Dates—Unable to Work boxes.

12. Enter the dates Tanaka was totally disabled in the Dates—Total Disability boxes.

13. Enter the dates Tanaka was partially disabled in the Dates—Partial Disability boxes.

14. Enter the dates Tanaka was hospitalized in the Dates—Hospitalization boxes.

15. Leave the Last X-Ray Date box blank.

16. Since Tanaka was not injured at work, the Workers' Compensation boxes should be left blank.

17. Check your work for accuracy.

18. Save the changes.

19. Do not close the Patient List dialog box.

MISCELLANEOUS TAB

The Miscellaneous tab records a variety of miscellaneous information about the patient and his or her treatment (see Figure 5-10).

Outside Lab Work   If the Outside Lab Work box is checked, the lab work was performed by a lab other than the physician's office. If the lab bills the provider rather than the patient, then the provider bills the patient for the lab work even though it was performed by an outside lab.

Lab Charges   The charges for lab work, whether performed inside or outside the practice, are entered in the Lab Charges box.

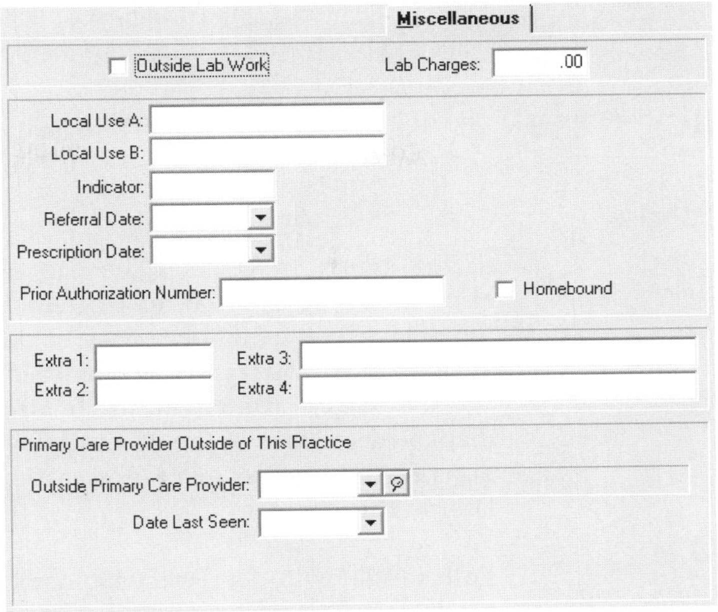

Figure 5-10 **Miscellaneous Tab**

Local Use A and B These boxes may be used by some medical practices to record information specific to the local office.

Indicator If an indicator code is used to categorize patients or services, it is entered in the Indicator box. For example, patients might be categorized according to the primary diagnosis. Services might be divided into such categories as lab work, consultations, and hospital visits.

Referral Date If the patient was referred to the provider, enter the date of the referral.

Prescription Date This field is required for hearing and vision claims.

Prior Authorization Number Before some services are performed, prior authorization must be obtained from the appropriate insurance carrier. If an insurance carrier has issued an authorization number for treatment that has not yet occurred, the number is entered in the Prior Authorization Number box.

Homebound Click this box if the patient is homebound.

Extra 1, 2, 3, and 4 The Extra 1, 2, 3, and 4 boxes are used for different purposes depending on the medical practice.

Outside Primary Care Provider If a patient is covered by a managed care plan and the patient's primary care provider is outside the medical practice, the name of the provider is selected from the drop-down list in this box.

Date Last Seen   The Date Last Seen box lists the date a patient was last seen by the outside primary care provider.

POLICY 1 TAB   The Policy 1 tab is where information about a patient's primary insurance carrier and coverage is recorded (see Figure 5-11).

Insurance 1   The Insurance 1 box lists the code number and name of the insurance carrier. The drop-down list shows the carriers already in the system. If the carrier is not listed, it must be added to the database. It is not necessary to close the Case dialog box to add an insurance carrier to the database. When Insurance Carriers is clicked on the Lists menu, the Insurance Carrier List dialog box is displayed in front of the other dialog boxes on the screen. Instructions for adding an insurance carrier to the database are covered later in this chapter.

Policy Holder 1   The Policy Holder 1 box lists the person who is the insured under a particular policy. For example, if the patient is a child covered under his or her parent's insurance plan, the parent's chart number would be entered in this box. The insured's chart number is selected from the choices on the drop-down list. (If the insured is not a patient of the practice, he or she must be entered as a guarantor in NDCMedisoft, and a chart number must be established.)

Relationship to Insured   This box describes a patient's relationship to the individual listed in the Policy Holder 1 box. The drop-down list offers the following choices: Child, Other, Self, and Spouse.

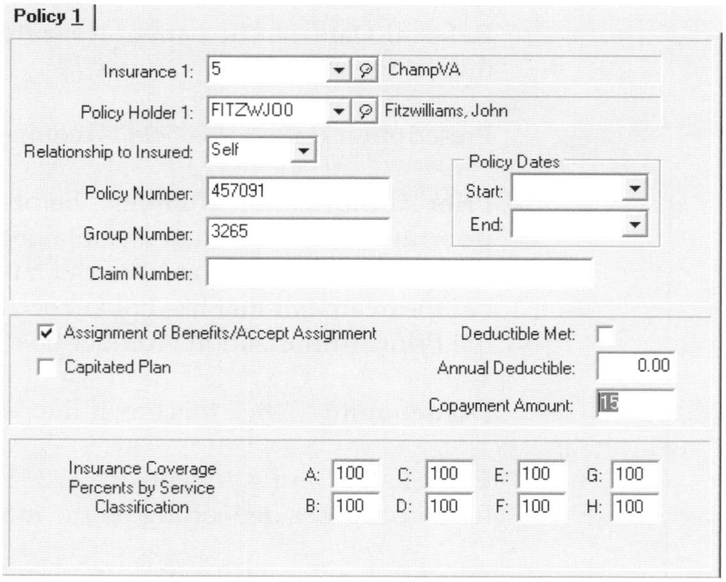

Figure 5-11 **Policy 1 Tab**

Policy Number   A patient's policy number is entered in the Policy Number box.

Group Number   The group number for a patient's policy is entered in the Group Number box.

Claim Number   This field is used on property, casualty, and auto claims. The number is assigned by the property and casualty payer, usually during eligibility determinations.

Policy Dates—Start/End   The date a patient's insurance policy went into effect is entered in the Policy Dates—Start box. If the date is not known, the date the patient first came to the practice for treatment can be entered. If the policy has ended, such as because the carrier changed or the coverage expired, the date on which coverage terminated is entered in the Policy Dates—End box.

Assignment of Benefits/Accept Assignment   For physicians who are participating in an insurance plan, a check mark in the Accept Assignment box indicates that the provider accepts payment directly from the insurance carrier.

Capitated Plan   In a **capitated plan,** payments are made to physicians from managed care companies for patients who select the physician as their primary care provider, regardless of whether they visit the physician or not. A check mark in this box indicates that this insurance plan is capitated.

Deductible Met   This box is checked when a patient has met the deductible for the current year.

Annual Deductible   The dollar amount of the insured's insurance plan deductible is entered in this box.

Copayment Amount   The dollar amount of a patient's copayment per visit is entered in the Copayment Amount box.

Insurance Coverage Percents by Service Classification   The percentage of fees that an insurance carrier covers is entered in the Insurance Coverage Percents by Service Classification box. Some insurance plans pay different percentages of charges based on the type of service provided. For example, a plan may pay 80 percent of necessary medical procedures, 100 percent of lab work, and 50 percent of outpatient mental health charges. A practice can assign a different category of service to each of the letters A through H. For example, "A" could represent necessary medical procedures performed in the office, "B" could represent lab tests, and "C" outpatient mental health. With some managed care plans, 100 percent is entered in boxes A through H, because the patient is required to pay a copayment only, not a percentage of the charges.

capitated plan an insurance plan in which payments are made to a physician by a managed care company for a patient who selects the physician as his or her primary care provider, regardless of whether he or she visits the physician.

Adding an Insurance Carrier to the Database

If an insurance carrier is not listed in the Insurance drop-down list in the Policy 1, 2, or 3 tabs, it needs to be added to the database. To add an insurance carrier, click Insurance Carriers on the Lists menu. The Insurance Carrier List dialog box shows all the carriers already in the system (see Figure 5-12). Clicking the New button brings up the Insurance Carrier (new) dialog box, where information on a carrier is entered (see Figure 5-13). The Insurance Carrier dialog box contains five tabs: Address; Options; EDI, Codes; Allowed; and PINs.

ADDRESS TAB The Address tab contains basic information about an insurance carrier (see Figure 5-13).

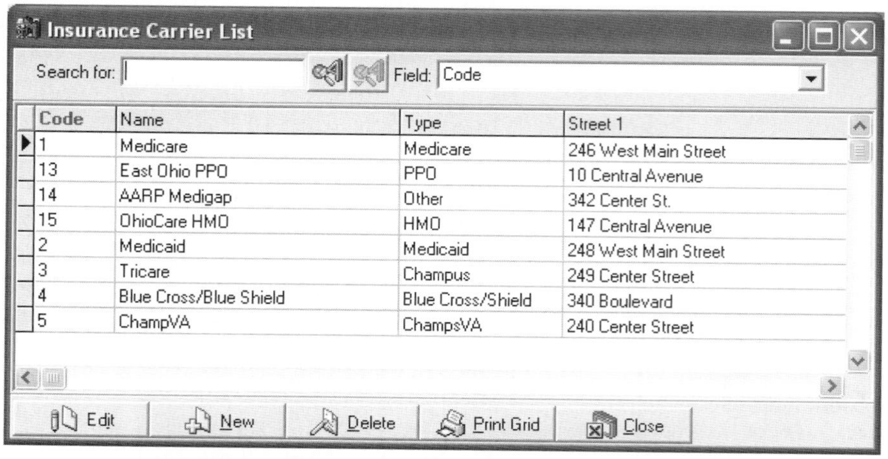

Figure 5-12 **Insurance Carrier List Dialog Box**

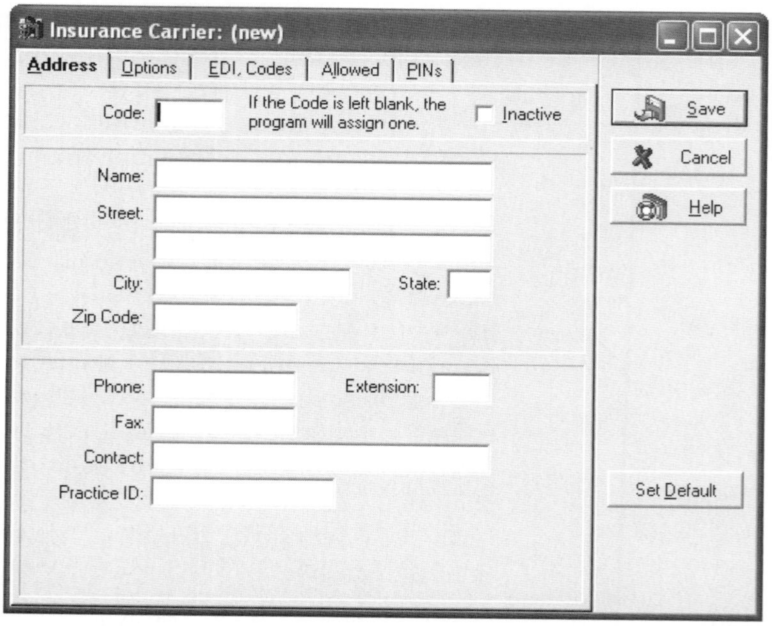

Figure 5-13 **Insurance Carrier Dialog Box**

Code The code is a unique identification number assigned to an insurance carrier. It can be up to five characters long. If a code is not entered in the Code box, the system will assign one. Once created, the code cannot be changed.

Inactive The Inactive check box is used when a carrier is no longer accepting new claims for any patients, but some outstanding claims have not been completed.

Name, Address, and Phone Numbers The Name, Street, City, State, Zip Code, Phone, Extension, and Fax boxes list basic information about a carrier.

Contact If there is a specific person at the insurance carrier who is assigned to handle the practice's claims, that person's name is entered in the Contact box.

Practice ID The Practice ID box lists the identification number assigned to the practice by the insurance carrier.

OPTIONS TAB The Options tab records detailed information about an insurance carrier (see Figure 5-14).

Plan Name The name of the insurance plan is entered in the Plan Name box.

Type The type of insurance plan is selected from a drop-down list of choices:

◆ Other

◆ Medicare

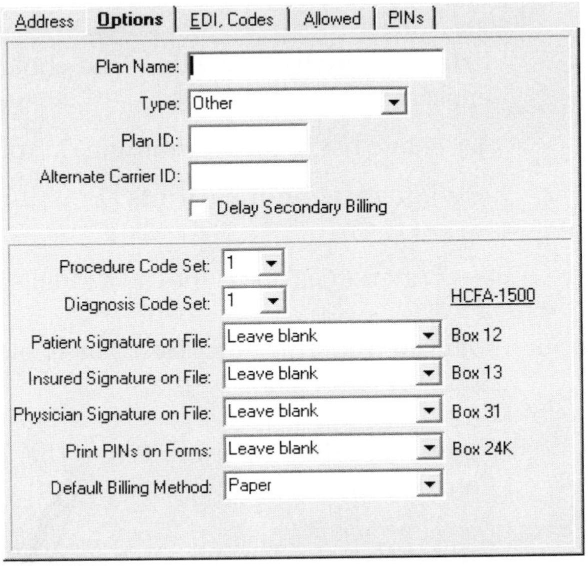

Figure 5-14 **Options Tab**

- Medicaid
- Tricare/Champus
- ChampsVA
- Group
- FECA
- Blue Cross/Shield
- Worker's Comp
- HMO
- PPO

Plan ID   The Plan ID field is provided to contain the Health Plan Identifier, which will be implemented by insurance carriers. It will identify a contract between the provider and carrier to conduct or process transactions of health plans in compliance with HIPAA requirements.

Alternate Carrier ID   This field is used if an alternate ID is required.

Delay Secondary Billing   A check in this box delays printing the secondary claim form until a response is recorded from the primary carrier.

Procedure Code Set   If a practice uses more than one set of procedure codes, enter the code number for the set used by the particular insurance carrier.

Diagnosis Code Set   If a practice uses more than one set of diagnosis codes, enter the code number for the set used by the particular insurance carrier.

Patient Signature on File   The choices in the Patient Signature on File drop-down list are:

- Leave blank (prints nothing on form)
- Signature on file (prints "Signature on file" in relevant box on form)
- Print name (prints the individual's name in relevant box on form)

Insured Signature on File   The choices are the same as for Patient Signature on File.

Physician Signature on File   The choices are the same as for Patient Signature on File.

Print PINs on Forms   The Print PINs on Forms box indicates whether the provider name and PIN are included in the claim file.

Default Billing Method The Default Billing Method box indicates whether claims are to be submitted electronically or on paper. For the purposes of this book, the default method for submitting claims is electronic.

EDI, CODES TAB The third tab in the Insurance Carrier (new) dialog box is the EDI, Codes tab. This tab contains data for electronic claim submissions (see Figure 5-15).

EDI Receiver The EDI Receiver box contains the name of the receiver of electronic claims for this insurance carrier.

EDI Payor Number The payer identification number assigned by the clearinghouse is entered in the EDI Payor Number box.

EDI Sub ID The EDI Sub ID box contains the sub ID number assigned by the clearinghouse.

EDI Extra 1/Medigap The EDI Extra 1/Medigap box can be used to enter additional information about the EDI setup.

EDI Extra 2 The EDI Extra 2 is another box that can be used to enter additional information about the EDI setup.

NDC Record Code The record code assigned to the insurance carrier by the clearinghouse is entered in the NDC (National Data Corporation) Record Code box.

EDI Max Transactions The EDI Max Transactions field is provided for carriers that limit the number of transactions per claim accepted

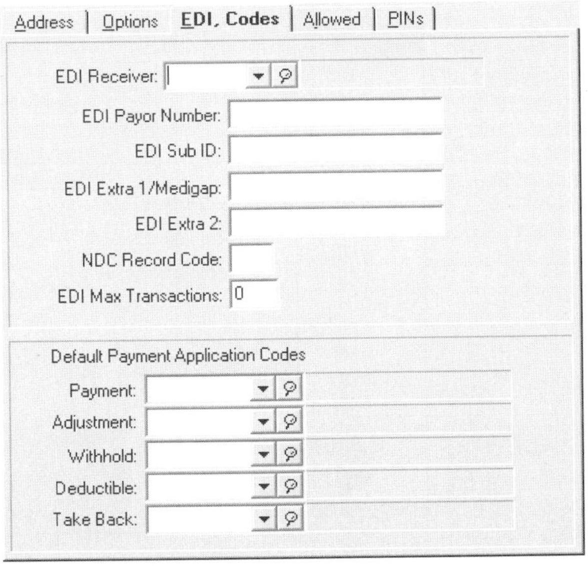

Figure 5-15 **EMC, Codes Tab**

electronically. If the carrier has a maximum, enter the maximum number of transactions accepted in this field. Then, when a claim is created that has more than the maximum number of transactions per claim, the program automatically splits the claim.

Default Payment Application Codes   These are the default codes (Payment, Adjustment, Withhold, Deductible, Take Back) that are used when entering deposit or payment information from the insurance carrier. These codes are set up in the Procedure/Payment/Adjustment Codes list.

When all the information about an insurance carrier has been entered and checked for accuracy, data are saved by clicking the Save button.

ALLOWED TAB

The next tab in the Insurance Carrier (new) dialog box is the Allowed tab (see Figure 5-16). The program provides an option to automatically calculate allowed amounts when insurance payments are applied to procedures (this is covered in Chapter 7). For the purposes of this book, this feature is not used.

PINS TAB

The last tab in the Insurance Carrier (new) dialog box is the PINs tab (see Figure 5-17). This tab lists the insurance carrier's assigned PIN and Group ID for each provider in the practice.

Address	Options	EDI, Codes	**Allowed**	PINs

Code	Procedure	Allowed
12011	Simple suture--face--local anes.	0.00
29125	Application of short arm splint; static	0.00
29425	Application of short leg cast, walking	0.00
45378	Colonoscopy--diagnostic	0.00
45380	Colonoscopy--with biopsy	0.00
50390	Aspiration of renal cyst by needle	0.00
71010	Chest x-ray, single view, frontal	0.00
71020	Chest x-ray, two views, frontal & lat...	0.00
71030	Chest x-ray, complete, four views	0.00
73070	Elbow x-ray, AP and lateral views	0.00
73090	Forearm x-ray, AP and lateral views	0.00
73100	Wrist x-ray, AP and lateral views	0.00
73510	Hip x-ray, complete, two views	0.00
73600	Ankle x-ray, AP and lateral views	0.00
80048	Basic metabolic panel	0.00
80061	Lipid panel	0.00
82270	Blood screening, occult; feces	0.00
82947	Glucose screening--quantitative	0.00
82951	Glucose tolerance test, three specimens	0.00

Figure 5-16 Allowed Tab

Address	Options	EDI, Codes	Allowed	**PINs**

Code	Provider	Pin	Group Id
1	Yan, Katherine	901	9870
2	Rudner, John	902	9870
3	Rudner, Jessica	903	9870
4	McGrath, Patricia	904	9870
5	Beach, Robert	905	9870
6	Banu, Dana	906	9870

Figure 5-17 PINS Tab

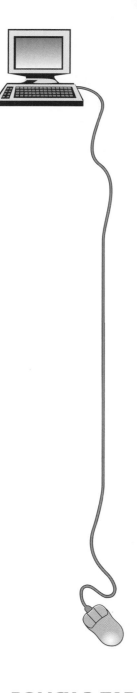

Exercise 5-5

Complete the Policy 1 tab for Hiro Tanaka. The information needed to complete this exercise is found on Source Document 1.

Date: October 4, 2010

1. Edit the case for Hiro Tanaka.

2. Make the Policy 1 tab active.

3. Select Tanaka's primary insurance carrier from the drop-down list in the Insurance 1 box. Press Tab.

4. The program completes the Policy Holder 1 field with the name of the patient. Since Tanaka is the policyholder, accept this entry.

5. Notice that the Relationship to Insured box already has "Self" entered. Since this is correct, do not make any changes.

6. Enter Tanaka's insurance policy number in the Policy Number box. Press Tab.

7. Enter Tanaka's group number in the Group Number box. Press Tab.

8. In the Policy Dates—Start box, key *01012010* as the start date of the policy. Press Tab. The program displays a Confirm message stating that the date entered is in the future, and asking whether you want to change it. Click No.

9. Dr. Yan accepts assignment for this carrier, so click the Assignment of Benefits/Accept Assignment box.

10. The insurance plan is capitated, so check the Capitated Plan box.

11. Key *30* in the Copayment box if it does not already appear. Press Tab.

12. Key *100* in each of the Insurance Coverage Percents by Service Classification boxes.

13. Check your work for accuracy.

14. Save the changes.

15. Do not close the Patient List dialog box.

POLICY 2 TAB   The boxes in the Policy 2 tab are the same as those in the Policy 1 tab, with a few exceptions. The Copayment Amount, Capitated Plan, and Annual Deductible boxes are only in the Policy 1 tab. Only the Policy 2 tab has a Crossover Claim box (see Figure 5-18 on page 106).

Crossover Claim   The Crossover Claim box is used when a patient has Medicare as the primary carrier and Medicaid as the secondary

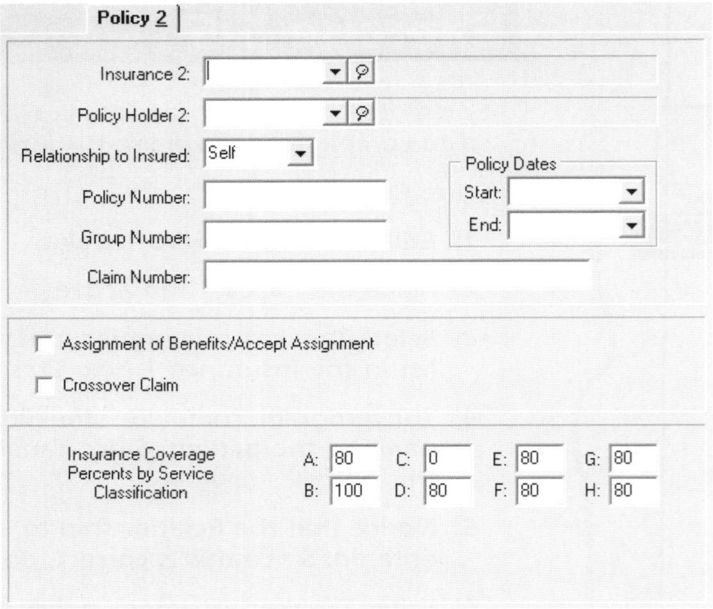

Figure 5-18 **Policy 2 Tab**

carrier. Because Medicare is the primary carrier, it pays first on a claim and then submits the claim to the Medicaid carrier.

POLICY 3 TAB   The Policy 3 tab does not contain the Copayment Amount, Capitated Plan, Annual Deductible, and Crossover Claim boxes. Otherwise, the boxes are the same as those in the Policy 1 and Policy 2 tabs (see Figure 5-19).

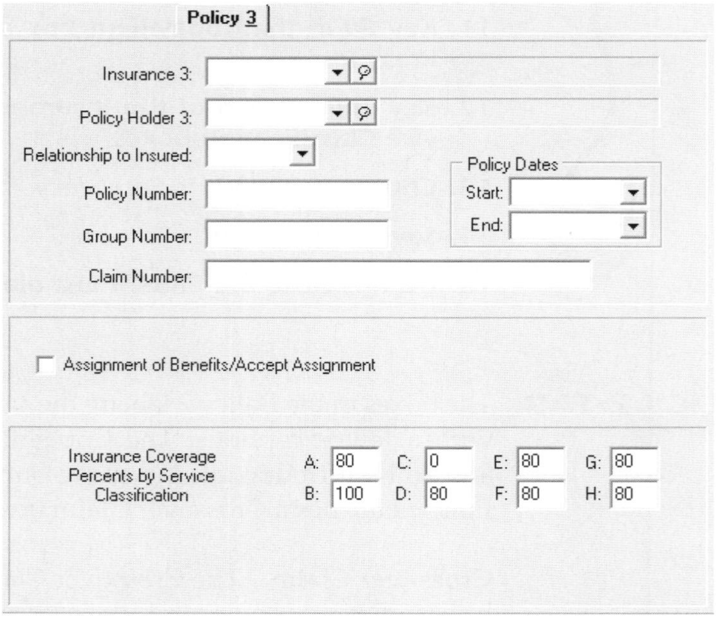

Figure 5-19 **Policy 3 Tab**

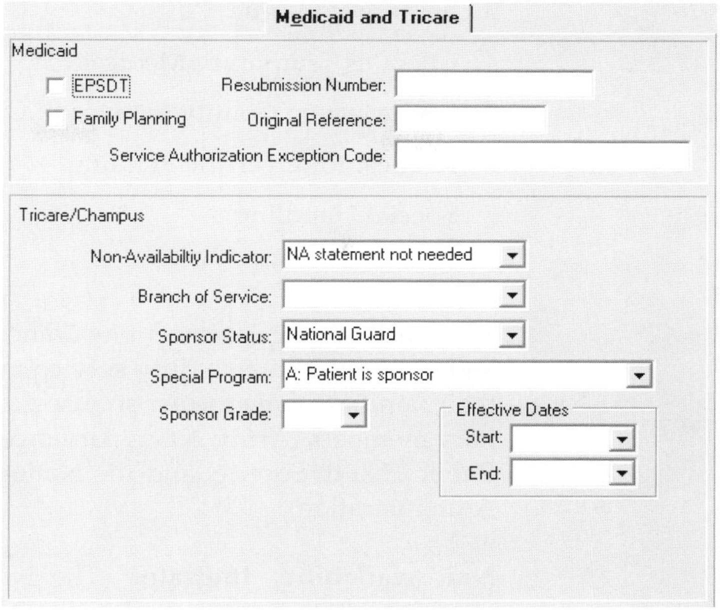

Figure 5-20 **Medicaid and Tricare Tab**

MEDICAID AND TRICARE TAB

For patients covered by Medicaid or TRICARE, the Medicaid and Tricare tab is used to enter additional information about the government programs (see Figure 5-20).

Medicaid

EPSDT   EPSDT stands for "Early and Periodic Screening, Diagnosis, and Treatment." This is a Medicaid program for patients under the age of twenty-one who need screening and diagnostic services to determine physical or mental problems as well as treatment for conditions discovered. It also includes well-baby checkup examinations. A check mark in the EPSDT box indicates that a patient's visit is part of the EPSDT program.

Family Planning   A check mark in the Family Planning box specifies that a patient's condition is related to family planning.

Resubmission Number   For claims being resubmitted to Medicaid, the resubmission number is entered in this box.

Original Reference   For claims being resubmitted to Medicaid, the original reference number is recorded in the Original Reference box.

Service Authorization Exception Code   This code is required on some Medicaid claims. If a service authorization code was not obtained before seeing the patient, select one of the following codes:

1   Immediate/Urgent Care

2   Services Rendered in a Retroactive Period

3   Emergency Care

4   Client as Temporary Medicaid

5   Request from County for Second Opinion to Recipient Can Work

6   Request for Override Pending

7   Special Handling

TRICARE

TRICARE is the government insurance program that serves spouses and children of active-duty service members, military retirees and their families, some former spouses, and survivors of deceased military members (Army, Navy, Air Force, Marine Corps, Coast Guard, Public Health Service, and the National Oceanic and Atmospheric Administration).

Non-Availability Indicator   The Non-Availability Indicator box specifies whether a nonavailability (NA) statement is required. The choices on the drop-down list are NA statement not needed, NA statement obtained, and Other carrier paid at least 75%.

Branch of Service   The Branch of Service box indicates the particular branch of service: Air Force, Army, Champ VA, Coast Guard, Marines, Navy, NOAA, and Public Health Service.

sponsor in TRICARE, the active-duty service member.

Sponsor Status   The **sponsor** is the active-duty service member. The sponsor's family members are covered by the TRICARE insurance plan. The drop-down list in the Sponsor Status box provides choices to indicate the sponsor's status in the service, such as Active, Medal of Honor, or Reserves.

Special Program   The Special Program drop-down list contains codes for special TRICARE programs.

Sponsor Grade   The two-character sponsor grade is entered in the Sponsor Grade box.

Effective Dates   The start date of the TRICARE policy is entered in the Effective Dates—Start box. If there is an end date, it is entered in the Effective Dates—End box. Specific dates can be entered, or a selection can be made from the pop-up calendar.

EDITING CASE INFORMATION ON AN ESTABLISHED PATIENT

Information in an existing case is modified by selecting the case to be edited and clicking the Edit Case button at the bottom of the Patient List dialog box. (The Case radio button must be clicked for the Edit Case button to be displayed.)

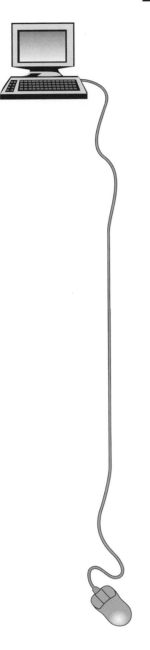

Exercise 5-6

John Fitzwilliams, an established patient, has just remarried. Edit the information in his Case dialog box to reflect this change.

Date: October 4, 2010

1. Click in the Search For field and press the backspace key to delete the "T" that was entered to search for Hiro Tanaka. The Patient List once again displays the complete list of patients.

2. Enter *F* in the Search For field. All patients who have last names beginning with the letter "F" are displayed. Click anywhere in the listing for John Fitzwilliams to select his entry.

3. Click the Case radio button. Verify that Acute Gastric Ulcer is listed in the Case area of the dialog box.

4. Click the Edit Case button.

5. In the Personal tab, change the entry in the Marital Status box from Divorced to Married.

6. Check your work for accuracy.

7. Save the changes.

8. Close the Patient List dialog box.

9. Create a backup of your work and exit NDCMedisoft by selecting Exit on the File menu. The Backup Reminder dialog box is displayed.

10. Click the Back Up Data Now button. The Backup dialog box appears.

11. Enter the file path and file name in the Destination File Path and Name or click the Find button and browse to the desired location. The file name should be FCC8-5.mbk (the database name followed by the chapter number). The file path will vary depending on your computer and network setup. Ask your instructor for the file path.

12. Click the Start Backup button. NDCMedisoft creates a backup file. When it is complete, an Information box is displayed, indicating that the backup is complete. Click OK. The Backup dialog box closes and the program is shut down.

CHAPTER REVIEW

USING TERMINOLOGY

Match the terms on the left with the definitions on the right.

_____ 1. capitated plan

_____ 2. case

_____ 3. chart

_____ 4. record of treatment and progress

_____ 5. referring provider

_____ 6. sponsor

a. A folder that contains a patient's medical records.

b. Physician's notes about a patient's condition and diagnosis.

c. A physician who recommends that a patient make an appointment with a particular doctor.

d. An insurance plan in which payments are made to primary care providers for patients whether they visit the office or not.

e. A grouping of transactions organized around a patient's condition.

f. The active-duty service member on the TRI-CARE government insurance program.

CHECKING YOUR UNDERSTANDING

Answer the questions below in the space provided.

7. Sarina Bell has no insurance of her own but is covered by her father's insurance policy. How would this be indicated in the Policy 1 tab for Sarina Bell?

_____

_____

8. Where in the Case dialog box can you find information about a patient's allergies?

_____

_____

9. Is it necessary to set up a new case when a patient changes insurance carriers? Why?

_____

_____

10. In the Case dialog box, where would you enter information about a work-related accident?

_____

_____

11. Where is information needed to complete the Diagnosis tab usually found?

_____

_____

12. A patient has been seeing the doctor regularly for treatment of diabetes. She was hospitalized yesterday, and the doctor saw her in the hospital for treatment. Do you need to set up a new case for the hospitalization?

_____

_____

APPLYING KNOWLEDGE

Answer the questions below in the space provided.

13. While you are entering case information for a new patient, you realize that the patient's referring provider is not one of the choices in the Referring Provider box in the Account tab. What should you do?

_____

_____

_____

14. One of the established patients has changed insurance carriers from Blue Cross and Blue Shield to OhioCare HMO. What specific boxes need to be changed in the Case dialog box?

_____

_____

_____

AT THE COMPUTER

Answer the following questions at the computer.

15. Using the information contained in the Case dialog box, list Randall Klein's primary and secondary insurance carriers.

16. Who is the guarantor for Janine Bell's account?

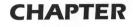

CHAPTER

6

Entering Charge Transactions

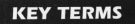

WHAT YOU NEED TO KNOW

To use this chapter, you need to know how to:

◆ Start NDCMedisoft, use menus, and enter and edit text.

◆ Edit information in an existing case.

◆ Work with chart and case numbers.

OBJECTIVES

When you finish this chapter, you will be able to:

◆ Enter charges for procedures.

◆ Enter copayment charges.

◆ Edit and delete charge transactions.

◆ Use NDCMedisoft's Search features to find specific transaction data.

KEY TERMS

adjustments   MultiLink codes
charges   payments
modifiers

TRANSACTION ENTRY OVERVIEW

charges *amounts a provider bills for the services performed.*

payments *monies received from patients and insurance carriers.*

adjustments *changes to patients' accounts that alter the amount charged or paid.*

Three types of transactions are recorded in NDCMedisoft: charges, payments, and adjustments. **Charges** are the amounts a provider bills for the services performed. **Payments** are monies received from patients and insurance carriers. **Adjustments** are changes to patients' accounts. Examples of adjustments include returned check fees, insurance write-offs, Medicare adjustments, and changes in treatment. This chapter covers charge transactions. Chapter 7 covers payment and adjustment transactions.

The primary document needed to enter charge transactions in NDCMedisoft is a patient's encounter form. Typically, the physician circles or checks the appropriate procedure and diagnosis codes on the encounter form during or just after the patient visit. Charges and payments listed on an encounter form are later entered in the Transaction Entry dialog box in NDCMedisoft by an insurance billing specialist. After the information is entered, it is checked for accuracy. If all the information is correct, the transaction data are saved and a walkout statement is printed for the patient. If it is incorrect, the data are edited and then saved.

THE TRANSACTION ENTRY DIALOG BOX

Transactions are entered in the Transaction Entry dialog box, which is accessed by clicking Enter Transactions on the Activities menu (see Figure 6-1). The Transaction Entry dialog box lists existing transactions and provides options for editing them and for creating new transactions. The following section provides an overview of the different areas of the Transaction Entry dialog box.

CHART AND CASE

All transactions entered in NDCMedisoft begin with two critical pieces of information: a patient's chart number and the case number, which is related to the procedures performed. The chart number and case number must be selected in the Transaction Entry dialog box before a transaction can be entered. Boxes for entering these numbers are found at the top left of the dialog box (see Figure 6-2).

Chart A patient's chart number is selected from the drop-down list in the Chart box. Many practices have long lists of chart numbers in NDCMedisoft. The fastest way to enter a chart number is to key the first few letters of the patient's last name, which then displays that location in the drop-down list of chart numbers.

Case After the chart number has been selected, the Case box displays a case number and description for a particular patient. The transactions for the most recent case are displayed (see Figure 6-3). Transactions for other cases can be displayed by changing the selection in the Case box. Only one case can be opened at a time.

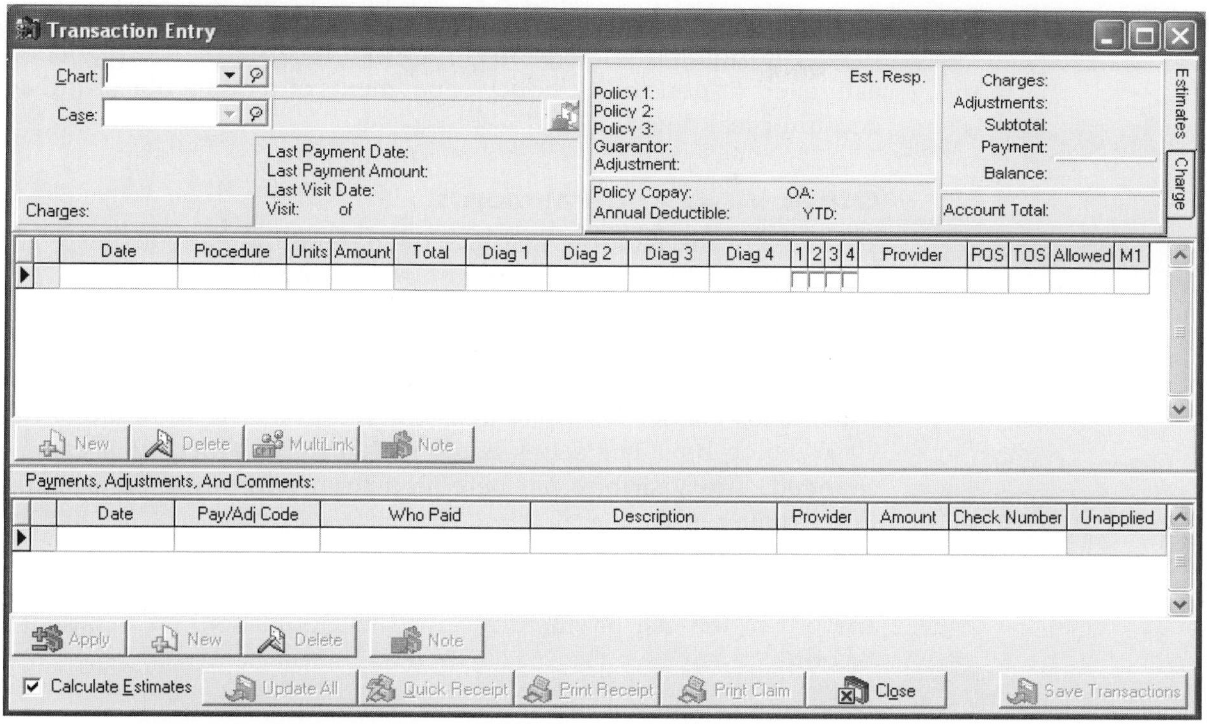

Figure 6-1 **Transaction Entry Dialog Box**

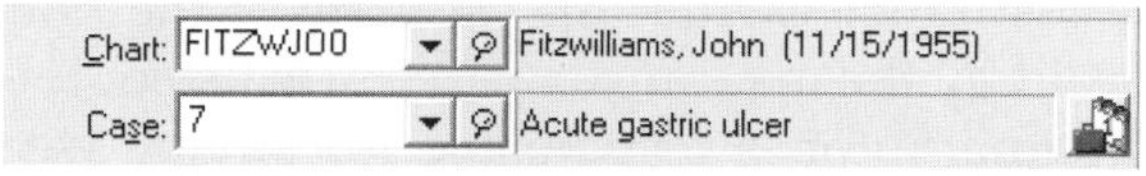

Figure 6-2 **Chart and Case Fields Within the Transaction Entry Dialog Box**

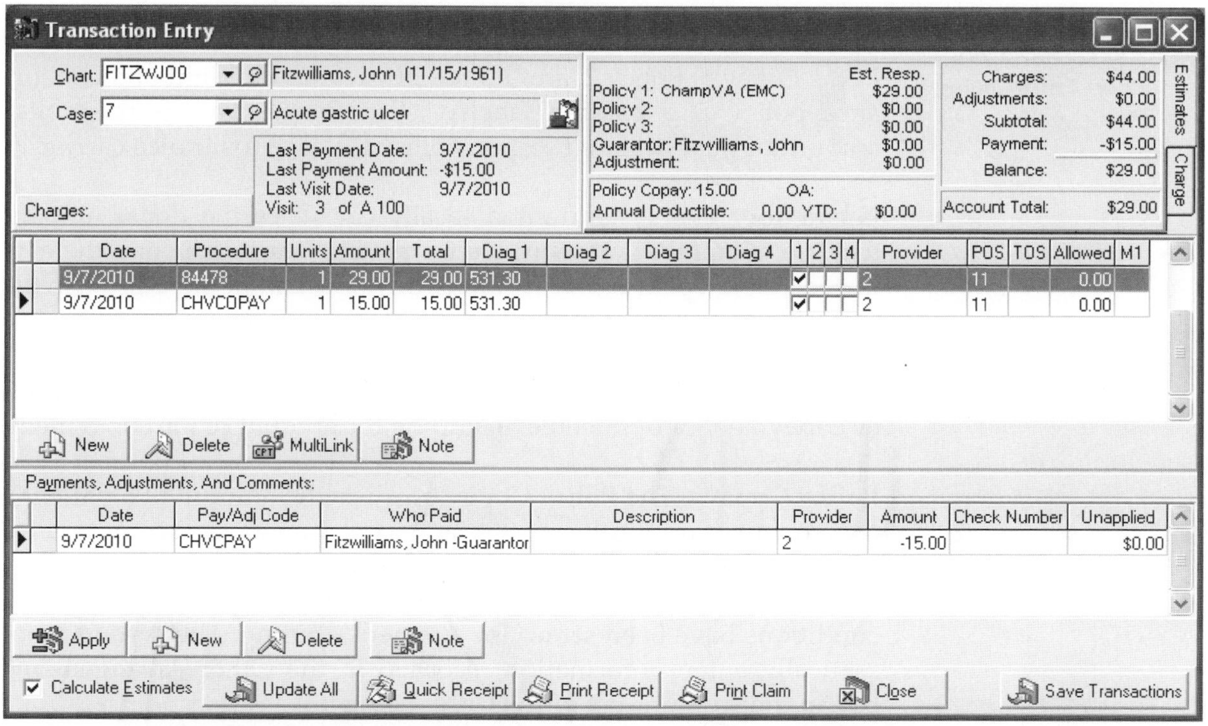

Figure 6-3 **Transaction Entry Dialog Box with Case Transactions Displayed**

ACCOUNT DETAIL

The account detail section of the Transaction Entry dialog box displays information related to number of office visits, last payment, estimated responsibility, policy copayments and deductibles, and an account breakdown.

Office Visits and Payments

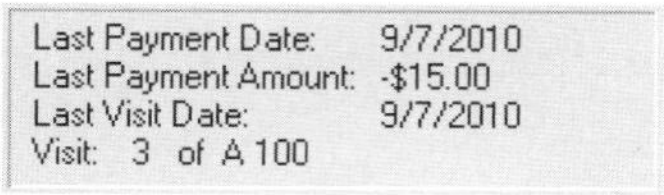

Figure 6-4 **Last Payment and Visit Area of Transaction Entry Dialog Box**

This area of the window displays the date of the patient's last visit for this case and the visit number (see Figure 6-4).

Last Visit   The Date box within the Last Visit area lists the date of a patient's most recent visit to a particular physician. The Visit box lists the visit series information as entered in the Account tab of the Case dialog box. The series is set to 100 by default, but it can be changed. The Visit box can be edited from within the Transaction Entry dialog box.

Last Payment   The Last Payment area lists the date (Date box) and amount of the last payment received (Amount box) on a patient's account.

Estimated Responsibility

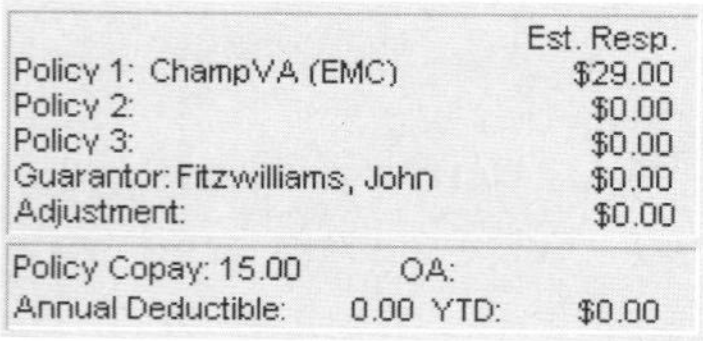

Figure 6-5 **Estimated Responsibility Section Within the Transaction Entry Dialog Box**

This section displays information about the financial responsibilities of the guarantor and the insurance carrier. An estimate of the portion of a bill that will be paid by the insurance carrier(s) is listed, followed by the amount the guarantor is responsible for paying (see Figure 6-5).

Policy 1, Policy 2, Policy 3   A patient's insurance carriers are listed in the Policy 1, Policy 2, and Policy 3 boxes. To the right of the insurance policy is a column labeled "Est. Resp." This is the dollar amount of the estimated responsibility for each insurance carrier.

Guarantor   The system automatically calculates the dollar amount that the guarantor is responsible for paying, after deducting the estimated amount paid by the insurance carrier. This amount is listed in the Guarantor box, followed by the guarantor's last name and first name.

This area of the window also lists information pertaining to the policy copayment or deductible, including the amount of the copayment.

Policy Copay   The Policy Copay box lists the amount of a patient's copayment, if applicable.

OA   The OA (Other Arrangements) box indicates whether special conditions have been set up for a patient's billing. The system automatically enters information recorded in the Other Arrangements box in the Account tab of the Case dialog box.

Annual Deductible The Annual Deductible box lists the amount of the patient's annual insurance deductible, if one exists. The YTD (Year-to-Date) box indicates how much of the annual deductible has been met so far in the current year.

Account Breakdown

This section of the dialog box contains a summary of a patient's account, including charges, adjustments, subtotal, payment, balance, and account total (see Figure 6-6).

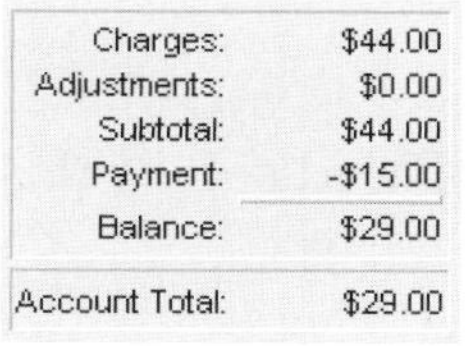

Charges The Charges box lists the total of the charges for a particular case.

Adjustments The Adjustments box lists the total of the adjustments for the case.

Subtotal The Subtotal box lists a subtotal of the amounts shown in the Charges and Adjustments boxes. If the amount in the Adjustments box is preceded by a minus sign, that amount is subtracted from the amount in the Charges box.

Payment The Payment box lists the total payments received to date for the case.

Balance The Balance box lists the amount owed for the case.

Account Total The Account Total box lists the amount owed for a particular patient for all cases, not just the case currently displayed in the Transaction Entry dialog box.

The amounts listed in the estimated responsibility area are updated whenever transactions are saved. These entries can also be updated by clicking the Update All button at the bottom of the Transaction Entry dialog box.

Charge Tab

It is also possible to view information about charges in the account detail section. On the far right side of the dialog box are two horizontal tabs: Estimates and Charge. All the information just discussed is located on the Estimates tab. Clicking the Charge tab displays summary information about the current charges. Also available in this same space is charge information. The Charge tab must be opened to display this information (see Figure 6-7).

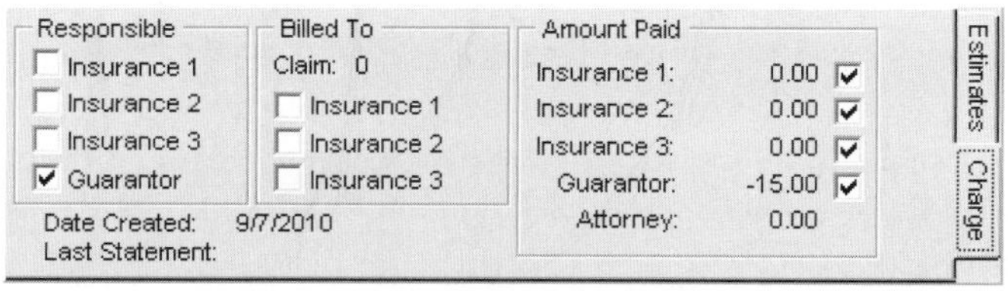

Figure 6-6 **Account Breakdown Area Within the Transaction Entry Dialog Box**

Figure 6-7 **Charge Tab Within the Transaction Entry Dialog Box**

ENTERING CHARGES

Charges are entered in the Charges section in the middle of the Transaction Entry dialog box (see Figure 6-8). Charges are entered for procedures performed by a provider and for copayments owed at the time of an office visit. (Payments and adjustments are discussed in Chapter 7.)

The process of creating a charge transaction in NDCMedisoft begins with clicking the New button.

Date   When the New button is clicked, the program automatically enters the current date (the date that the NDCMedisoft Program Date is set to) in the Date box (see Figure 6-9).

If this is not the date on which the procedures were performed, the date must be changed to the actual date of the procedures. To change the default date for these boxes, either of these methods is used:

◆   The Set Program Date command on the File menu is clicked.

◆   The date button in the bottom right corner of the screen is clicked. (This must be done before the New button is clicked in the Transaction Entry dialog box.)

The date can also be changed by keying over the information that is already in the Date box.

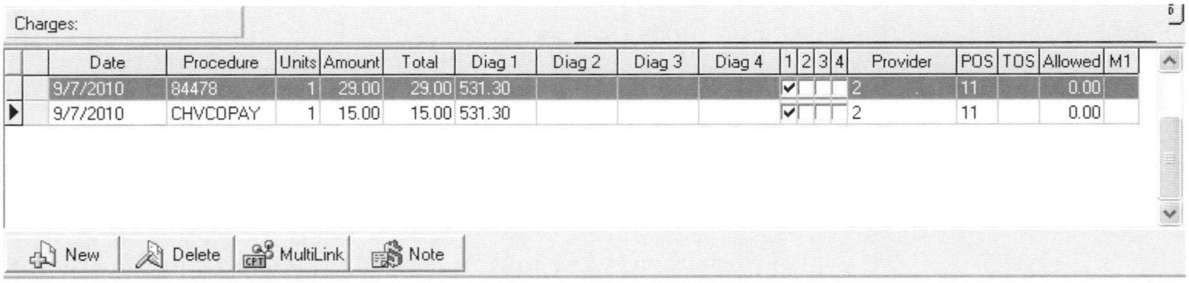

		Date	Procedure	Units	Amount	Total	Diag 1	Diag 2	Diag 3	Diag 4	1	2	3	4	Provider	POS	TOS	Allowed	M1	
		9/7/2010	84478	1	29.00	29.00	531.30				✔				2	11		0.00		
▶		9/7/2010	CHVCOPAY	1	15.00	15.00	531.30				✔				2	11		0.00		

Figure 6-8 **Charges Area in the Transaction Entry Dialog Box**

		Date	Procedure	Units	Amount	Total	Diag 1	Diag 2	Diag 3	Diag 4	1	2	3	4	Provider	POS	TOS	Allowed	M1	
		9/7/2010	84478	1	29.00	29.00	531.30				✔				2	11		0.00		
		9/7/2010	CHVCOPAY	1	15.00	15.00	531.30				✔				2	11		0.00		
*		9/7/2010 ▼		1	0.00	0.00	531.30				✔				2			0.00		

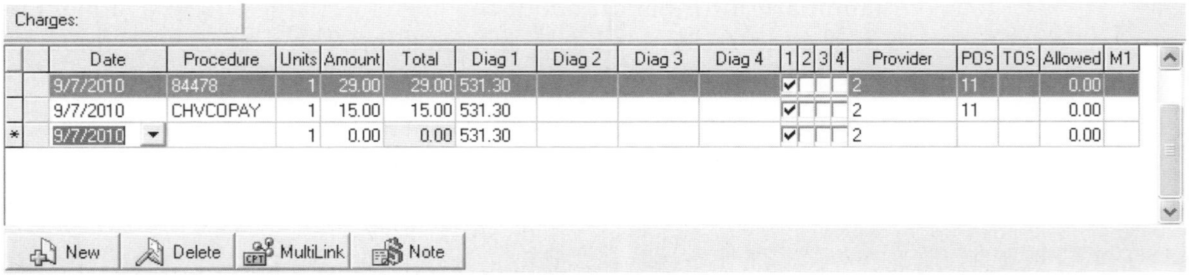

Figure 6-9 **Charges Area After Clicking the New Button**

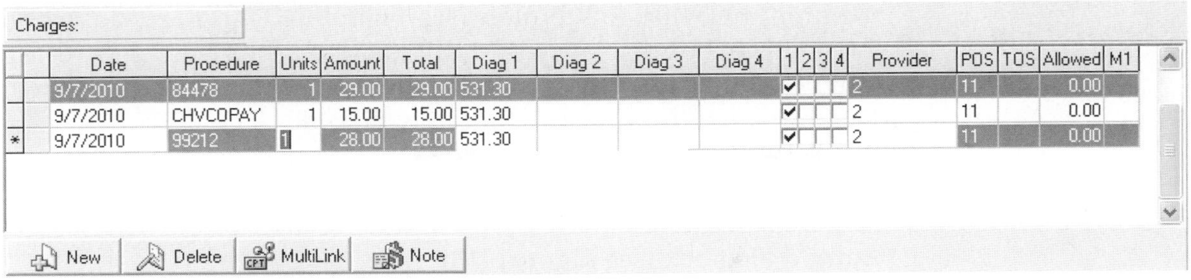

Charges:

	Date	Procedure	Units	Amount	Total	Diag 1	Diag 2	Diag 3	Diag 4	1	2	3	4	Provider	POS	TOS	Allowed	M1
	9/7/2010	84478	1	29.00	29.00	531.30				✓				2	11		0.00	
	9/7/2010	CHVCOPAY	1	15.00	15.00	531.30				✓				2	11		0.00	
*	9/7/2010	99212	1	28.00	28.00	531.30				✓				2	11		0.00	

New   Delete   MultiLink   Note

Figure 6-10 *Charges Area After Entering Procedure Code*

Procedure Once the correct date is entered, pressing the Tab key moves the cursor to the Procedure box. The procedure code for a service performed is selected by entering the code number or by selecting it from the drop-down list of CPT codes already entered in the system.

If a CPT code is not listed, it will need to be added to the database by pressing the F8 key or by clicking Procedure/Payment/Adjustment Codes on the Lists menu. This may be done without exiting the Transaction Entry dialog box.

Only one procedure code can be selected for each transaction. If multiple procedures were performed for a patient, each must be entered as a separate transaction, or a MultiLink code, which is discussed below, must be used.

After the code is selected and the Tab key is pressed, the charge for a procedure is displayed in the Amount box (see Figure 6-10).

MULTILINK CODES

MultiLink codes groups of procedure code entries that relate to a single activity.

NDCMediSoft provides a feature that saves time when entering multiple CPT codes that are related. **MultiLink codes** are groups of procedure code entries that relate to a single activity. Using MultiLink codes saves time by eliminating the need to enter related multiple procedure codes one at a time. For example, suppose a MultiLink code is created for the procedures related to diagnosing a strep throat. The MultiLink code STREPM is created. STREPM includes three procedures: 99211 OF—Established patient, minimal; 87430—Strep test, quick; and 85018—Hemogram, automated and manual.

When the MultiLink code STREPM is selected, all three procedure codes are automatically entered by the system. The MultiLink feature saves time by reducing the number of procedure code entries, and it also reduces omission errors. When procedure codes are entered as a MultiLink, it is impossible to forget to enter a procedure, since all the codes that are in the MultiLink group are entered automatically.

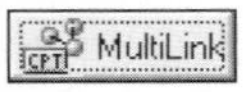

Figure 6-11
MultiLink Button

Clicking the MultiLink button (see Figure 6-11) in the Transaction Entry dialog box displays the MultiLink dialog box (see Figure 6-12). After a MultiLink code is selected from the MultiLink drop-down list, the Create Transactions button is clicked.

The codes and charges for each procedure are automatically added to the list of transactions in the middle section of the Transaction Entry dialog box (see Figure 6-13).

Units   The Units box indicates the quantity of the procedure. Normally, the number of units is one. In some cases, however, it may be more than one. For example, if a physician made three hospital visits to a patient and the charge linked to the CPT code is for one visit, "3" would be entered in the Units box.

Amount   The Amount box lists the charge amount for a procedure. The amount is entered automatically by the system based on the CPT code and insurance carrier. Each CPT code stored in the system has a charge amount associated with it for each insurance carrier. The charge amount can be edited if necessary.

Total   To the right of the Amount box is the Total box. This field displays the total charges for the procedure(s) performed. To calculate the amount, the system multiplies the number in the Units box by the number in the Amount box. For example, suppose a patient had three X-rays at a charge of $45.00 each. The Units box would read "3," and the Amount box would read "$45.00." The Total box would read "$135.00," which is 3 × $45.00.

Diagnosis   The Diag 1, 2, 3, and 4 boxes correspond to the information in the Diagnosis tab of the Case folder. If a patient has several different diagnoses, the diagnosis that is most relevant to the procedure is used.

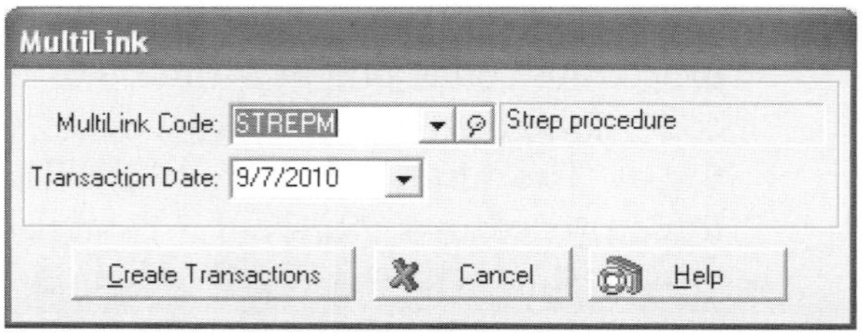

Figure 6-12 **MultiLink Dialog Box**

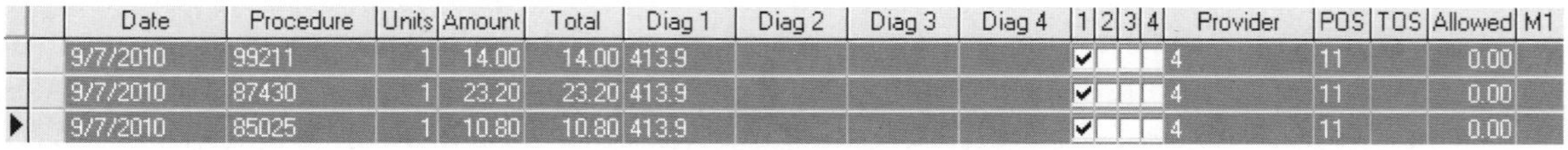

	Date	Procedure	Units	Amount	Total	Diag 1	Diag 2	Diag 3	Diag 4	1	2	3	4	Provider	POS	TOS	Allowed	M1
	9/7/2010	99211	1	14.00	14.00	413.9				✔				4	11		0.00	
	9/7/2010	87430	1	23.20	23.20	413.9				✔				4	11		0.00	
▶	9/7/2010	85025	1	10.80	10.80	413.9				✔				4	11		0.00	

Figure 6-13 **Charge Transactions Created with STREPM MultiLink Code**

1, 2, 3, 4   The 1, 2, 3, and 4 boxes to the right of the Diag 1, 2, 3, and 4 boxes indicate which diagnoses should be used for this charge. A check mark appears in each Diagnosis box for which a diagnosis was entered in the Diag 1, 2, 3, and 4 boxes. Some insurance carriers do not permit more than one diagnosis per procedure. Diagnoses can be checked or unchecked as needed.

Provider   The Provider box lists the code number for a patient's assigned provider. If a patient sees a different provider, the Provider box can be changed to list the code number for that provider instead. Clicking the triangle button to the right of the box displays a list of providers and code numbers in the database.

POS   The POS, or Place of Service box, indicates where services were performed. Standard numerical codes are:

11   Provider's office

21   Inpatient hospital

22   Outpatient hospital

23   Hospital emergency room

When NDCMedisoft is set up for use in a practice, an option is provided to set a default POS code. In addition, POS codes can be assigned to specific procedure codes when they are set up in the Procedure/ Payment/Adjustment List. For the purposes of this book, the default code has been set to 11 for Provider's office.

TOS   TOS stands for "type of service." Medical offices may set up a list of codes to indicate the type of service performed. For example, 1 may indicate an examination, 2 a lab test, and so on. The TOS code is specified in the Procedure/Payment/Adjustment entry for each CPT code.

modifiers one- or two-digit codes that allow more specific descriptions to be entered for services the physician performed.

M1   The M1 box is for a CPT code modifier. **Modifiers** are two-digit codes that allow more specific descriptions to be entered for the services the physician performed. For example, a modifier needs to be used when the circumstances require services beyond those normally associated with a particular procedure code. A common modifier is −90, which indicates that the procedure is performed by an outside laboratory. If a modifier is indicated on an encounter form, it is entered in the M1 box.

BUTTONS IN THE CHARGES AREA OF THE TRANSACTION ENTRY DIALOG BOX

Four buttons are provided at the bottom of the Charges area: New, Delete, MultiLink, and Note. The New and MultiLink buttons have already been discussed. The Delete button is used to delete a transaction. The Note button is used to store notes about a particular transaction.

| Update All | Quick Receipt | Print Receipt | Print Claim | Close | Save Transactions |

Figure 6-14 *Transaction Entry Buttons*

SAVING CHARGES

When all the charge information has been entered and checked for accuracy, it needs to be saved. Transactions are saved in NDCMedisoft by clicking the Save Transactions button, which is located at the bottom of the Transaction Entry dialog box (see Figure 6-14). Once saved, the transactions will be shaded gray to indicate that they have been saved.

Transactions can also be saved by clicking the Update All button, located in the same row of buttons. When Update All is clicked, the transactions are saved, and the program checks all fields for missing or invalid information and displays various messages, such as warning that the date entered is in the future.

The other buttons located in this row (Quick Receipt, Print Receipt, and Print Claim) will be discussed in Chapter 7, Entering Payments and Adjustments.

Exercise 6-1

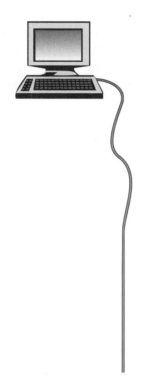

Using Source Document 2, enter a charge transaction for Hiro Tanaka's accident case.

> Note: Steps 1 through 3 are required for the first exercise in each chapter. These steps start NDCMedisoft, set the path to the correct location, and restore the data saved at the end of the last work session.

Date: October 4, 2010

1. Hold down the F7 key and start NDCMedisoft. Enter the location of the NDCMedisoft data in the Find NDCMedisoft Directory box and click OK. (If you are unsure what to enter, ask your instructor.) When the Open practice dialog box appears, verify that Family Care Center is highlighted and click OK.

2. Restore the data from your last work session by selecting Restore Data on the File menu. When a Warning box appears, click OK. Enter the file path and file name in the File Destination Path and Name box or click the Find button and browse to the desired location. The file name should be FCC8–5.mbk (the database name followed by the chapter number that you last worked on). The file path will vary depending on your computer and network set up. Ask your instructor for the file path.

3. Click the Start Restore button. When a Confirm dialog box appears, click OK. NDCMedisoft restores the data. When it is complete, an Information box is displayed, indicating that the restore is complete. Click OK. The Restore box closes and the main NDCMedisoft window is displayed.

4. Change the NDCMedisoft Program Date to October 4, 2010, if it is not already set to that date.

5. On the Activities menu, click Enter Transactions. The Transaction Entry dialog box is displayed.

6. Key *T* in the Chart box and press Tab to select Hiro Tanaka. An Information dialog box is displayed with a message about Tanaka's allergies. Click the OK button to close the box.

7. Verify that the Accident—back pain case is active in the Case box.

8. In the Charges section of the dialog box, click the New button.

9. Verify that the entry in the Date box is 10/4/2010. Notice that the diagnosis box and the Units box have been automatically completed. If necessary, these entries could be edited by clicking in the box and entering new data.

10. Click in the Procedure box and enter *99202* to select the procedure code for the service checked off on the encounter form. Press Tab. The Amount box is automatically completed ($62.00).

11. Review the entries in the Provider (1) and POS (11) boxes. Since there are no modifiers to the procedure code, the M1 box is left blank.

12. Click the New button again, this time to enter a charge for the OhioCare HMO copayment. An Information box is displayed, reminding you that the case requires a $30.00 copayment for each visit. You will enter this copayment in Chapter 7, Entering Payments and Adjustments. For now, click the OK button, and then click the New button again.

13. In the Procedure field, click the drop-down list and scroll down to find the correct code for the OhioCare HMO copayment charge. When you locate it, click to select it. The program enters it in the procedure field. Press Tab. Notice that the Amount box is completed by the program.

14. Check your entries for accuracy.

15. Click the Save Transactions button to save your work. A Date of Service Validation box is displayed, stating that the date is in the future and asking whether the transaction should be saved. Click Yes. Since you entered two transactions, the Date of Service Validation appears again. Click Yes. The transactions are saved.

16. Do not close the Transaction Entry dialog box.

Exercise 6-2

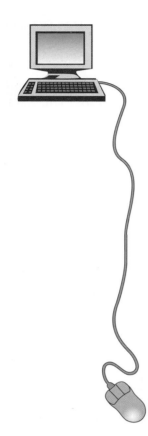

Using Source Document 4, enter a charge transaction for Elizabeth Jones' diabetes case.

Date: October 4, 2010

1. If necessary, open the Transaction Entry dialog box.

2. Click in the Chart field, key *JO* in the Chart box, and press Tab to select Elizabeth Jones. Verify that the Diabetes case is active in the Case box. If it is not active, click the Case drop-down list and click Diabetes to select it.

3. Click the New button in the Charges section of the window.

4. Accept the default in the Date box (10/4/2010).

5. Key *99213* in the Procedure box to select the procedure code for the services checked off on the encounter form. Press Tab.

6. Keep "1" in the Units box.

7. Accept the charge for the procedure that is displayed in the Amount box ($39.00).

8. Review the entries in the other boxes, and check your entries for accuracy.

9. Click the Save Transactions button. When the Date of Service Validation box appears, click Yes.

10. Do not close the Transaction Entry dialog box.

Exercise 6-3

Using Source Document 5, enter the procedure charges for John Fitzwilliams' acute gastric ulcer case.

Date: October 4, 2010

1. Click in the Chart box and key *F.* Notice that the chart number for John Fitzwilliams is highlighted on the drop-down list. Press the Tab key. Verify that Acute gastric ulcer is the active case in the Case box. Notice there are already two procedure charges displayed in the Charges section of the dialog box.

2. Click the New button in the Charges section of the dialog box.

3. Accept the default in the Date box (10/4/2010).

4. Select the procedure code for the services checked off on the encounter form. There is more than one procedure. Enter the first procedure code (99212). Press Tab.

5. Accept the default entries in the other boxes.

6. Check your entries for accuracy.

Now enter the second procedure code marked on the encounter form by completing the remaining steps.

7. Click the New button. If an Information box appears about a copayment that is due, click the OK button, and then click the New button again.

8. Accept the default in the Date box.

9. Select the procedure code for the second service checked off on the encounter form (82270). Press Tab. Since a modifier (−90) is listed on the encounter form for this procedure, click in the M1 box. Enter *90* and press Tab.

10. Accept the default entries in the other boxes.

11. Click New and enter a copayment charge for this office visit. *Hint:* Look at the Estimated Responsibility section at the top of the Transaction Entry dialog box to determine Fitzwilliams' insurance company and copay amount.

12. Check your entries for accuracy.

13. Click the Save Transactions button. Three Date of Service Validation boxes appear, one for each transaction. Click Yes each time a box is displayed.

14. Close the Transaction Entry dialog box.

EDITING AND DELETING TRANSACTIONS

All transactions can be edited and deleted from within the Transaction Entry dialog box. Caution should be exercised in both cases, but especially when using the Delete feature. **Deleted data cannot be recovered!!**

EDITING TRANSACTIONS

The most efficient way to edit a transaction is to click in the field that needs to be changed. For example, to change the procedure code, click in the Procedure box and either key a new code or select a new code from the drop-down list. After changes are made, the data must be saved. To view the updated amounts in the Estimates tab, click the Update All button near the bottom of the Transaction Entry dialog box.

Depending on the type of edit, the program may display several message boxes. For example, if an attempt is made to change the Payment Type or Who Paid fields, a message is displayed to confirm the change. If someone tries to change a diagnosis code that is already included in a claim, the program asks whether to remove the transaction from the existing claim and create a new claim, or to replace the original diagnosis code in the transaction.

DELETING TRANSACTIONS

Transactions can also be deleted from the Transaction Entry dialog box. To delete a transaction, click anywhere in the transaction record and then click the Delete button. A confirmation box will be displayed, asking "Are you sure you want to delete this charge?" Clicking the Yes button deletes the transaction; clicking the No button cancels the action.

Exercise 6-4

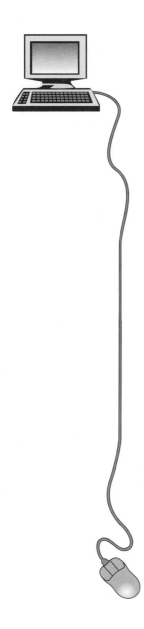

Make a change to a procedure code in John Fitzwilliams' acute gastric ulcer case. The code 99212 was marked incorrectly on the encounter form. The correct code is 99213.

Date: October 4, 2010

1. Open the Transaction Entry dialog box.

2. Select John Fitzwilliams as the patient.

3. Confirm that the Acute gastric ulcer case is selected.

4. Click in the Procedure box for the 99212 code on 10/4/2010.

5. Select the correct code—99213—from the drop-down list. Press Tab.

6. Click the Save Transactions button. A box appears reminding you that the case requires a $15.00 copayment. Click OK. Click the Save Transactions button again. A Date of Service Validation box appears. Click Yes.

7. Close the Transaction Entry dialog box.

8. Create a backup of your work and exit NDCMedisoft by selecting Exit on the File menu. The Backup Reminder dialog box is displayed.

9. Click the Back Up Data Now button. The Backup dialog box appears.

10. Enter the file path and file name in the Destination File Path and Name box or click the Find button and browse to the desired location. The file name should be FCC8–6.mbk (the database name followed by the chapter number). The file path will vary depending on your computer and network setup. Ask your instructor for the file path.

11. Click the Start Backup button. NDCMedisoft creates a backup file. When it is complete, an Information box is displayed, indicating that the backup is complete. Click OK. The Backup dialog box closes and the program is shut down.

CHAPTER REVIEW

USING TERMINOLOGY

Match the terms on the left with the definitions on the right.

_____ **1.** adjustments

_____ **2.** charges

_____ **3.** modifiers

_____ **4.** MultiLink codes

_____ **5.** payments

a. One- or two-digit codes that add a specific description to a procedure code.

b. Changes to patients' accounts that alter the amount charged or paid.

c. The amounts billed by a provider for particular services.

d. Monies paid to a medical practice by patients and insurance carriers.

e. Groups of procedure code entries that are related to a single activity.

CHECKING YOUR UNDERSTANDING

Answer the questions below in the space provided.

6. What are the two key pieces of information you must have before entering a procedure charge?

_____

_____

7. List two advantages of using MultiLink codes.

_____

_____

APPLYING KNOWLEDGE

Answer the questions below in the space provided.

8. After you have entered a charge for procedure code 99393, you realize that it should have been 99394. What should you do?

_____

_____

_____

9. The receptionist working at the front desk phones to tell you that Maritza Ramos has just seen the physician and would like to know what the charges were for her September 8, 2010, office visit. You are in the middle of entering charges from an encounter form for another patient. What should you do first? What is your reasoning?

_____

_____

_____

AT THE COMPUTER

Answer the following questions at the computer.

10. What are the procedure codes and charges for Randall Klein on September 7, 2010?

11. What is the amount of the procedure charge entered on July 12, 2010, for patient Jo Wong?

WHAT YOU NEED TO KNOW

To use this chapter, you need to know how to:
- ◆ Start NDCMedisoft, use menus, and enter and edit text.
- ◆ Edit information in an existing case.
- ◆ Work with chart and case numbers.
- ◆ Select patients and cases for transaction entry.

OBJECTIVES

When you finish this chapter, you will be able to:
- ◆ Record and apply payments received from patients.
- ◆ Print walkout statements.
- ◆ Record and apply payments received from insurance carriers.
- ◆ Record insurance adjustments.

KEY TERM

capitation payments

ENTERING PAYMENTS IN NDCMEDISOFT

Payments are entered in two different areas of the NDCMedisoft program: the Transaction Entry dialog box, which was introduced in Chapter 6, and the Deposit List dialog box, which will be discussed shortly. Practices may have different preferences for entering payments, depending on their billing procedures. In this book, you will be introduced to both methods.

Payments made at the time of an office visit are entered in the Transaction Entry dialog box. This method is convenient for entering patient copayments that are made at the conclusion of an office visit. Payments that are received after the conclusion of an office visit, such as insurance payments received electronically or by mail as well as patient payments received by mail, are entered in the Deposit List dialog box. The Deposit List feature is very efficient for entering large insurance payments that must be split up and applied to a number of different patients.

ENTERING PAYMENTS MADE DURING OFFICE VISITS

A payment made at the end of an office visit is entered in the Transaction Entry dialog box. Just as when entering charges, a patient's chart number and case number must be selected before a transaction can be entered.

After the chart and case numbers have been entered, a new payment transaction can be created or an existing transaction can be edited. Payments are entered in the Payments, Adjustments, And Comments section in the lower portion of the Transaction Entry dialog box (see Figure 7-1).

The process of creating a payment transaction begins with clicking the New button. When the New button is clicked, the program automatically enters the current date (the date that the NDCMedisoft Program Date is set to) in the Date box (see Figure 7-2).

If this is not the date on which the payment was received, the date must be changed. To change the default date for these boxes, either of these methods is used:

◆ The Set Program Date command on the File menu is clicked.

◆ The date button in the bottom-right corner of the screen is clicked. (This must be done before the New button is clicked in the Transaction Entry dialog box.)

The date can also be changed by keying over the information that is already in the Date box.

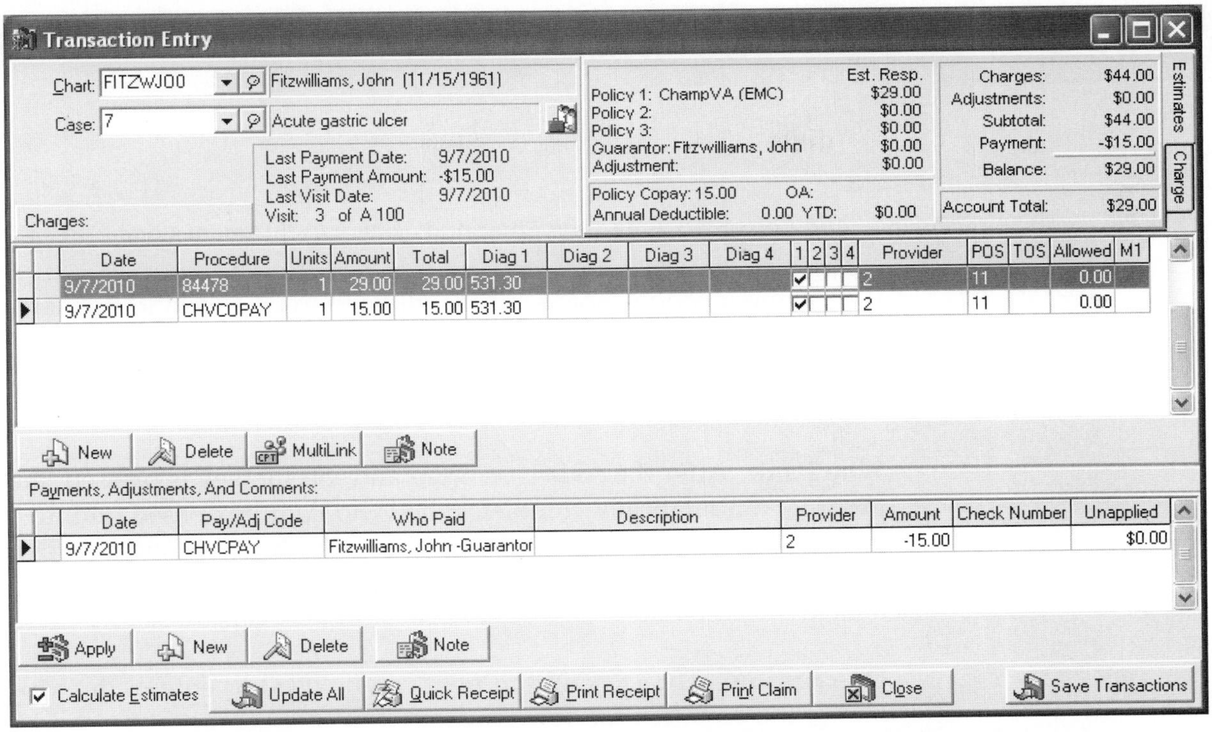

Figure 7-1 Payments, Adjustments, And Comments Area in the Transaction Entry Dialog Box

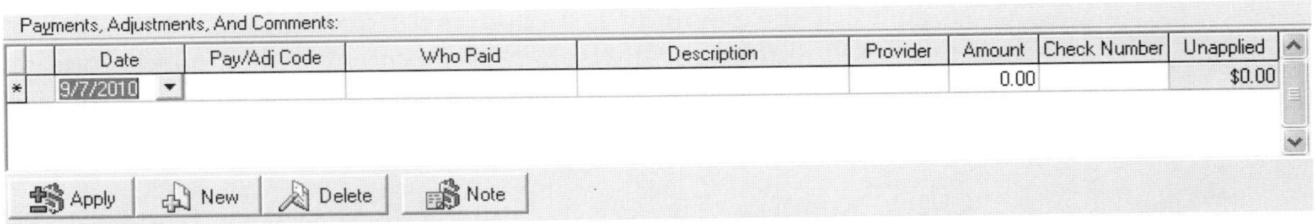

Figure 7-2 Payments, Adjustments, And Comments Area After Clicking the New Button

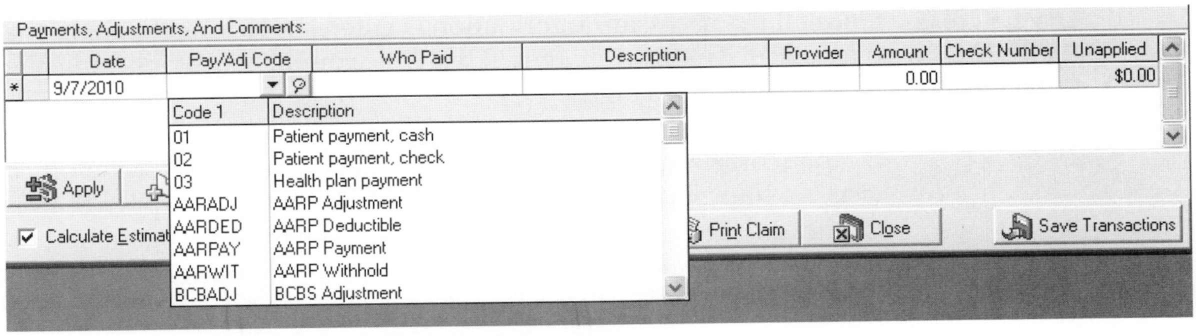

Figure 7-3 Payment/Adjustment Code Drop-Down List

Payment/Adjustment Code Once the correct date is entered, pressing the Tab key moves the cursor to the Payment/Adjustment Code box. The code for a payment is selected by entering the code number or by selecting it from the drop-down list of payment codes already entered in the system (see Figure 7-3).

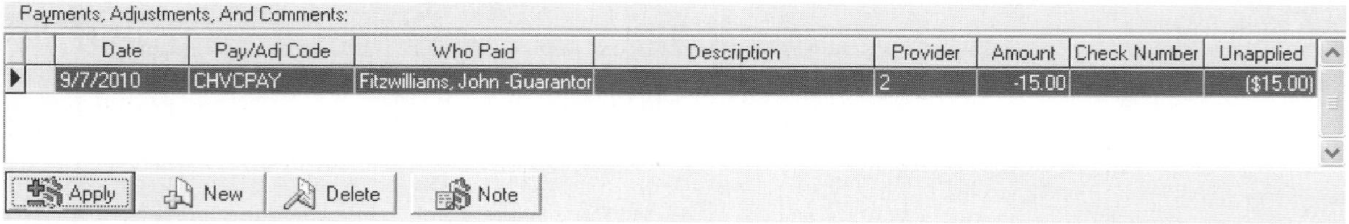

Figure 7-4 Payments, Adjustments, And Comments Area After Entering Payment/Adjustment Code

If a payment code is not listed, it will need to be added to the database by pressing the F8 key or by clicking Procedure/Payment/Adjustment Codes on the Lists menu. This may be done without exiting the Transaction Entry dialog box.

Who Paid After the code is selected and the Tab key is pressed, the program automatically completes the Who Paid box based on information stored in the database (see Figure 7-4). The Who Paid field displays a drop-down list of guarantors and carriers that are assigned in the patient case folder.

Description The Description field can be used to enter a description of the payment received, if desired.

Amount The Amount field contains the amount of payment received. If the payment is a copayment from a patient, this box is completed automatically when a Payment/Adjustment code is selected. Again, the program uses information stored in the program databases.

Check Number The Check Number field is used to record the number of the check used for payment.

APPLYING PAYMENTS TO CHARGES

Once all the necessary information is entered, it is time to apply the payment to specific charges. This is accomplished by clicking the Apply button (see Figure 7-5).

Figure 7-5 Apply Button

If a patient is required to pay a copayment at the time of the office visit, an Information dialog box is displayed after the Apply button is clicked. This box provides a reminder that a copayment is required (see Figure 7-6). After clicking the OK button, the Apply Payment to Charges dialog box appears.

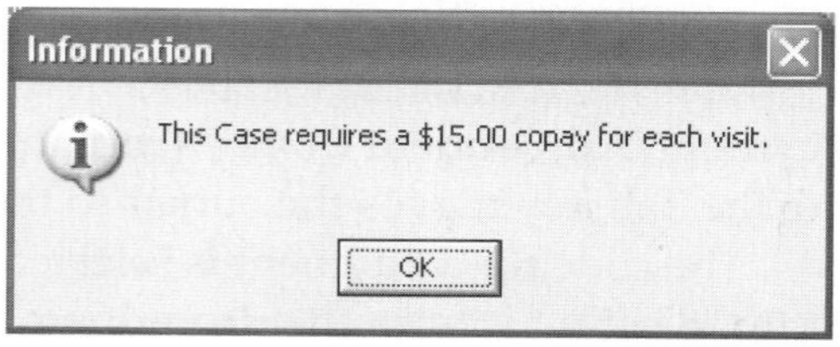

Figure 7-6 Information Dialog Box with Copayment Reminder

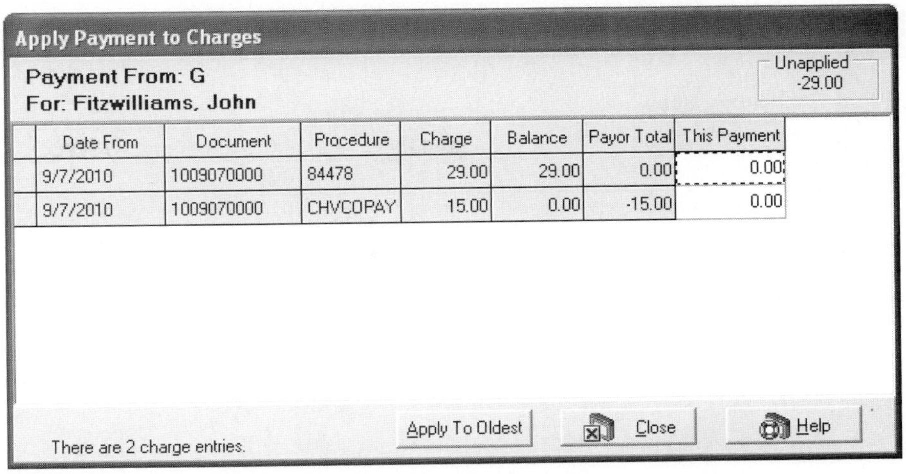

Date From	Document	Procedure	Charge	Balance	Payor Total	This Payment
9/7/2010	1009070000	84478	29.00	29.00	0.00	0.00
9/7/2010	1009070000	CHVCOPAY	15.00	0.00	-15.00	0.00

Figure 7-7 **Apply Payment to Charges Dialog Box**

The Apply Payment to Charges dialog box lists information about all unpaid charges for a patient, including the date of the procedure, the document number, the procedure code, the charge, the balance, and the total amount paid (see Figure 7-7).

In the top-right corner of the dialog box, the amount of payment that has not yet been applied to charges appears in the Unapplied box. The first step in applying a payment is to determine the charge to which the payment should be applied. For example, if the payment is a copayment for an office visit on 9/7/2010, it would be necessary to locate that charge before applying the payment.

When the Apply Payment to Charges box is opened, the cursor appears in the top box of the column labeled "This Payment." If this is not the charge to which the payment should be applied, another box must be selected. If the payment is to be applied to the oldest charge, the Apply To Oldest button at the bottom of the dialog box can be used. To select a box, click in it; a dotted rectangle appears around the outside of the box. Once the box has been selected, click in the box again. This moves the zeros to the top-left corner of the box, indicating that the box is active and ready for payment entry. The amount of a payment that is to be applied to a charge is then entered without a decimal point, and the Tab key is pressed. The system inserts a decimal point automatically (see Figure 7-8 on page 134).

Once the box is closed, the payment appears in the Payments, Adjustments, And Comments area of the Transaction Entry dialog box (see Figure 7-9 on page 134).

Apply Payment to Charges

Payment From: G
For: Fitzwilliams, John

Unapplied
15.00

Date From	Document	Procedure	Charge	Balance	Payor Total	This Payment
9/7/2010	1009070000	84478	29.00	0.00	-29.00	
9/7/2010	1009070000	CHVCOPAY	15.00	0.00	-15.00	15.00

There are 2 charge entries.

Apply To Oldest   Close   Help

Figure 7-8 Apply Payment to Charges with Payment Entered

Payments, Adjustments, And Comments:

	Date	Pay/Adj Code	Who Paid	Description	Provider	Amount	Check Number	Unapplied	
▶	9/7/2010	CHVCPAY	Fitzwilliams, John -Guarantor		2	-15.00		$0.00	

Apply   New   Delete   Note

Figure 7-9 Payments, Adjustments, And Comments Area with Payment Listed

Payments can be applied to more than one charge. For example, suppose that the payment is $200 and there are three unpaid charges. The $200 payment can be applied to one of the charges, two of the charges, or all three charges. It is not even necessary to apply the entire payment amount. A balance can remain in the Unapplied box, or the balance can be used to reduce the amount due on another charge.

SAVING PAYMENT INFORMATION

When all the information on a payment has been entered and checked for accuracy, it must be saved. Payment transactions are saved in the manner described earlier for charge transactions, by clicking the Save Transactions button.

Exercise 7-1

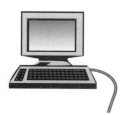

Using Source Document 2, enter the copayment made by Hiro Tanaka for her October 4, 2010, office visit.

Note: Steps 1 through 3 are required at the beginning of each chapter. These steps start NDCMedisoft, set the path to the correct data location, and restore the data saved at the end of the last work session.

Date: October 4, 2010

1. Hold down the F7 key and start NDCMedisoft. Enter the location of the NDCMedisoft data in the Find NDCMedisoft Directory box and click OK. (If you are unsure what to enter, ask your instructor.) When the Open practice dialog box appears, verify that Family Care Center is highlighted and click OK.

2. Restore the data from your last work session by selecting Restore Data on the File menu. When a Warning box appears, click OK. Enter the file path and file name in the File Destination Path and Name box or click the Find button and browse to the desired location. The file name should be FCC8–6.mbk (the database name followed by the chapter number that you last worked on). The file path will vary depending on your computer and network setup. Ask your instructor for the file path.

3. Click the Start Restore button. When a Confirm dialog box appears, click OK. NDCMedisoft restores the data. When it is complete, an Information box is displayed, indicating that the restore is complete. Click OK. The Restore box closes and the main NDCMedisoft window is displayed.

4. Change the NDCMedisoft Program Date to October 4, 2010, if it is not already set to that date, and open the Transaction Entry dialog box.

5. In the Chart box, key *T* and press Tab to select Hiro Tanaka. An Information box is displayed with information about Tanaka's allergies. Click the OK button.

6. Verify that Accident—back pain is the active case in the Case box.

7. Click the New button in the Payments, Adjustments, And Comments section of the dialog box.

8. Accept the default entry of 10/4/2010 in the Date box.

9. Click in the Pay/Adj Code box. Select OHCCOPAY (the code for OhioCare HMO copayment) and press Tab. Notice that all the boxes except Description and Check Number have been completed by the program.

10. Verify that Tanaka, Hiro—Guarantor, is listed in the Who Paid box.

11. Notice that −30.00 has already been entered in the Amount box. Confirm that this is correct.

12. The Unapplied Amount box should read (30.00).

13. Click in the Check Number box, enter *123*, and press Tab.

14. Click the Apply button. The Apply Payment to Charges dialog box is displayed.

15. Notice that the amount of this payment (−30.00) is listed in the Unapplied box at the top right of the dialog box.

16. Double-click the box in the This Payment column that corresponds to the charge for the copayment.

17. Enter *30* in this box. Press Tab. The system inserts a decimal point automatically.

18. Click the Close button. A reminder that the case requires a $30.00 copayment appears. Click OK. The Transaction Entry box is visible again.

19. Notice that the amount listed in the Unapplied column is now zero. Also notice that the line listing the charge for the copayment is now white rather than gray, indicating that the charge has been paid.

20. Click the Save Transactions button. When the date warning boxes appear, click Yes.

21. Do not close the Transaction Entry dialog box.

Exercise 7-2

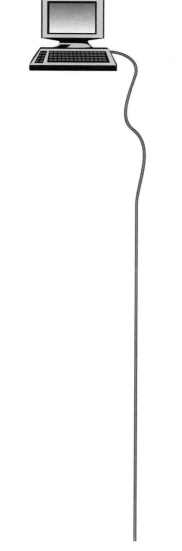

Using Source Document 5, enter the copayment made by John Fitzwilliams for his October 4, 2010, office visit.

Date: October 4, 2010

1. Click in the Chart box and enter *F* to locate John Fitzwilliams. Then press Tab to select John Fitzwilliams. Verify that Acute gastric ulcer is active in the Case box.

2. Click the New button in the Payments, Adjustments, And Comments section of the dialog box.

3. Accept the default entry of 10/4/2010 in the Date box.

4. On the Pay/Adj Code drop-down list, click CHVCPAY (ChampVA Copayment) and press Tab. Check number and the Description box. Verify that the entries are correct.

5. Enter *456* in the Check Number box and press Tab.

6. Click the Apply button. The Apply Payment to Charges dialog box is displayed.

7. Notice that the amount of this payment (−15.00) is listed in the Unapplied box at the top right of the dialog box.

8. In the list of charges that appears, locate the copayment charge for Fitzwilliams' October 4, 2010, office visit. Double-click in the This Payment box located on the same line as this charge.

9. Enter *15* in the This Payment box. Press the Tab key. The system inserts a decimal point automatically.

10. Click the Close button. The Transaction Entry dialog box reappears.

11. Notice that the amount listed in the Unapplied Amount column is now zero. Also notice that the line listing the charge for the copayment is now white rather than gray, indicating that the charge has been paid.

12. **Click the Save Transactions button. When the date warning boxes are displayed, click the Yes button.**

13. **Do not close the Transaction Entry dialog box.**

PRINTING WALKOUT STATEMENTS

After a patient payment has been entered in the Transaction Entry dialog box, a walkout statement is printed and given to the patient before he or she leaves the office. A walkout statement includes information on the procedures, diagnosis, charges, and payments for a visit. If there is a balance due, the statement serves as a reminder of the amount owed.

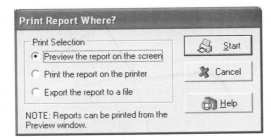

Figure 7-10 **Quick Receipt Button**

In the Transaction Entry dialog box, the most efficient way to print a walkout statement is to click the Quick Receipt button (see Figure 7-10). The Quick Receipt option eliminates several steps that are required when using the standard Print Receipt button. (A Print Claims button also appears in the Transaction Entry dialog box; claim management is discussed in detail in Chapter 9.)

When the Quick Receipt button is clicked, the Print Report Where? dialog box is displayed, providing three options (see Figure 7-11):

◆ Previewing the report on the screen

◆ Sending the report directly to the printer

◆ Exporting the report to a file

Once a printing choice is made, clicking the Start button sends the report to its destination.

Figure 7-11 **Print Report Where? Dialog Box**

Exercise 7-3

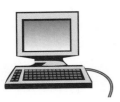

Create a walkout statement for John Fitzwilliams.

Date: October 4, 2010

1. **With the Transaction Entry dialog box open to John Fitzwilliams' Acute gastric ulcer case, click the Quick Receipt button. The Open Report dialog box may appear. If it does appear, accept the**

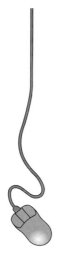

default selection of Walkout Receipt (All Transactions). Click OK. The Print Report Where? dialog box is displayed.

2. In the Print Report Where? dialog box, accept the default selection to preview the report on the screen. Click the Start button. The Walkout Receipt: Data Selection Questions dialog box appears. Accept the default entries. Click OK. The Preview Report window opens, displaying the walkout statement.

3. Review the charge and payment entries listed on the top half of the statement.

4. Scroll down and review the total charges, payments, and adjustments listed in the lower right area of the statement.

5. Click the Close button to exit the Preview Report window.

6. Close the Transaction Entry dialog box.

ENTERING INSURANCE CARRIER PAYMENTS

Information about payments from insurance carriers is sent to a physician through a remittance advice (RA). A remittance advice lists patients, dates of service, charges, and the amount paid or denied by the insurance carrier. Most RAs also provide an explanation of unpaid charges. In most cases, the payment is electronically deposited in the practice's bank account; sometimes a paper check is attached to the RA and must be manually deposited.

Payment information located on the RA is entered in the Deposit List dialog box. This dialog box is opened by clicking Enter Deposits/Payments on the Activities menu or by clicking the Enter Deposits and Apply Payments shortcut button. The Deposit List dialog box displays a list of all deposits already entered in the program for the current date (see Figure 7-12).

Deposit List

Deposit Date: 9/7/2010   ☐ Show All Deposits   Sort By: Date-Payor   Detail...
                          ☐ Show Unapplied Only

Deposit Date	Description	Payor Name	Payor Type	Payment
9/7/2010	1009070000	Fitzwilliams, John	Patient	15.00
9/7/2010	1009070000	Fitzwilliams, Sarah	Patient	15.00
▶ 9/7/2010	1009070000	Gardiner, John	Patient	30.00

Edit   New   Apply   Print   Delete   Export   Close

Figure 7-12 Deposit List Dialog Box

The Deposit List dialog box contains the following information:

Deposit Date The program displays the current date (the NDCMedisoft Program Date). The date can be changed by keying over the default date.

Show All Deposits If this box is checked, all payments are displayed, regardless of the date entered.

Show Unapplied Only If the Show Unapplied Only box is checked, only payments that have not been fully applied to charge transactions are displayed. If the box is not checked, all payments—both applied and unapplied—are listed.

Sort By The Sort By drop-down list offers several choices for how payment information is listed: the default is sorting payments by amount, from lowest to highest. Payments can also be sorted by other data fields (see Figure 7-13).

Locate Buttons The Locate and Locate Next buttons, indicated by the two magnifying glass icons, are used to search for a deposit.

Detail To view a specific deposit in more detail, highlight the deposit and click the Detail button. A dialog box opens with more information about the selected deposit (see Figure 7-14 on page 140).

In the middle section of the Deposit List window, information is listed for each deposit and payment, including:

Deposit Date Lists the date of the deposit or payment.

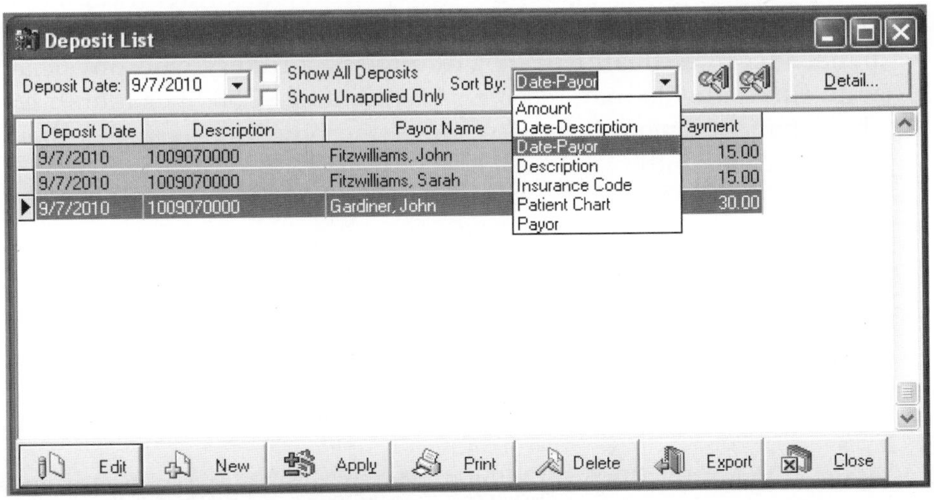

Figure 7-13 **Deposit List Dialog Box with Sort By Drop-Down List Displayed**

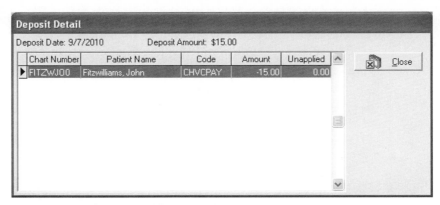

Figure 7-14 **Deposit Detail Dialog Box**

Description   Displays whatever was entered in the Description or Check Number box in the Deposit dialog box. The Deposit dialog box is where new payments and deposits are recorded (see Figure 7-15). It is accessed by clicking the New button in the Deposit List dialog box.

Payor Name   Lists the name of the insurance carrier or individual who made the payment.

Payor Type   A classification column that lists whether the payment is an insurance payment, a patient payment, or a capitation payment. **Capitation payments** are made to physicians on a regular basis (such as monthly) for providing services to patients in a managed care insurance plan. In traditional insurance plans, physicians are paid based on the specific procedures they perform and the number of times the procedures are performed. Under a capitated plan, a flat fee is paid to the physician no matter how many times a patient receives treatment. For example, a primary care physician with fifty patients may receive a payment of $2,500 per month for those patients, regardless of whether the physician has seen them during that month.

capitation payments *payments made to physicians on a regular basis (such as monthly) for providing services to patients in a managed care insurance plan.*

Payment   Lists the amount of the payment.

At the bottom of the Deposit List dialog box are buttons that perform the following actions:

Edit   Opens the highlighted payment or deposit for editing.

New   Opens the Deposit dialog box, where new payments and deposits are recorded.

Apply   Applies payments to specific charge transactions.

Print   Sends a command to print the deposit list.

Delete   Deletes the highlighted transaction.

Export   Exports the data in either Quicken or Quick Books program format.

Close   Exits the Deposit List dialog box.

ENTERING INSURANCE PAYMENTS

The entry of new insurance carrier payments begins when the New button is clicked in the Deposit List dialog box. This causes the Deposit dialog box to appear (see Figure 7-15).

Deposit Date   The program's current date is displayed by default, and must be changed if it is not the date of the deposit.

Payor Type   This box indicates whether the payer is an insurance carrier, a capitation plan, or a patient. Some of the boxes at the bottom of the Deposit dialog box change based on the selection in this box. If Insurance is selected, the dialog box is as illustrated in Figure 7-15. If capitation is selected, all the boxes below Insurance disappear. If Patient is chosen, the boxes listed below Deposit Code become Chart Number, Payment Code, and Adjustment Code.

Payment Method   This box lists whether the payment is check, cash, credit card, or electronic.

Check Number   The number of the check (if a check payment) is selected in this box.

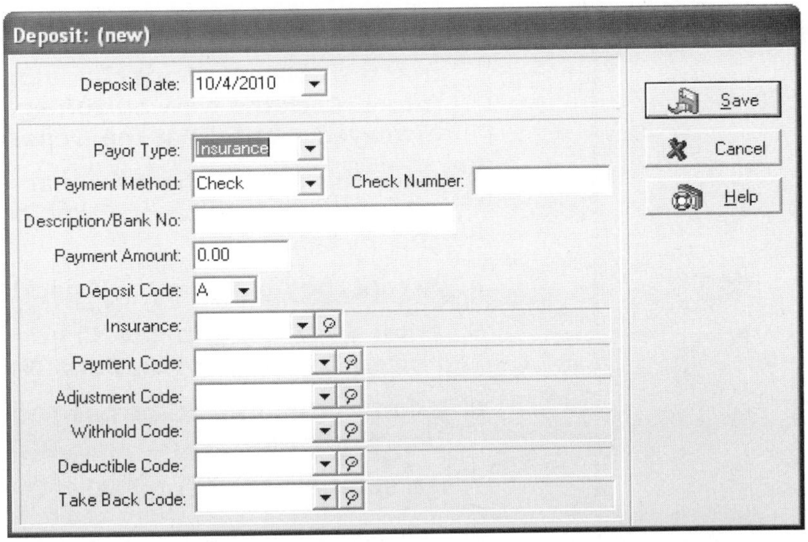

Figure 7-15 **Deposit Dialog Box with Insurance Selected as Payor Type**

Description/Bank No. This box can be used to enter a description of the payment, if desired.

Payment Amount The total amount of the payment is entered in this box.

Deposit Code This field can be used by practices to sort deposits according to user-defined categories.

Insurance The insurance carrier that is making the payment is selected.

Payment Code, Adjustment Code, Withhold Code, Deductible Code, Take Back Code The appropriate codes for the insurance carrier are selected.

Once all the information has been entered and checked for accuracy, the deposit is saved by clicking the Save button. The Deposit List dialog box reappears, with the new deposit listed.

Exercise 7-4

Using Source Document 6, enter the payment received from John Fitzwilliams' insurance carrier for services provided on September 7, 2010. Note that since John is guarantor for his daughter Sarah, her charges and payments are included on the remittance advice (RA).

Date: October 4, 2010

1. Click Enter Deposits/Payments on the Activities menu. The Deposit List dialog box is displayed. Verify that 10/4/2010 is displayed in the Deposit Date box and that Date-Payor is displayed in the Sort By box. If it is not displayed, change it to Date-Payor.

2. Click the New button. Click No in response to the message that is displayed about changing the date because it is in the future. Click the New button again. The Deposit dialog box is displayed. Verify that the Deposit Date is 10/4/2010.

3. Since this is a payment from an insurance carrier, change the selection in the Payor Type box to Insurance if it is not already selected.

4. Accept the default entry (Check) in the Payment Method box.

5. Enter *214778924* in the Check Number box and press Tab twice. (The Description/Bank No. field can be left blank.)

6. Enter the amount of the payment (*70*) in the Payment Amount box. Press Tab.

7. Accept the default entry (A) in the Deposit Code box. Press Tab.

8. Select the insurance carrier that is making the payment (5—ChampVA) from the Insurance drop-down list. NDCMedisoft

automatically enters the defaults for ChampVA in the Payment, Adjustment, Withhold, Deductible, and Take Back Code boxes.

9. Click the Save button to save the entry and close the Deposit dialog box.

10. The Deposit List box reappears. The insurance payment appears in the list of deposits.

11. Now the payment must be applied to the specific procedure charges to which it corresponds. With the ChampVA payment entry highlighted, click the Apply button. The Apply Payment/Adjustments to Charges dialog box appears.

12. Key *F* in the For box and press Tab to select John Fitzwilliams, since a portion of this payment is for his account. All the charge entries for John Fitzwilliams that have not been paid in full are listed. Notice that the amount listed in the Unapplied box in the top-right corner shows the full deposit amount, since nothing has been applied yet.

13. Since this payment is for the 84478 procedure completed on 09/07/2010, that is the line in which the payment will be applied. Notice that the cursor is blinking in the Payment box for this charge. (By default, the cursor blinks in the Payment box of the oldest unpaid transaction.)

14. Enter *29* in the Payment box and press Tab. NDCMedisoft automatically places a minus sign before the amount. Notice that once the payment was applied, the Complete box to the right of the dialog box was checked. This indicates that the transaction is complete—the entire amount of the charge has been paid. Also notice that the Unapplied amount has been reduced by $29.00.

15. Click the Print Statement Now box at the bottom of the dialog box so the "x" in the box disappears.

16. Click the Save Payments/Adjustments button to save your entry. When you click this button, the dialog box is cleared of the current transactions and is ready for a new transaction.

17. Now enter the payments for Sarah Fitzwilliams, using the same method as for John Fitzwilliams. When you are finished, click the Save Payments/Adjustments button.

18. Click the Close button to exit the Apply Payment/Adjustments to Charges dialog box.

19. Without closing the Deposit List dialog box, open the Transaction Entry dialog box, select John Fitzwilliams, and verify that an insurance carrier payment appears in the list of transactions. Payments entered in the Deposit List dialog box also appear in the Transaction Entry dialog box. In the Estimates area of the dialog box, notice that there is still a balance due on Fitzwilliams' account, from his office visit on 10/4/2010.

20. Now select Sarah Fitzwilliams. The payments from ChampVA appear in the Payments, Adjustments, And Comments section,

and the balance in the Estimates area is now 0.00. The account is current.

21. Close the Transaction Entry dialog box.

Exercise 7-5

The medical office has just received an electronic RA from East Ohio PPO (see Source Document 7). The total amount of the electronic funds transfer (EFT) is $526.60. This amount includes payments for a number of patients. Enter the insurance carrier payment and apply it to the appropriate patients.

Date: October 4, 2010

1. Verify that the entry in the Deposit Date box in the Deposit List dialog box is 10/04/2010.

2. Click the New button. Click No in response to the message that is displayed about changing the date because it is in the future. Click the New button again. The Deposit dialog box is displayed. Verify that the Deposit Date is 10/4/2010.

3. Select Insurance in the Payor Type box.

4. Select Electronic in the Payment Method box. Press Tab twice.

5. Enter the RA ID number, *00146972*, in the Description/Bank No. box.

6. Enter *526.60* in the Payment Amount box and press Tab.

7. Accept the default entry in the Deposit Code box.

8. Select 13—East Ohio PPO in the Insurance box. NDCMedisoft automatically completes the Payment, Adjustment, Withhold, Deductible, and Take Back Code boxes.

9. Click the Save button.

10. The payment entry appears in the Deposit List dialog box.

11. Now apply the payment to the specific transaction charges.

12. With the East Ohio PPO line highlighted, click the Apply button. The Apply Payment/Adjustments to Charges dialog box is displayed.

13. Key *A* in the For box and press Tab to select Susan Arlen.

14. Locate the charge for procedure code 99212 on 09/06/2010. Key the amount of the payment, *46.00*, in the Payment box and press Tab. Notice that NDCMedisoft automatically checks the Complete box, since Susan Arlen has only one insurance carrier (there is no payment forthcoming from any other carrier, so the charge is complete).

15. Click the Save Payments/Adjustments button. The data for Susan Arlen that was visible in the Apply Payment/Adjustments to Charges dialog box is cleared and the dialog box is ready for the next payment or adjustment. Notice also that the amount

listed in the Unapplied column for East Ohio PPO has been reduced by the amount of the Arlen payment.

16. Now enter the payment for the next patient listed on the RA, Herbert Bell.

17. Key *BE* in the For box and press Tab to select Herbert Bell.

18. Enter the payment of *30.00* in the This Payment box for the 99211 charge on 09/06/2010. Press Tab.

19. Click the Save Payments/Adjustments button.

20. Key *BELLJ* in the For box and press Tab to select Janine Bell.

21. Enter the payment of *62.00* in the This Payment box for the 99213 charge on 09/06/2010. Press Tab.

22. Enter the payment of *103.00* in the This Payment box for the 73510 charge on 09/06/2010. Press Tab.

23. Click the Save Payments/Adjustments button.

24. Continue to apply the insurance payments for Jonathan Bell, Samuel Bell, and Sarina Bell using the information on Source Document 7. Click the Save Payments/Adjustments button after you complete the payment entries for each patient. When you have applied all the payments, the amount in the Unapplied box for the East Ohio PPO payment should be 0.00.

25. Close the Apply Payment/Adjustments to Charges dialog box.

ENTERING INSURANCE PAYMENTS WITH ADJUSTMENTS

Many times insurance carriers do not pay claims in full. Charges may be denied by insurance carriers for a number of reasons. For example, a procedure may not be covered by the patient's plan, or a procedure or diagnosis may be coded incorrectly.

If the claim denial was the result of an error by the billing department, the error can be corrected and the claim resubmitted to the insurance carrier. If the denial was not the result of an error, an adjustment must be entered in NDCMedisoft.

Exercise 7-6

The medical office has just received an electronic RA from Blue Cross and Blue Shield (see Source Document 8). The total amount of the remittance is $214.40. This amount includes payments for a number of patients. Enter the insurance carrier payment for each patient. You will need to enter an adjustment for Sheila Giles, as one of her charges was denied.

Date: November 4, 2010

1. In the Deposit List dialog box, use the drop-down calendar to change the date in the Deposit Date box to 11/04/2010 and press the Tab key. A Confirm box is displayed, stating that the

date entered is in the future, and asking if you want to change the date. Click the No button.

2. Click the New button in the Deposit List dialog box.

3. Select Insurance in the Payor Type box. Press Tab.

4. Change the entry in the Payment Method box to Electronic, since this payment was sent electronically to the practice's bank account.

5. Enter the RA number, *001234*, in the Description/Bank No. box.

6. Enter *214.40* in the Payment Amount box. Press Tab.

7. Accept the default entry in the Deposit Code box. Press Tab.

8. Select 4—Blue Cross/Blue Shield in the Insurance box. NDCMedisoft automatically completes the Payment, Adjustment, Withhold, Deductible, and Take Back Code boxes.

9. Click the Save button.

10. The payment entry appears in the Deposit List dialog box.

11. Now apply the payment to the specific transaction charges.

12. With the Blue Cross/Blue Shield line highlighted, click the Apply button. The Apply Payment/Adjustments to Charges dialog box is displayed.

13. Key *GI* in the For box to select Sheila Giles, and then press Tab.

14. Three charges are listed. Locate the charge for procedure code 99213 on 10/29/2010. Key the amount of the payment, *57.60*, in the Payment box and press Tab. NDCMedisoft automatically checks the Complete box, since Giles has only one insurance carrier (no payment is forthcoming from any other carrier, so the charge is complete).

15. Now enter the payment for the next procedure listed on the RA (71010). Notice that when you click in the Payment box for the second payment entry, NDCMedisoft calculates the amount still owed on the first procedure charge—the remainder—and displays it in the Remainder column for that charge. In this instance, the remainder is $14.40.

16. Look again at Source Document 8. Notice that the amount paid for the third procedure, 87430, is $0.00. Read the note listed to determine why the charge was not paid. This denial of payment must be entered in NDCMedisoft, so the practice billing staff are aware that Giles is responsible for the entire amount of that charge, $58.00.

17. Click in the Payment box for the charge for procedure 87430. Enter *0* and press Tab. Notice that the amount listed in the Remainder column is the full amount of the charge, $58.00. The charge has also been marked as complete, since the insurance carrier is not responsible for the remainder amount.

18. Click the Save Payments/Adjustments button. (*Note:* If the Open Report dialog box appears, click Cancel.)

19. Close the Apply Payments/Adjustments to Charges dialog

box; then, without closing the Deposit List dialog box, open the Transaction Entry dialog box.

20. **Locate Sheila Giles' Upper respiratory infection case. In the Charges area, notice that two of the charges appear in an aqua color, which indicates they have been partially paid. The charge that was denied by the insurance carrier—87430—is still in gray, indicating that no payment has been made.**

21. **Now look at the Est. Resp. area in the Transaction Entry dialog box. Sheila Giles is listed as being responsible for paying $90.60, which breaks down as follows:**

Code	Charge	Amount Patient Responsible for
99213	$72.00	$14.40 (20% of charge)
71010	$91.00	$18.20 (20% of charge)
87430	$58.00	$58.00 (100% of charge)
Totals	$221.00	$90.60

22. **Close the Transaction Entry dialog box.**

23. **Back in the Deposit List dialog box, make sure the Blue Cross/ Blue Shield line is still highlighted, and click Apply Payments/ Adjustments to Charges. Enter the payments for the next patient listed on the RA, Jill Simmons.**

24. **Key S in the For box and press Tab to select Jill Simmons.**

25. **Enter the payment of *43.20* in the Payment box for the 99212 charge on 10/29/2010. Press Tab.**

26. **Enter the other payment for Jill Simmons.**

27. **Click the Save Payments/Adjustments button. (*Note:* If the Open Report dialog box appears, click Cancel.) Notice that the amount listed in the Unapplied area is now 0.00, indicating that the entire payment has been entered.**

28. **Close the Apply Payment/ Adjustments to Charges dialog box.**

29. **The Deposit List dialog box reappears, with the Blue Cross/Blue Shield deposit listed.**

ENTERING CAPITATION PAYMENTS AND ADJUSTMENTS

Many health care practices have agreements with managed care organizations that offer capitated plans. In this type of insurance plan, the practice is paid a set fee to cover all of the HMO members who choose the practice for health care services. This fixed payment is made on a regular schedule (usually monthly), regardless of whether any of the patients visit the practice or regardless of how often they visit. In addition, the patient pays a set copayment amount at the time of an office visit.

When a capitation payment is entered in NDCMedisoft, the payment is not applied to the charges of individual patients (see Figure 7-16). However, the charges in each patient's account must be adjusted to

Deposit List

Deposit Date	Description	Payor Name	Payor Type	Payment
10/4/2010		ChampVA	Insurance	70.00
10/4/2010	00146972	East Ohio PPO	Insurance	526.60
10/4/2010	1010040000	Fitzwilliams, John	Patient	15.00
▶ 10/4/2010	78901234	OhioCare HMO	Capitation	2,500.00
10/4/2010	1010040000	Tanaka, Hiro	Patient	30.00

Deposit Date: 10/4/2010 ☐ Show All Deposits ☐ Show Unapplied Only   Sort By: Date-Payor   Detail...

Edit   New   Apply   Print   Delete   Export   Close

Figure 7-16 **Deposit List Dialog Box for a Capitation Payment**

indicate that the insurance company has met its obligation (through the capitation payment), and that the patient has also done so (by paying a copayment at the time of the office visit).

In order to adjust the patient accounts of those covered by the plan, adjustments are entered in the Transaction Entry dialog box for each patient covered by the capitation payment who has an outstanding balance. After the adjustments, the patient should have a zero balance on the account.

Exercise 7-7

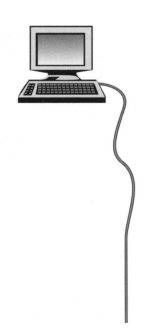

Using Source Document 9, enter a capitation payment from Ohio-Care HMO for the month of September 2010. The total amount of the electronic funds transfer (EFT) is $2,500.00.

Date: October 4, 2010

1. In the Deposit List dialog box, change the date in the Deposit Date box to 10/04/2010. Click the New button. A Confirm box appears with a message about entering a future date. Click No. Click the New button again. The Deposit dialog box appears.

2. In the Payor Type box, select Capitation. Press Tab.

3. Select Electronic in the Payment Method box. Notice that the Check Number box becomes an EFT Tracer box. Press Tab twice.

4. Key *001006003* in the Description/Bank No. box. This is the ID number that is listed on the RA. Press Tab.

5. Key *2500* in the Payment Amount box and press Tab.

6. Accept the default entry of A in the Deposit Code box. Press Tab.

7. Click 15—OhioCare HMO in the Insurance drop-down list.

8. Click the Save button.

9. The Deposit List window reappears, displaying the payment just entered. Unlike other insurance payments, capitation payments are not applied to individual charges in the Deposit List dialog box. However, amounts do need to be adjusted in the patient accounts in the Transaction Entry dialog box. Close the Deposit List dialog box.

Exercise 7-8

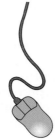

Enter adjustments to John Gardiner and Leila Patterson's accounts so that their account balances are zero. These are the two Ohio-Care HMO patients who have outstanding charges on their accounts for office visits during the month of September 2010.

Date: October 4, 2010

1. Open the Transaction Entry dialog box.

2. Enter *G* in the Chart field and press Tab to select John Gardiner. Notice that the Account Total is listed as $24.00, reflecting the unpaid $24.00 charge for procedure 99211 on 9/7/2010 (listed in the Charges area of the dialog box).

3. Click the New button in the Payments, Adjustments, And Comments area.

4. Click in the Pay/Adj Code box and select CAPADJ (Capitation Adjustment) from the drop-down list. Press Tab.

5. Leave the Who Paid box blank.

6. Enter *24* in the Amount box and press Tab.

7. Click the Apply button to apply the payment to the appropriate charge.

8. Locate the $24.00 charge and enter *24* in the This Adjust column. Press Tab.

9. Click the Close button. If a message is displayed about a $30.00 copayment requirement, click OK.

10. Click the Save Transactions button. Click Yes in response to the future date messages that are displayed.

11. Notice that the Account Total is now listed as zero, and all charges are displayed in white, indicating that they have been paid in full.

12. Now follow the same procedure to bring Leila Patterson's account to a zero balance.

13. Close the Transaction Entry dialog box.

14. Create a backup of your work and exit NDCMedisoft by selecting Exit on the File menu. The Backup Reminder dialog box is displayed.

15. Click the Back Up Data Now button. The Backup dialog box appears.

16. Enter the file path and file name in the File Destination Path and Name box or click the Find button and browse to the desired location. The file name should be FCC8–7.mbk (the database name followed by the chapter number). The file path will vary depending on your computer and network setup. Ask your instructor for the file path.

17. Click the Start Backup button. NDCMedisoft creates a backup file. When it is complete, an Information box is displayed, indicating that the backup is complete. Click OK. The Backup dialog box closes and the program is shut down.

CHAPTER REVIEW

USING TERMINOLOGY

Define the term in the space provided.

1. capitation payments

_____

_____

CHECKING YOUR UNDERSTANDING

Answer the questions below in the space provided.

2. When is it appropriate to print a walkout statement?

_____

_____

3. Why is it easier to enter large insurance payments in the Deposit List dialog box than in the Transaction Entry dialog box?

_____

_____

4. When all payments on a remittance advice have been successfully entered and applied to charges, what should appear in the Unapplied box in the upper-right corner of the Deposit List dialog box?

_____

_____

5. When a capitated payment is entered in the Deposit List dialog box, what amount appears in the Unapplied Amount box?

_____

_____

6. Why do charges need to be adjusted for patients who are covered under a capitated insurance plan?

_____

_____

APPLYING KNOWLEDGE

Answer the questions below in the space provided.

7. After you have entered a patient copayment for $20, you realize it should have been $30. What should you do?

_____

_____

_____

8. Randall Klein calls. He would like to know whether Medicare has paid any of the charges for his September office visit. How would you look up this information in NDCMedisoft?

_____

_____

_____

AT THE COMPUTER

Answer the following questions at the computer.

9. What is the total amount that John Fitzwilliams paid in copayments in September 2010? (*Hint:* Include his daughter Sarah in the calculation.)

10. On September 10, 2010, a payment of $168.00 was received from Blue Cross/Blue Shield as payment for James Smith's facial nerve function studies performed on September 9, 2010. What is the remaining amount of the charge that is James Smith's responsibility to pay, assuming he has met his annual deductible? (Do not actually enter the payment in the computer; use NDCMedisoft to look up the necessary information and then calculate the remaining amount.)

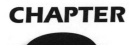

CHAPTER 8

Scheduling

WHAT YOU NEED TO KNOW

To use this chapter, you need to know how to:
- ◆ Start NDCMedisoft, use menus, and enter and edit text.
- ◆ Work with chart numbers and codes.

OBJECTIVES

When you finish this chapter, you will be able to:
- ◆ Start Office Hours.
- ◆ View the appointment schedule.
- ◆ Enter an appointment.
- ◆ Change or delete an appointment.
- ◆ Search for an appointment.
- ◆ Create a recall list.
- ◆ Enter a break in a provider's schedule.
- ◆ Print appointment schedules.

KEY TERMS

Office Hours break

Office Hours schedule

INTRODUCTION TO OFFICE HOURS

Appointment scheduling is one of the most important tasks in a medical office. Different medical procedures take different lengths of time, and each appointment must be the right length. On the one hand, physicians want to be able to go from one appointment to another without unnecessary breaks. On the other hand, patients should not be kept waiting more than a few minutes for a physician. Managing and juggling the schedule are usually the job of a medical office assistant working at the front desk. NDCMedisoft provides a special program called Office Hours to handle appointment scheduling.

OVERVIEW OF THE OFFICE HOURS WINDOW

The Office Hours program has its own window (see Figure 8-1), including its own menu bar and toolbar. The Office Hours menu bar lists the menus available: File, Edit, View, Lists, Reports, Tools, and Help (see Figure 8-2). Under the menu bar is a toolbar with shortcut

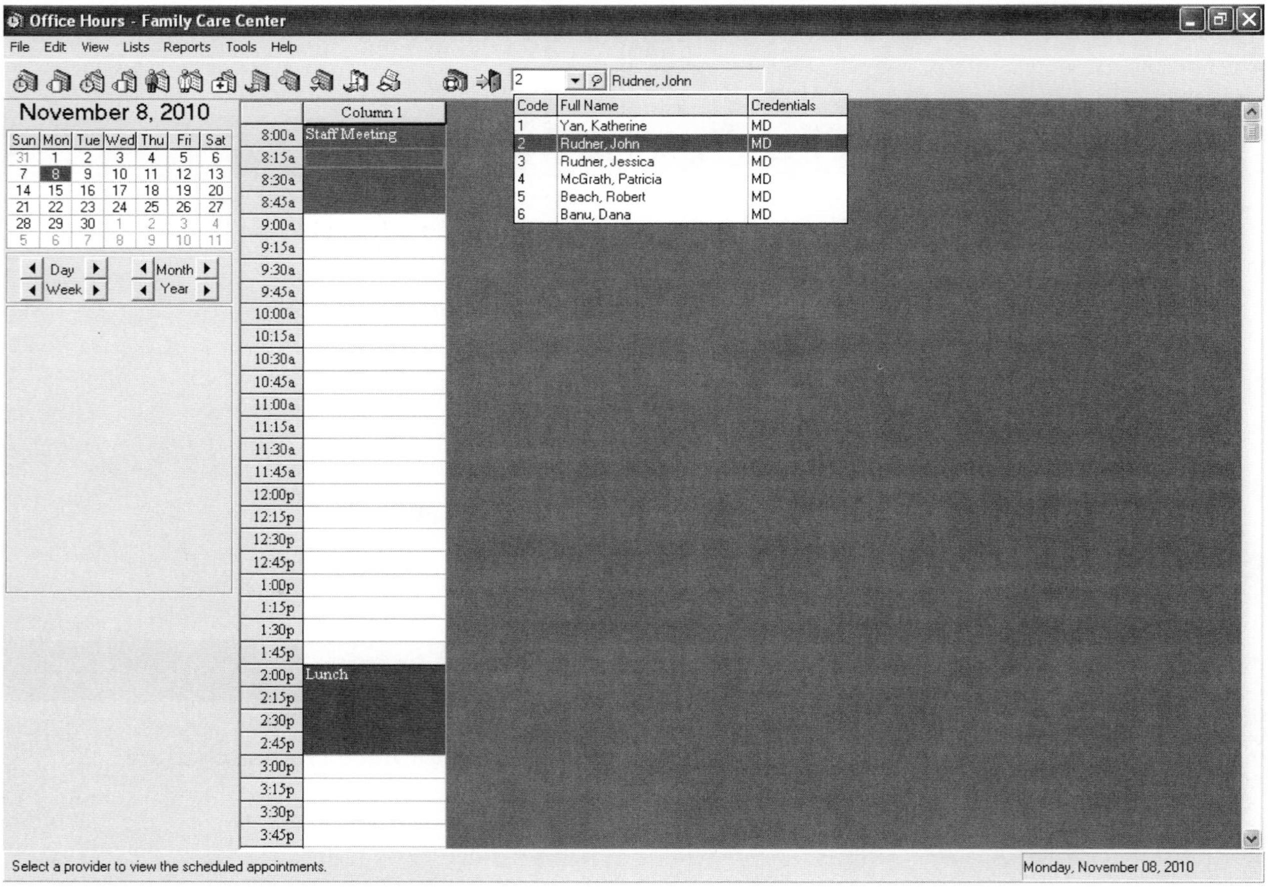

Figure 8-1 **The Office Hours Window**

Figure 8-2 **The Office Hours Menu Bar**

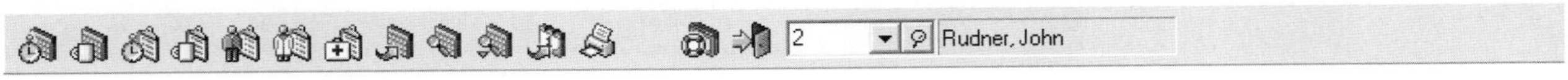

Figure 8-3 **The Office Hours Toolbar**

Table 8-1   Office Hours Toolbar Buttons

Button	Button Name	Associated Function	Activity
	Appointment Entry	New Appointment Entry dialog box	Enter appointments
	Break Entry	New Break Entry dialog box	Enter break
	Appointment List	Appointment List dialog box	Display list of appointments
	Break List	Break List dialog box	Display list of breaks
	Patient List	Patient List dialog box	Display list of patients
	Provider List	Provider List dialog box	Display list of providers
	Resource List	Resource List dialog box	Display list of resources
	Go to a Date	Go to a Date dialog box	Change calendar to a different date
	Search for Open Time Slot	Find Open Time dialog box	Locate first available time slot
	Search Again	Find Open Time dialog box	Locate next available time slot
	Go to Today		Return calendar to current date
	Print Appointment List		Print appointment list
	Help	Office Hours Help	Display Office Hours Help contents
	Exit	Exit	Exit the Office Hours program

buttons. The functions of Office Hours are accessed by selecting a choice from one of the menus or by clicking a button on the toolbar.

Located just below the menu bar, the toolbar contains a series of buttons that represent the most common activities performed in Office Hours. These buttons are shortcuts for frequently used menu commands. The toolbar displays fourteen buttons (see Figure 8-3 and Table 8-1).

The left half of the Office Hours screen displays the current date and a calendar of the current month (see Figure 8-4 on page 156). The current date is highlighted on the calendar. When a different date is clicked on the calendar, the calendar switches to the new date.

Office Hours schedule a listing of time slots for a particular day for a specific provider.

The **Office Hours schedule,** shown in the right half of the screen, is a listing of time slots for a particular day for a specific provider. The provider's name and number is displayed at the top to the right of the shortcut buttons. The provider can be easily changed by clicking the triangle button in the Provider box.

PROGRAM OPTIONS

When Office Hours is installed in a medical practice, it is set up to reflect the needs of that particular practice. Most offices that use NDCMedisoft already have Office Hours set up and running. However, if NDCMedisoft is just being installed, the options to set up the

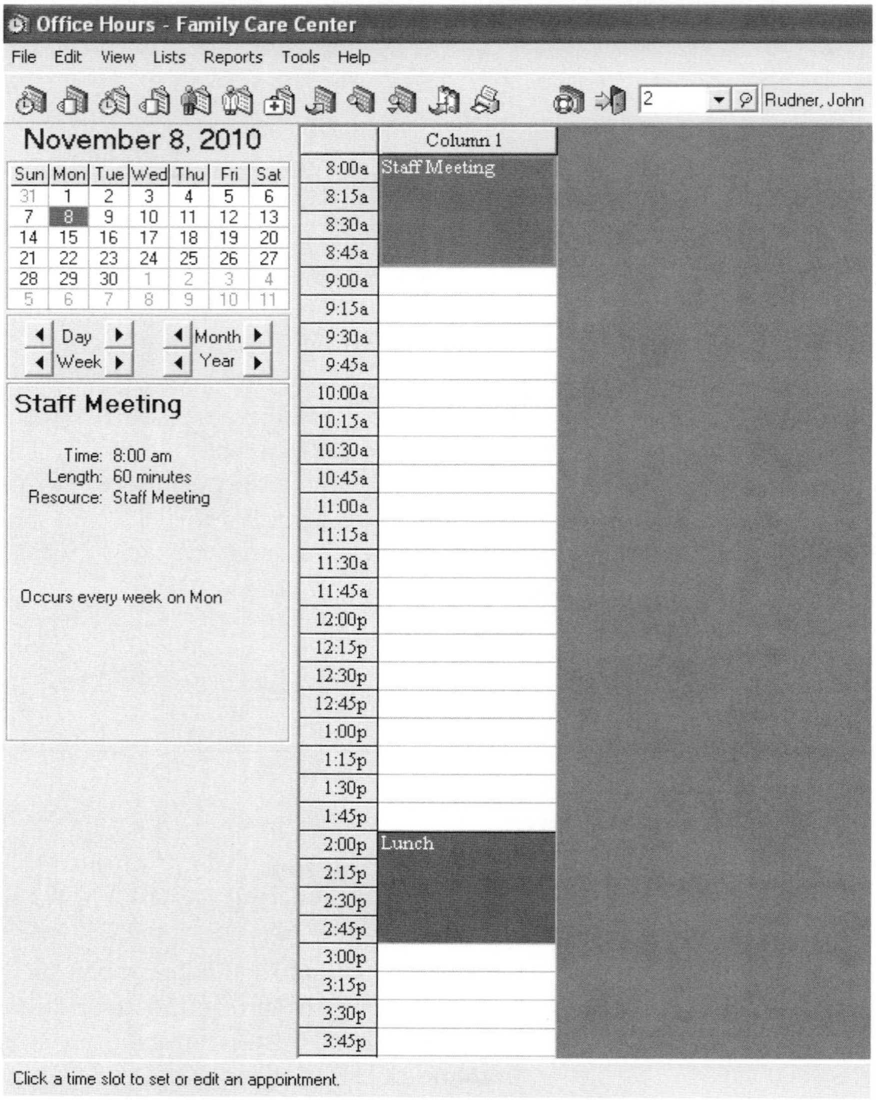

Figure 8-4 *The left side of the Office Hours window displays the date and a monthly calendar. The right side of the window contains the selected provider's schedule for the day selected in the calendar.*

Office Hours program can be found in the Program Options dialog box, which is accessed by clicking Program Options on the Office Hours File menu.

ENTERING AND EXITING OFFICE HOURS

Office Hours can be started from within NDCMedisoft or directly from Windows. To access Office Hours from within NDCMedisoft, Appointment Book is clicked on the Activities menu. Office Hours can also be started by clicking the corresponding shortcut button on the toolbar.

To start Office Hours without entering NDCMedisoft first:

1. Click Start > All Programs.

2. Click NDCMedisoft on the Programs submenu.

3. Click Office Hours on the NDCMedisoft submenu.

The Office Hours program is closed by clicking Exit on the Office Hours File menu, or by clicking the Exit button on its toolbar. If Office Hours was started from within NDCMedisoft, exiting will return you to NDCMedisoft. If Office Hours was started directly from Windows, clicking Exit will return you to the Windows desktop.

ENTERING APPOINTMENTS

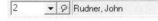

Figure 8-5 **Provider Box**

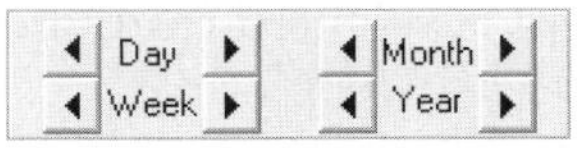

Entering an appointment begins with selecting the provider for whom the appointment is being scheduled. The current provider is listed in the Provider box at the top right of the screen (see Figure 8-5). Clicking the triangle button displays a drop-down list of providers in the system. To choose a different provider, click the name of the provider on the drop-down list.

Figure 8-6 **Day, Week, Month, and Year Triangle Buttons**

After the provider is selected, the date of the desired appointment must be chosen. Dates are changed by clicking the Day, Week, Month, and Year right and left arrow buttons located under the calendar (see Figure 8-6). After the provider and date have been selected, patient appointments can be entered.

Appointments are entered by clicking the Appointment Entry shortcut button or by double-clicking in a time slot on the schedule. When either action is taken, the New Appointment Entry dialog box is displayed (see Figure 8-7).

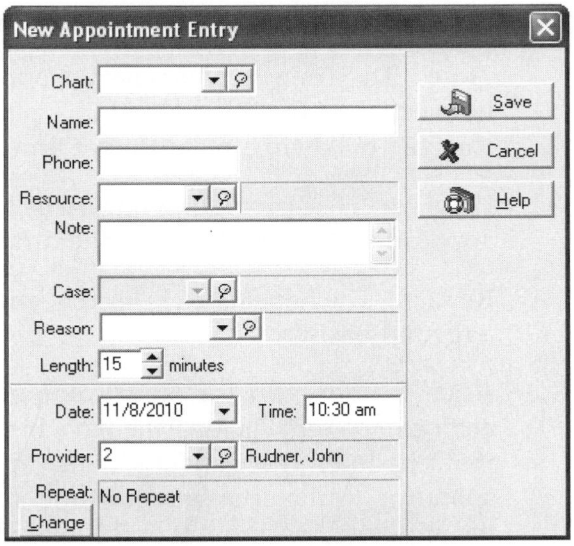

Figure 8-7 **New Appointment Entry Dialog Box**

The New Appointment Entry dialog box contains the following fields:

Chart   A patient's chart number is chosen from the Chart drop-down list. To select the desired patient, click on the name and press Tab. If you are setting up an appointment for a new patient who has not been assigned a chart number, skip this box and key the patient's name in the Name box.

Name   Once a patient's chart is selected from the Chart drop-down list and the Tab key is pressed, NDCMedisoft displays the patient's name in the Name box. If a patient does not have a chart number, key the patient's name in this box.

Phone   After a patient's chart is selected, that patient's phone number is automatically entered in the Phone box.

Resource   This box is used if the practice assigns codes to resources, such as exam rooms or equipment.

Note   Any special information about an appointment is entered in the Note box.

Case   The case that pertains to the appointment is selected from the drop-down list of cases.

Reason   Reason codes can be set up in the program to reflect the reason for an appointment.

Length   The amount of time an appointment will take (in minutes) is entered in the Length box by keying the number of minutes or using the up and down arrows.

Date   The Date box displays the date that is currently displayed on the calendar. If this is not the desired date, it may be changed by keying in a different date or by clicking the triangle button and selecting a date from the pop-up calendar that appears.

Time   The Time box displays the appointment time that is currently selected on the schedule. If this is not the desired time, it may be changed by keying in a different time.

Provider   The provider who will be treating the patient during this appointment is selected from the drop-down list of providers.

Repeat   The Repeat box is used to enter appointments that recur on a regular basis.

After the boxes in the New Appointment Entry dialog box have been completed, clicking the Save button enters the information on the schedule. The patient's name appears in the time slot corresponding to the appointment time. In addition, information about the appointment appears in the lower left corner of the Office Hours window.

LOOKING FOR A FUTURE DATE

Often a patient will need a follow-up appointment at a certain time in the future. For example, suppose a physician would like a patient to return for a checkup in three weeks. The most efficient way to search for a future appointment in Office Hours is to use the Go to a Date shortcut button on the toolbar. (This feature can also be accessed on the Edit menu.)

Clicking the Go to a Date shortcut button displays the Go to Date dialog box (see Figure 8-8). Within the dialog box, five boxes offer options for choosing a future date.

Date From   This box indicates the current date in the appointment search.

Go ___ Days   This box is used to locate a date that is a specific number of days in the future. For example, if a patient needs an appointment ten days from the current day, "10" would be entered in this box.

Go ___ Weeks   This box is used when a patient needs an appointment a specific number of weeks in the future, such as six weeks from the current day.

Go ___ Months   This box is used when a patient needs an appointment a specific number of months in the future, such as three months from the current day.

Go ___ Years   Similar to the weeks and months options, this box is used when an appointment is needed in one year, or several years in the future.

After a future date option has been selected, clicking the Go button closes the dialog box and begins the search. The system locates the future date and displays the calendar schedule for that date.

Figure 8-8 Go to Date Dialog Box

Exercise 8-1

Enter an appointment for Herbert Bell at 3:00 p.m. on Monday, November 15, 2010. The appointment is fifteen minutes in length and is with Dr. John Rudner.

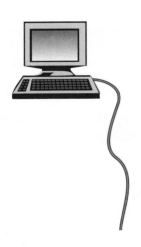

> Note: Steps 1 through 3 are required at the beginning of each chapter. These steps start NDCMedisoft, set the path to the correct data location, and restore the data saved at the end of the last work session.

1. Hold down the F7 key and start NDCMedisoft. Enter the location of the NDCMedisoft data in the Find NDCMedisoft Directory box and click OK. (If you are unsure what to enter, ask your instructor.) When the Open practice dialog box appears, verify that Family Care Center is highlighted and click OK.

2. Restore the data from your last work session by selecting Restore Data on the File menu. When a warning box appears, click OK. Enter the file path and file name in the File Destination Path and Name or click the Find button and browse to the desired location. The file name should be FCC8-7.mbk (the database name followed by the chapter number that you last worked on). The file path will vary depending on your computer and network setup. Ask your instructor for the file path.

3. Click the Start Restore button. When a Confirm dialog box appears, click OK. NDCMedisoft restores the data. When it is complete, an Information box is displayed, indicating that the restore is complete. Click OK. The Restore box closes and the main NDCMedisoft window is displayed.

4. Start Office Hours by clicking the Appointment Book shortcut button on the toolbar.

5. If John Rudner is not already selected, click 2, John Rudner, on the drop-down list in the Provider box to select him.

6. Change the date on the calendar to Monday, November 15, 2010. Use the arrow keys to change the month and year, and then click the day on the calendar.

7. In the schedule, double-click the 3:00 P.M. time slot. (You may need to use the scroll bar to view 3:00 P.M.) The New Appointment Entry dialog box is displayed.

8. Click Herbert Bell from the list of names on the drop-down list in the Chart box and press Tab. The system automatically fills in a number of boxes in the dialog box, such as the patient's name and phone number.

9. Accept the default entry in the Case box.

10. Notice that the Length box already contains an entry of fifteen minutes. This is the default appointment length. Since Herbert Bell's appointment is for an annual exam, this entry must be changed to sixty minutes. Key *60* in the Length box, or use the up arrow next to the Length box to change the appointment length to sixty minutes.

11. Verify the entries in the Date, Time, and Provider boxes, and then click the Save button. Office Hours saves the appointment, closes the dialog box, and displays the appointment on the schedule, as well as in the lower-left corner of the Office Hours window. Herbert Bell's name is displayed in the 3:00 P.M. time slot on the schedule.

Exercise 8-2

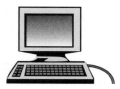

Enter the following appointments with Dr. John Rudner.

1. The first appointment is Monday (November 15, 2010) at 4:00 P.M. for John Fitzwilliams, thirty minutes in length. Verify that "2 Rudner, John" is displayed in the Provider box.

2. In the schedule, double-click the 4:00 P.M. time-slot box.

3. Select John Fitzwilliams on the Chart drop-down list.

4. Press the Tab key. The program automatically completes several boxes in the dialog box.

5. Press the Tab key until the entry in the Length box is highlighted.

6. Key *30* in the Length box, or click the up arrow once to change the length to thirty minutes.

7. Click the Save button. Verify that the appointment for John Fitzwilliams appears on the schedule for November 15, 2010, at 4:00 P.M. for a length of thirty minutes.

8. Enter an appointment on Monday, November 15, 2010, at 4:30 P.M. for Leila Patterson, fifteen minutes in length.

9. Enter an appointment on Tuesday, November 16, 2010, at 12:15 P.M. for James Smith, thirty minutes in length.

10. To schedule an appointment for James Smith two weeks after November 16, 2010, at 12:15 P.M., fifteen minutes in length, click the Go To a Date shortcut button.

11. Key *2* in the Go ___ Weeks box. Click the Go button. The program closes the Go To Date box and displays the appointment schedule for November 30, 2010.

12. Enter James Smith's appointment.

Exercise 8-3

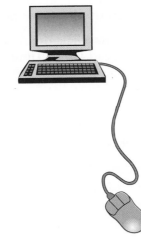

Enter these appointments with Dr. Jessica Rudner.

1. Click Dr. Jessica Rudner from the list of providers in the Provider drop-down list.

2. Enter an appointment for Friday, November 19, 2010, at 3:00 P.M. for Janine Bell, fifteen minutes in length.

3. Use Office Hours' Go to a Date feature to schedule an appointment three weeks from November 19, 2010 at 1:15 P.M. for Sarina Bell, thirty minutes in length.

4. Schedule an appointment for Sarah Fitzwilliams one week from November 19, 2010, at 9:00 A.M., fifteen minutes in length.

5. Temporarily leave Office Hours by clicking the minimize button in the upper-right corner of the window.

Exercise 8-4

Enter an appointment on Thursday, November 11, 2010, at 9:00 A.M. for John Gardiner, thirty minutes in length. You do not know his provider, so this information must be looked up in NDCMedisoft before you enter the appointment.

1. Go to the Patient List dialog box.

2. Select John Gardiner as the patient.

3. Click the Other Information tab to find his assigned provider.

4. Click the Office Hours button on the Windows task bar (bottom of screen). Notice that the Patient/Guarantor dialog box is still partially visible underneath the Office Hours window.

5. Select Gardiner's provider in the Provider box in Office Hours.

6. Enter the appointment.

7. Minimize Office Hours.

8. In NDCMedisoft, close the open dialog boxes.

SEARCHING FOR AVAILABLE APPOINTMENT TIME

Often it is necessary to search for available appointment space on a particular day of the week and at a specific time. For example, a patient needs a thirty-minute appointment and would like it to be during his lunch hour, which is from 12:00 P.M. to 1:00 P.M. He can get away from the office only on Mondays and Fridays. Office Hours makes it easy to locate an appointment slot that meets these requirements with the Search for Open Time Slot shortcut button.

Exercise 8-5

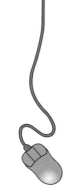

Search for the next available appointment slot beginning November 11, 2010, with Dr. Yan, on a Tuesday, between the hours of 11:00 A.M. and 2:00 P.M.

1. Click the Office Hours button on the Windows taskbar. Verify that Dr. Katherine Yan is displayed next to the Provider box.

2. On the Edit menu, click Find Open Time, or click the Search for Open Time Slot shortcut button. The Find Open Time dialog box is displayed (see Figure 8-9).

3. Key *30* in the Length box. Press the Tab key.

4. Key *11* in the Start Time box. Press the Tab key.

5. Key *2* in the End Time box. Press the Tab key.

6. To search for an appointment on Tuesday, click the Tuesday box in the Day of Week area of the dialog box.

7. Click the Search button to begin looking for an appointment slot. NDCMedisoft closes the dialog box and locates the first

Find Open Time

Length: 15

Start Time: 8:00 am

End Time: 5:00 pm

Day of Week
- Sun
- Mon
- Tue
- Wed
- Thu
- Fri
- Sat

Search
Cancel
Help

Figure 8-9 **Find Open Time Dialog Box**

available time slot that meets these specifications. The time slot is outlined on the schedule.

8. Double-click the selected time slot. Click Maritza Ramos on the drop-down list in the Name box.

9. Press the Tab key until the cursor is in the Length box.

10. Key *30* and press the Tab key.

11. Click the Save button.

12. Verify that the appointment has been entered by looking at the schedule.

Exercise 8-6

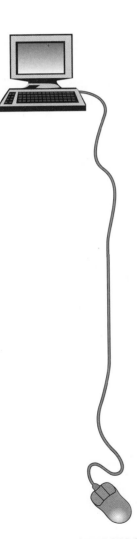

Schedule Randall Klein for a thirty-minute appointment with Dr. John Rudner on November 15, 2010. Mr. Klein is available only between 3:00 P.M. and 5:00 P.M.

1. Click the desired provider in the Provider box.

2. Change the calendar to November 15, 2010.

3. Click Find Open Time on the Edit menu to display the Find Open Time dialog box.

4. In the Length box, highlight the number already entered and key *30.* Press the Tab key to move the cursor to the Start Time box.

5. Key *3* in the Start Time box. Press Tab. Click on *am* to highlight it and then key *p* to change am to pm. Press Tab to move to the End Time box.

6. Key *5* in the End Time box. Press Tab.

7. In the Day of Week boxes, select Monday. Click the Tuesday box to deselect that day.

8. Click the Search button. The first available slot that meets the requirements is outlined on the schedule.

9. Double-click in the time slot to open the New Appointment Entry dialog box.

10. Click Randall Klein from the drop-down list in the Chart box. Press tab several times to move the cursor to the Length box.

11. Key *30* in the Length box, and press the Tab key.

12. Click the Save button. The dialog box closes and Randall Klein's appointment appears on the schedule.

ENTERING APPOINTMENTS FOR NEW PATIENTS
When a new patient phones the office for an appointment, the appointment can be scheduled in Office Hours before the patient information is entered in NDCMedisoft. However, while the prospective patient is still on the phone, most offices obtain basic data and enter it in the appropriate NDCMedisoft dialog boxes (Patient/Guarantor and Case).

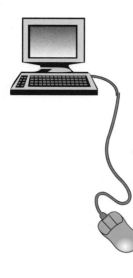

Exercise 8-7

Schedule Lisa Green, a new patient, for a forty-five-minute appointment with Dr. John Rudner on November 15, 2010, at 1:15 P.M.

1. Verify that November 15, 2010, is displayed on the schedule and that Dr. John Rudner is selected as the provider.

2. Double-click the 1:15 P.M. time slot.

3. Click in the Name box and key *Green, Lisa.* Press the Tab key to move the cursor to the Phone box.

4. Key *6145553604* in the Phone box, and press Tab until the cursor is in the Length box.

5. Key *45* in the Length box.

6. Click the Save button. The appointment is displayed on the November 15, 2010 schedule.

BOOKING REPEATED APPOINTMENTS

Some patients require appointments on a repeated basis, such as every Thursday for eight weeks. Repeated appointments are also set up in the New Appointment Entry dialog box. The Repeat feature is located at the bottom of the dialog box. When the Change button is clicked, the Repeat Change dialog box is displayed. The Repeat Change dialog box provides a number of choices for setting up repeating appointments (see Figure 8-10).

The left side of the dialog box contains information about the frequency of the appointments. The default is set to None. Other options include Daily, Weekly, Monthly, and Yearly. When an option other than None is selected, the center section of the dialog box changes and displays additional options for setting up the appointments (see Figure 8-11).

In the center section, an option is provided to indicate how often the appointments should be scheduled, such as every one week. Below

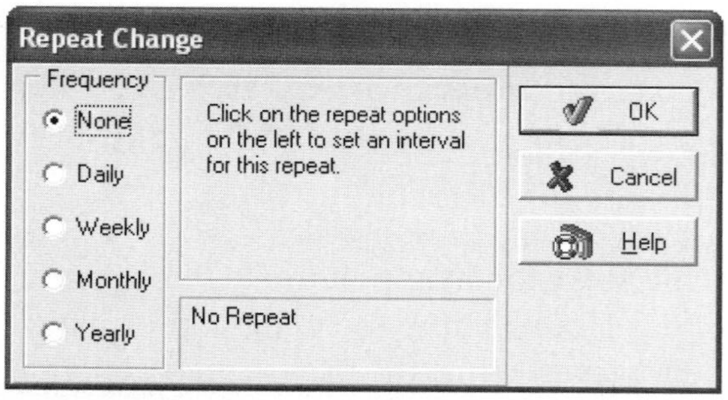

Figure 8-10 *Repeat Change Dialog Box When None Is Selected*

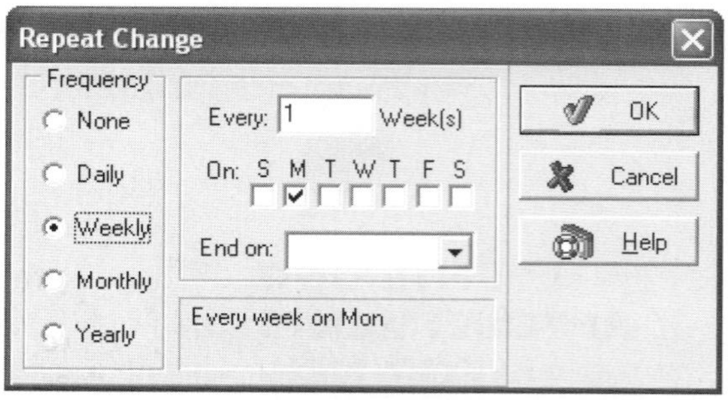

Figure 8-11 *Repeat Change Dialog Box When an Option Other Than None Is Selected*

that there is an option to indicate the day of the week on which the appointment should be scheduled. Finally, there is a box to indicate when the repeating appointments should stop. When all the information has been entered, clicking the OK button closes the Repeat Change dialog box and the New Appointment Entry dialog box is once again visible. Clicking the Save button enters the repeating appointments on the schedule.

Exercise 8-8

Schedule Li Y. Wong for a fifteen-minute appointment with Dr. Katherine Yan, once a week for six weeks. Mrs. Wong has requested that the appointments be at the same time every week, preferably in the early morning, beginning with Wednesday, November 17, 2010.

1. Click the desired provider on the Provider drop-down list.

2. Change the schedule to November 17, 2010.

3. Double-click in the 8:00 A.M. time slot. The New Appointment Entry dialog box is displayed.

4. Select Li Y. Wong from the Chart drop-down list. Press the Tab key.

5. Confirm that the entry in the Length box is fifteen minutes.

6. Click the Change button to schedule the repeating appointments.

7. In the Frequency column, select Weekly.

8. Accept the default entry of 1 in the Every ___ Week(s) box.

9. Accept the default entry of W to accept Wednesday as the day of the week.

10. Click the arrow for the drop-down list in the End On box. A calendar pops up. Count six weeks from November 17, 2010. When you find the sixth Wednesday (counting November 17 as the first week), click in the calendar box for that day. 12/22/2010 appears in the End On box.

11. Click the OK button. Notice that "Every week on Wed" is displayed in the Repeat area of the New Appointment Entry dialog box.

12. Click the Save button to enter the appointments. Notice that "Occurs every week on Wed" appears in the lower left corner of the Office Hours window.

13. Go to December 22, 2010, to verify that Mrs. Wong is scheduled for an appointment at 8:00 A.M.

14. Go to December 29, 2010, and confirm that Mrs. Wong is not scheduled. This is the seventh week, and her repeating appointments were scheduled for six weeks, so no appointment should appear on December 29, 2010.

CHANGING OR DELETING APPOINTMENTS

It is often necessary to change or cancel a patient's appointment. Changing an appointment is accomplished with the Cut and Paste commands on the Office Hours Edit menu.

The following steps are used to reschedule an appointment:

1. Locate the appointment that needs to be changed. Make sure the appointment slot is visible on the schedule.

2. Click on the existing time-slot box. A black border surrounds the slot to indicate that it is selected.

3. Click Cut on the Edit menu. The appointment disappears from the schedule.

4. Click the date on the calendar when the appointment is to be rescheduled.

5. Click the desired time-slot box on the schedule. The slot becomes active.

6. Click Paste on the Edit menu. The patient's name appears in the new time-slot box.

The following steps are used to cancel an appointment without rescheduling:

1. Locate the appointment on the schedule.

2. Click the time-slot box to select the appointment.

3. Click Cut on the Edit menu. The appointment disappears from the schedule.

TIP Instead of using the Cut and Paste commands to change or delete an appointment, select the appointment and press the right mouse button. A shortcut menu appears with several options, including Cut, Copy, and Delete.

Exercise 8-9

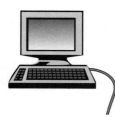

Change Janine Bell's and John Gardiner's appointments.

1. Click Jessica Rudner on the Provider box drop-down list.

2. Go to Friday, November 19, 2010, on the calendar.

3. Locate Janine Bell's 3:00 P.M. appointment on the schedule. Click the 3:00 P.M. time-slot box.

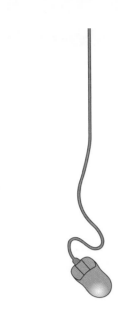

4. Click Cut on the Edit menu. Janine Bell's appointment is removed from the 3:00 P.M. time-slot box. (You may also use the right-mouse-click shortcut.)

5. Click the 4:00 P.M. time-slot box.

6. Click Paste on the Edit menu. Janine Bell's name is displayed in the 4:00 P.M. time-slot box.

7. Click Katherine Yan on the Provider drop-down list.

8. Go to Thursday, November 11, 2010, on the calendar.

9. Locate John Gardiner's 9:00 A.M. appointment. Remove his appointment from the 9:00 A.M. time slot.

10. Go to Friday, November 19, 2010, on the calendar.

11. Enter John Gardiner's appointment in the 9:15 A.M. time slot.

12. Exit Office Hours.

CREATING A RECALL LIST

Medical offices frequently must keep track of patients who need to return for future appointments. Some offices schedule future appointments when the patient is leaving the office. For example, if a patient has just seen a physician and needs to return for a follow-up appointment in six weeks, the appointment is usually made before the patient leaves the office. However, when the appointment is needed farther in the future, such as one year later, it is not always practical to set up the appointment. It is difficult for the patient and the physician to know their schedules a year in advance. For this reason, many offices keep lists of patients who need to be contacted for future appointments.

In NDCMedisoft, a recall list can be created and maintained by clicking Patient Recall on the Lists menu. Patients can also be added to the recall list by clicking the Patient Recall Entry shortcut button on the toolbar. When Patient Recall is selected from the Lists menu, the Patient Recall List dialog box is displayed (see Figure 8-12 on page 168). This dialog box organizes the recall information in a column format. The scroll bar is used to display the last three columns on the right.

◆ **Date of Recall** Lists the date on which the recall is scheduled.

◆ **Name** Displays the patient's name.

◆ **Phone** Lists the patient's phone number, making it easy to call patients for appointments without having to look up phone numbers in another dialog box.

◆ **Extension** Lists the patient's phone extension.

◆ **Status** Indicates the patient's recall status: Call, Call Again, Appointment Set, No Appointment.

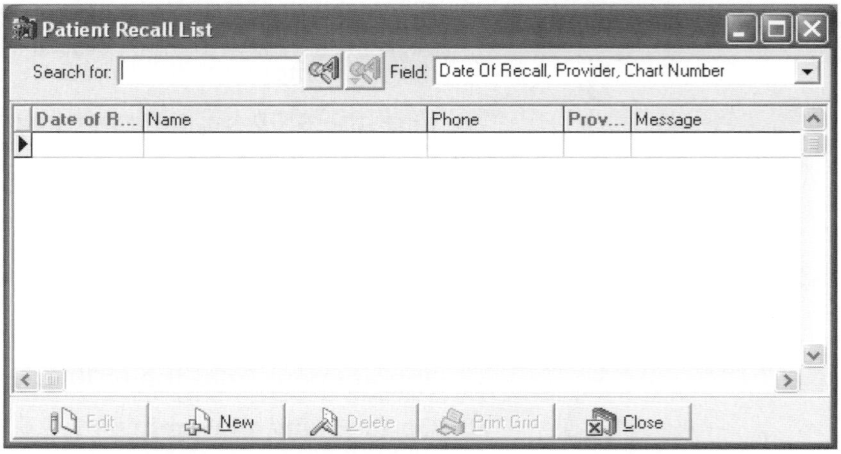

Figure 8-12 Patient Recall List Dialog Box

- ◆ **Provider** Displays the provider code for the patient's provider.
- ◆ **Message** Displays the entry made in the Message box of the Patient Recall dialog box.
- ◆ **Chart Number** Displays the patient's chart number.
- ◆ **Procedure Code** Lists the procedure code for the procedure for which the patient is being recalled.

The Patient Recall List dialog box contains the following boxes:

Search For   The Search For box is used to locate a specific patient on the recall list. Entering the first few letters or numbers in the Search For box displays the selection that is the closest match to the search criteria.

Field   The choices in the Field box determine the order in which patients are listed in the dialog box. There are three sorting options:

- ◆ Date of Recall, Provider, Chart Number
- ◆ Chart Number, Date of Recall
- ◆ Provider, Date of Recall

The Patient Recall List dialog box also contains these buttons: Edit, New, Delete, Print Grid, and Close.

Edit   Clicking the Edit button displays the Patient Recall dialog box for the patient whose entry is highlighted. The information on the patient can then be edited by making different selections in the boxes.

New   Clicking the New button displays an empty Patient Recall dialog box, in which data on a new recall patient can be entered.

Delete   Clicking the Delete button deletes from the patient recall list data on the patient whose entry is highlighted.

Print Grid   The Print Grid button is used to print a list of the data in each field listed in the dialog box.

Close   The Close button is used to exit the Patient Recall List dialog box.

ADDING A PATIENT TO THE RECALL LIST

Patients are added to the recall list by clicking the New button in the Patient Recall List dialog box or by clicking the Patient Recall Entry shortcut button. When either of these actions is performed, the Patient Recall dialog box is displayed (see Figure 8-13).

The Patient Recall dialog box contains the following boxes:

Recall Date   The date a patient needs to return to see a physician is entered in the Recall Date box.

Provider   A patient's provider is selected from the drop-down list.

Chart   A patient's chart number is selected from the drop-down list, or the first few letters of a patient's chart number are entered in the Chart box.

Name, Phone, Extension   After a chart number is entered, the system automatically completes the Name, Phone, and Extension boxes.

Procedure   If the procedure for which a patient is returning is known, it is entered in the Procedure box in one of two ways. The procedure code can be selected from the drop-down list, or the first few numbers can be entered and the drop-down list will display the entry that most closely matches the entered numbers. This is especially valuable in practices in which there are hundreds of procedure

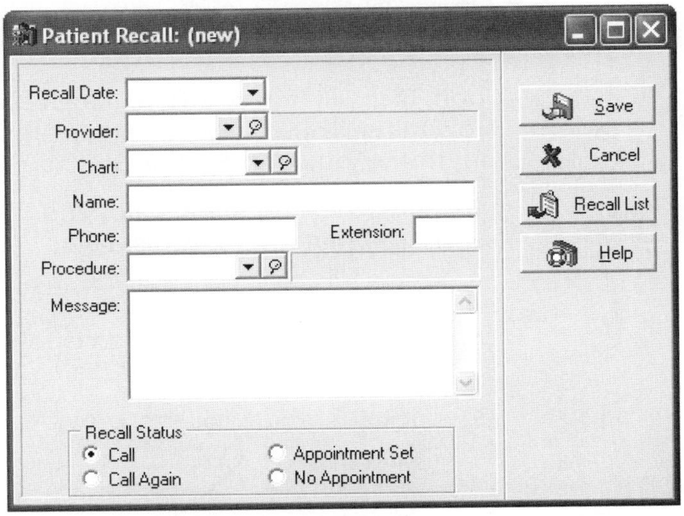

Figure 8-13 **Patient Recall (new) Dialog Box**

codes, because it eliminates the need to scroll through several hundred codes to locate the desired one.

Message   The Message box is used to record any special notes, reminders, or instructions about a patient and his or her appointment.

Recall Status   The choices in the Recall Status box are used to indicate the action that needs to be taken. They include:

Call   The Call button is used when a patient needs to be telephoned about a future appointment.

Call Again   The Call Again button is used when a patient has been called once, but contact was not made and an additional call is necessary.

Appointment Set   The Appointment Set button is used when a patient has an appointment already scheduled.

No Appointment   The No Appointment button is used when a patient has been contacted for an appointment but has declined for some reason.

After the information has been entered in the dialog box, clicking the Save button saves the data and adds the patient to the recall list. In addition to the Save button, the Patient Recall dialog box contains these buttons: Cancel, Recall List, and Help. The Cancel button exits the dialog box without saving the data entered. The Recall List button in the Patient Recall dialog box is used to display the Patient Recall List dialog box. The Help button displays NDCMedisoft's online help for the Patient Recall dialog box.

Exercise 8-10

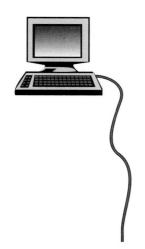

John Fitzwilliams needs to receive a phone call one year from November 15, 2010, to set up an appointment for an annual physical. Add John Fitzwilliams to the recall list.

1. **Click the Patient Recall Entry shortcut button. The Patient Recall dialog box is displayed.**

2. **In the Recall Date box, enter November 15, 2011. Press Tab.**

3. **Determine which physician is John Fitzwilliams's provider. (Look in the Patient/Guarantor dialog box for this information.)**

4. **Click John Fitzwilliams' provider on the drop-down list in the Provider box. Press Tab.**

5. **Enter John Fitzwilliams' chart number in the Chart box by keying the first few letters of his last name. Notice that the system**

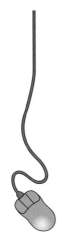

automatically completes the Name and Phone box. (The Extension box would also be completed if there were an extension.)

6. Enter the procedure code in the Procedure box by keying *99396* (Preventive est., 40–64 years).

7. Verify that the Call radio button in the Recall Status box is selected.

8. Click the Save button to save the entry.

9. Click Patient Recall on the Lists menu.

10. Verify that the entry for John Fitzwilliams has been added to the recall list.

11. Close the Patient Recall List dialog box.

CREATING BREAKS

Office Hours break a block of time when a physician is unavailable for appointments with patients.

Office Hours provides features for inserting standard breaks in providers' schedules. The **Office Hours break** is a block of time when a physician is unavailable for appointments with patients. Some examples of breaks include Lunch, Meeting, Personal, Emergency, Break, Vacation, Seminar, Holiday, Trip, and Surgery. In Office Hours, breaks can be created one at a time or on a recurring basis for all providers. One-time breaks, such as those for vacation, are set up for individual providers. Other breaks, such as staff meetings, can be entered once for multiple providers.

Often breaks need to be inserted into a provider's schedule when he or she is not available for appointments with patients. For example, if a physician will be in surgery on Thursday from 9 A.M. until 12:00 P.M., that time period must be marked as unavailable on his or her schedule.

To set up a break for a current provider (that is, the provider listed in the Office Hours Provider box), click the Break Entry shortcut button. This action causes the New Break Entry dialog box to appear (see Figure 8-14).

Figure 8-14 **New Break Entry Dialog Box**

The dialog box contains the following options:

Name The name field is used to store a name or description of the break.

Date The date field displays the current date on the Office Hours calendar. If this is not the correct date for the break entry, a different date can be entered.

Time The starting time of the break is entered in this box.

Length This box indicates the length of the break in minutes (from 0 to 720).

Resource The drop-down list entries in the Resource box display the different types of breaks already set up in Office Hours.

Change The Change button next to the Repeat box is used to enter breaks that recur at a regular interval.

Color By selecting a different color from the drop-down list, the color of the break time slot in the schedule can be changed.

Provider(s) The Provider(s) buttons are used to indicate whether the break is to be set for the current provider (the provider selected in the Provider box in Office Hours), some providers, or all providers. If some is selected, a Provider Selection dialog box will be displayed when the Save button is clicked. The appropriate providers can then be selected.

When all the information has been entered, clicking the Save button closes the dialog box and enters the break(s) in Office Hours.

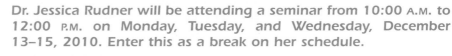

Exercise 8-11

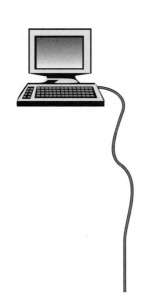

Dr. Jessica Rudner will be attending a seminar from 10:00 A.M. to 12:00 P.M. on Monday, Tuesday, and Wednesday, December 13–15, 2010. Enter this as a break on her schedule.

1. **Start Office Hours.**

2. **Select Jessica Rudner from the Provider drop-down list.**

3. **Change the date on the calendar to December 13, 2010.**

4. **Click in the 10:00 A.M. time slot.**

5. **Click the Break Entry shortcut button. The New Break Entry dialog box appears.**

6. **Enter *HIPAA Update Seminar* in the Name box.**

7. **Confirm that the date and time are correct.**

8. **Click the up arrow in the Length box and change the length of time to 120 minutes.**

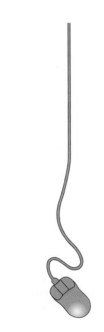

9. Select Seminar Break in the Resource box.

10. Press the Change button (to repeat the break for two additional days). The Repeat Change dialog box is displayed.

11. If it is not already selected, click the Daily button in the Frequency column.

12. Accept the default entry of 1 in the Every___Day(s) box, since the break occurs every day for a period of three days.

13. Key *12152010* in the End On box.

14. Click the OK button. You are returned to the New Break Entry dialog box.

15. Click the Save button to enter the break in Office Hours. Notice that the time slot from 10:00 A.M. to 12:00 P.M. on December 13, 2010, has been filled in on the calendar.

16. Change the calendar to December 14 and 15, 2010, to verify that the break has been entered correctly.

PREVIEWING AND PRINTING SCHEDULES

In most medical offices, providers' schedules are printed on a daily basis. To view a list of all appointments for a provider for a given day, click Appointment List from the Office Hours Reports menu. The report can be previewed on-screen or sent directly to the printer. If the preview option is selected, the appointment list is displayed in a preview window (see Figure 8-15 on page 174). Various buttons are used to view the schedule at different sizes, to move from page to page, to print the schedule, and to save the schedule as a file. Clicking the Close button closes the preview window.

The schedule can also be printed by clicking the Print Appointment List shortcut button, without using the Preview option. (Office Hours prints the schedule for the provider who is listed in the Provider box. To print the schedule of a different provider, change the entry in the Provider box before printing the schedule.)

Exercise 8-12

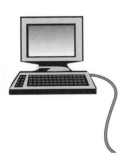

Print Dr. John Rudner's schedule for November 15, 2010.

1. Select Dr. John Rudner as the provider.

2. Go to Monday, November 15, 2010, on the calendar.

3. Click Appointment List on the Office Hours Reports menu. The Report Setup dialog box appears.

4. Under Print Selection, click the button that sends the report directly to the printer.

5. Click the Start button. The Data Selection box is displayed.

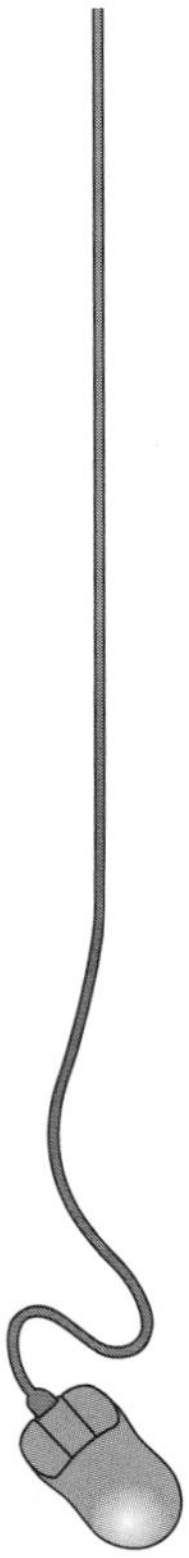

6. Enter *11152010* in both Dates boxes.

7. Select John Rudner in both Providers boxes.

8. Click the OK button. The Print dialog box appears.

9. Click OK to print the report.

10. Close Office Hours.

11. Create a backup of your work and exit NDCMedisoft by selecting Exit on the File menu. The Backup Reminder dialog box is displayed.

12. Click the Back Up Data Now button. The Backup dialog box appears.

13. Enter the file path and file name in the Destination File Path and Name box or click the Find button and browse to the desired location. The file name should be FCC8-8.mbk (the database name followed by the chapter number). The file path will vary depending on your computer and network setup. Ask your instructor for the file path.

14. Click the Start Backup button. NDCMedisoft creates a backup file. When it is complete, an Information box is displayed, indicating that the backup is complete. Click OK. The Backup dialog box closes and the program is shut down.

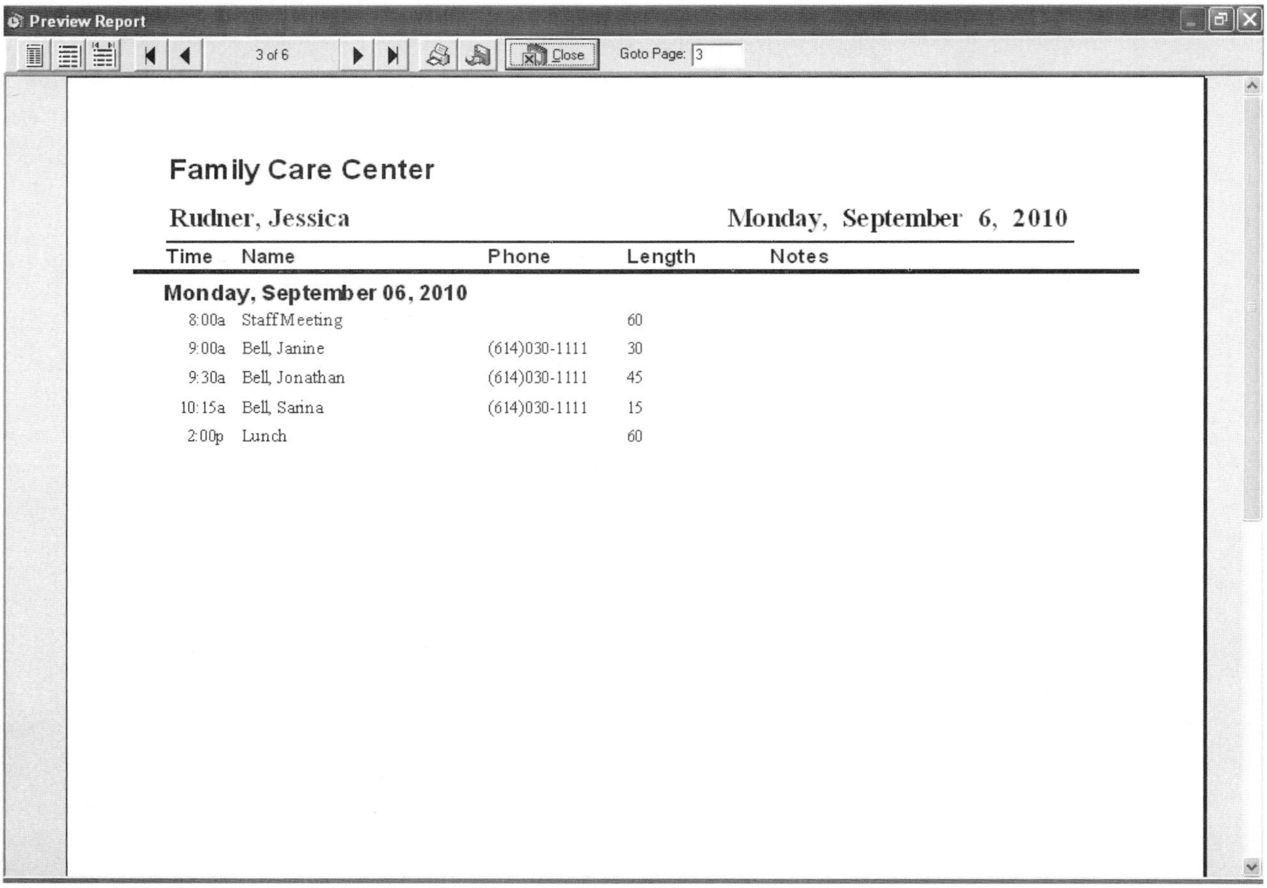

Preview Report   3 of 6   Close   Goto Page: 3

Family Care Center

Rudner, Jessica   Monday, September 6, 2010

Time	Name	Phone	Length	Notes
Monday, September 06, 2010				
8:00a	Staff Meeting		60	
9:00a	Bell, Janine	(614)030-1111	30	
9:30a	Bell, Jonathan	(614)030-1111	45	
10:15a	Bell, Sarina	(614)030-1111	15	
2:00p	Lunch		60	

Figure 8-15 **Preview Report Window with Appointment List Displayed**

CHAPTER REVIEW

USING TERMINOLOGY

Define the terms below as they apply to Office Hours.

1. Office Hours schedule

   _____

   _____

2. Office Hours break

   _____

   _____

CHECKING YOUR UNDERSTANDING

Answer the questions below in the space provided.

3. What are the different ways of starting Office Hours?

   _____

   _____

4. How do you display the schedule for a specific date?

   _____

   _____

5. If the Office Hours calendar shows October 6, how do you move to November 6?

   _____

   _____

6. How do you display the schedule for a specific provider?

   _____

   _____

7. How do you schedule a new appointment in Office Hours?

_____

_____

8. How is an appointment deleted?

_____

_____

9. How is an appointment moved from one time slot to another?

_____

_____

10. Suppose your office has set up Office Hours so that the default appointment length is fifteen minutes. If you need to make a one-hour appointment for a patient, in what box do you change 15 to 60?

_____

_____

APPLYING KNOWLEDGE

Answer the questions below in the space provided.

11. After you entered a personal break for Dr. Katherine Yan on February 24, she tells you that she gave you the wrong date. The break should be February 25. How do you correct the schedule?

_____

_____

_____

12. A patient calls to request an appointment on a specific day next week. You determine that the appointment is for a routine checkup, not an emergency. What steps should you follow to schedule the appointment?

_____

_____

_____

AT THE COMPUTER

Answer the following questions at the computer.

13. Today is Friday, September 3, 2010. Dr. Katherine Yan asks you to find out when Sarah Fitzwilliams is coming in for her next two appointments. Locate the appointments in Office Hours. (*Hint:* Use the Appointment List option on the Office Hours Lists menu, or click the Appointment List button on the Office Hours toolbar.)

14. Today is November 15, 2010. Samuel Bell needs to be scheduled as soon as possible for a thirty-minute appointment with Dr. John Rudner, between 10:00 A.M. and 12:00 P.M. When is the next available time slot that meets these requirements? How did you locate the open slot?

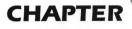

CHAPTER 9

Creating Claims and Statements

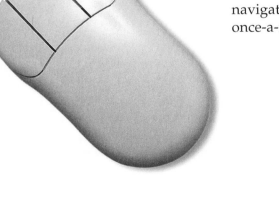

WHAT YOU NEED TO KNOW

To use this chapter, you need to know how to:
- ◆ Start NDCMedisoft, use menus, and enter and edit text.
- ◆ Work with chart numbers and codes.

OBJECTIVES

When you finish this chapter, you will be able to:
- ◆ Create electronic claims.
- ◆ Review claims for errors and omissions.
- ◆ Review an audit/edit report.
- ◆ Create statements.
- ◆ Edit statements.
- ◆ Print statements.

KEY TERMS

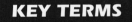

cycle billing
filter
navigator buttons
once-a-month billing

patient statement
remainder statements
standard statements

CREATING CLAIMS

Within the Claim Management area of NDCMedisoft, insurance claims are created, edited, and submitted for payment. Claims are created from transactions previously entered in NDCMedisoft. After claims are created, they can either be printed and mailed or transmitted electronically.

Figure 9-1 **Claim Management Shortcut Button**

The Claim Management dialog box is displayed by clicking Claim Management on the Activities menu or by clicking the Claim Management shortcut button on the toolbar (see Figure 9-1). The dialog box (see Figure 9-2) lists all claims that have already been created. In this dialog box, several actions can be performed: existing claims can be reviewed and edited, new claims can be created, the status of existing claims can be changed, and claims can be printed or submitted electronically.

navigator buttons buttons that simplify the task of moving from one entry to another.

First Previous Next Last Refresh
claim claim claim claim data

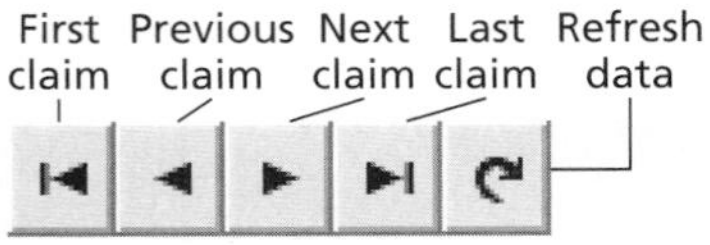

Figure 9-3 **Navigator Buttons**

The Claim Management dialog box contains five **navigator buttons** that simplify the task of moving from one entry to another (see Figure 9-3). The First Claim button selects the first claim in the list and makes it active. The Previous Claim button reactivates the claim that was most recently active. The Next Claim button makes the next claim in the list active. The Last Claim button makes the last claim in the list active. The Refresh Data button is used to restore data when necessary.

CREATE CLAIMS DIALOG BOX

filter a condition that data must meet to be included in the selection of data.

Claims are created in the Create Claims dialog box. This dialog box (see Figure 9-4) is accessed by clicking the Create Claims button in the Claim Management dialog box. It provides several filters to customize the creation of claims. A **filter** is a condition that data must meet to be included in the selection of data. For example, claims can be created for services performed between the first and the fifteenth of the month. If this were the case, the filter would be the condition that services must have been performed between the first and fifteenth of the month. Transactions that meet this criterion would be included in the selec-

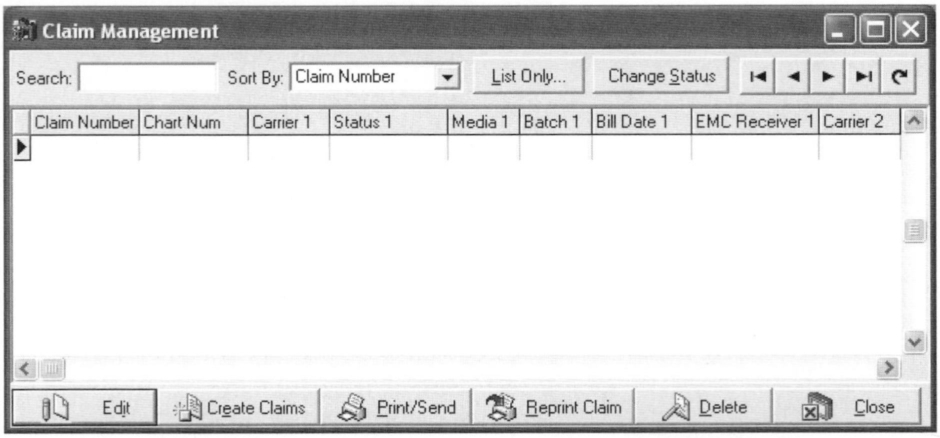

Figure 9-2 **Claim Management Dialog Box**

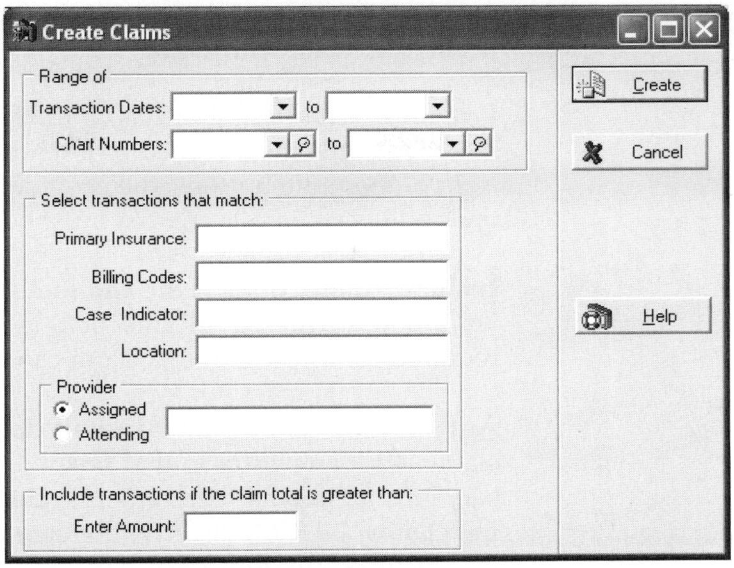

Figure 9-4 **Create Claims Dialog Box**

tion; transactions that do not fall within that date range would not be included. Filters can be used to create claims for a specific patient, for a specific insurance carrier, and for transactions that exceed a certain dollar amount, among others. The following filters can be applied within the Create Claims dialog box.

Range of   The options in this section of the dialog box provide filters for establishing the starting and ending dates as well as the starting and ending chart numbers for the claims that will be created.

Transaction Dates   The Transaction Dates boxes are used to specify the starting and ending dates for which claims will be created. If the boxes are left blank, transactions for all dates will be included.

Chart Numbers   In the Chart Numbers boxes, the starting and ending chart numbers for which claims will be created are entered. If the boxes are left blank, all chart numbers will be included.

Select Transactions That Match   The options in this section of the dialog box provide filters for matching the exact primary insurance carrier(s), billing code(s), case indicator(s), and location(s). In each case, when more than one item is entered, a comma must be placed between the entries.

Note: For the Primary Insurance filter, the carrier code for the insurance company is entered in the Primary Insurance box. If claims are being sent to a clearinghouse, more than one insurance carrier code can be entered. When more than one code is entered, a comma must be placed between the codes. If claims are being sent directly to the carrier, only that carrier's code is entered. For case indicators used to classify patients (such as by type of illness for workers' compensation cases), the case indicator can be listed in the Case Indicator box.

Provider   The radio buttons in the Provider box indicate whether the provider is the assigned or attending provider. In the box to the right of the radio buttons, the provider code is entered. If more than one code is entered, a comma must be placed between the codes.

Include Transactions if the Claim Total is Greater Than   The dollar amount entered in this box is the minimum total amount required for a case before a claim can be created.

Any box that is not filled in will default to include all data, and claims with any entry in that box will be included. When all necessary information has been entered, clicking the Create button creates the claims. NDCMedisoft will create a file of matching claims but will include only those that have not yet been billed.

Exercise 9-1

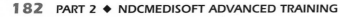

Create insurance claims for all patients who have transactions not already placed on a claim.

> Note: Steps 1 through 3 are required at the beginning of each chapter. These steps start NDCMedisoft, set the path to the correct data location, and restore the data saved at the end of the last work session.

Date: November 5, 2010

1. Hold down the F7 key and start NDCMedisoft. Enter the location of the NDCMedisoft data in the Find NDCMedisoft Directory box and click OK. (If you are unsure what to enter, ask your instructor.) When the Open practice dialog box appears, verify that Family Care Center is highlighted and click OK.

2. Restore the data from your last work session by selecting Restore Data on the File menu. When a Warning box appears, click OK. Enter the file path and file name in the File Destination Path and Name or click the Find button and browse to the disired location. The file name should be FCC8-8.mbk (the database name followed by the chapter number that you last worked on). The file path will vary depending on your computer and network setup. Ask your instructor for the file path.

3. Click the Start Restore button. When a Confirm dialog box appears, click OK. NDCMedisoft restores the data. When it is complete, an Information box is displayed, indicating that the restore is complete. Click OK. The Restore box closes and the main NDCMedisoft window is displayed.

4. Set the NDCMedisoft Program Date to November 5, 2010.

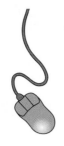

5. On the Activities menu, click Claim Management. The Claim Management dialog box is displayed.

6. Click the Create Claims button.

7. Leave all boxes in the Create Claims dialog box blank to select all transactions.

8. Click the Create button.

9. Use the scroll bars to view the claims just created.

10. Click the Close button.

CLAIM SELECTION

At times it is necessary to select and view specific claims that have already been created. For example, any claims prepared for submission to an insurance carrier must be selected and then reviewed for completeness and accuracy. In addition, all claims that have been rejected by insurance carriers are selected and reviewed before resubmission.

NDCMedisoft's List Only feature is used when it is necessary to list claims that match certain criteria. Filters are applied in the List Only Claims That Match dialog box. They can be used to view claims selectively, such as claims for a specific insurance carrier and claims created on a certain date. Unlike the filters in the Create Claims dialog box, those in the List Only Claims That Match dialog box do not create claims; they simply list existing claims that meet the specified criteria.

Once the filters have been applied, only those claims that match the criteria are listed at the bottom of the main Claim Management dialog box. Claims can be sorted by chart number, date the claim was created, insurance carrier, electronic claim (EDI) receiver, billing method, billing date, batch number, and claim status. Not all the boxes need to be filled in, only the ones that will be used to select the desired claims.

The List Only feature is activated by clicking the List Only . . . button in the Claim Management dialog box. This causes the List Only Claims That Match dialog box to be displayed (see Figure 9-5 on page 184).

The following filters are available in the List Only Claims That Match dialog box.

Chart Number   A patient's chart number is selected from the drop-down list of patients' chart numbers.

Claim Created   The date that a claim was created is entered in MMDDCCYY format.

Select Claims for Only   A radio button is clicked for either all insurance carriers, primary insurance carrier only, secondary insurance carrier only, or tertiary insurance carrier only. When a patient has insurance coverage with more than one carrier, the primary carrier is

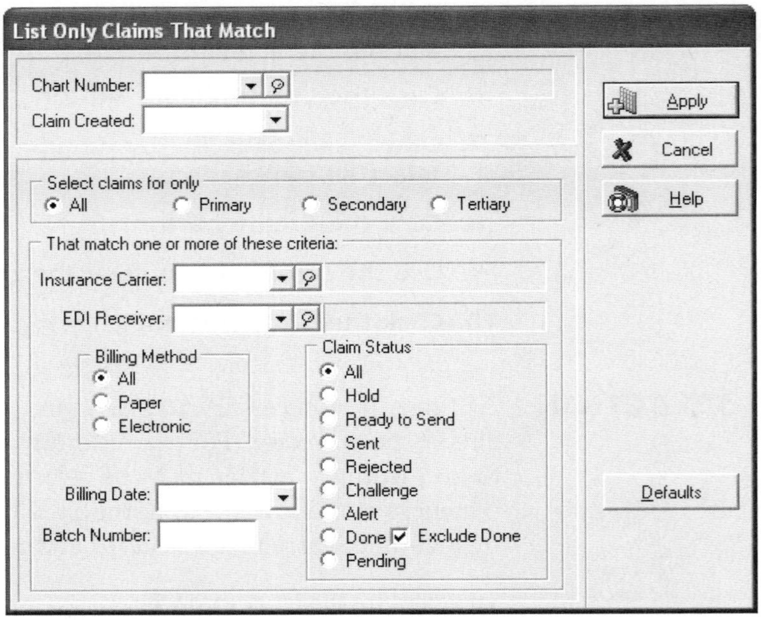

Figure 9-5 **List Only Claims That Match Dialog Box**

billed first, and then, if appropriate, the second and third (tertiary) carriers are billed.

Insurance Carrier An insurance carrier is selected from the drop-down list of choices.

EDI Receiver An EDI receiver is selected from the choices on the drop-down list.

Billing Method In the Billing Method box, the radio button for All, Paper, or Electronic is clicked.

Billing Date The date of billing is entered in the Billing Date box.

Batch Number A batch number is entered in the Batch Number box.

Claim Status A claim status is selected from the list of radio buttons provided. If claims that have been billed and accepted (not rejected) are to be excluded from the search, the Exclude Done box is clicked. This causes a check mark to be displayed beside the option.

When the desired boxes have been filled in, clicking the Apply button applies the selected filters to the claims data. The Claim Management dialog box is displayed, listing only those claims that match the criteria selected in the List Only Claims That Match dialog box. From the Claim Management dialog box, the claims can now be edited, printed, and mailed or transmitted electronically.

To restore the List Only Claims That Match dialog box to its original settings (that is, to remove the filters selected), this dialog box is reopened, the Defaults button is clicked, and then the Apply button is clicked. All the boxes in the dialog box will become blank, and the full list of claims is displayed again in the Claim Management dialog box.

EDITING CLAIMS

NDCMedisoft's Claim Edit feature allows claims to be reviewed and verified on screen before they are submitted to insurance carriers for payment. With careful checking, problems can be solved before claims are sent to insurance carriers. When a claim is active in the Claim Management dialog box, it can be edited by clicking the Edit button or by double-clicking the claim itself. The Claim dialog box is displayed (see Figure 9-6). The top section of the Claim dialog box lists the claim number, the date the claim was created, the chart number, the patient's name, and the case number. This information cannot be edited, although the information in the five tabs can be edited.

CARRIER 1 TAB The Carrier 1 tab displays information about claims being submitted to a patient's primary insurance carrier.

The following boxes are listed in the Carrier 1 tab:

Claim Status   The Claim Status box indicates the status of a particular claim: Hold, Ready to send, Sent, Rejected, Challenge, Alert, Done, and Pending. The radio button that reflects a claim's status should be clicked.

Billing Method   The Billing Method box displays two choices: Paper or Electronic. The radio button that describes the billing method should be clicked.

Initial Billing Date   If the bill was sent more than once, this box automatically displays the initial billing date.

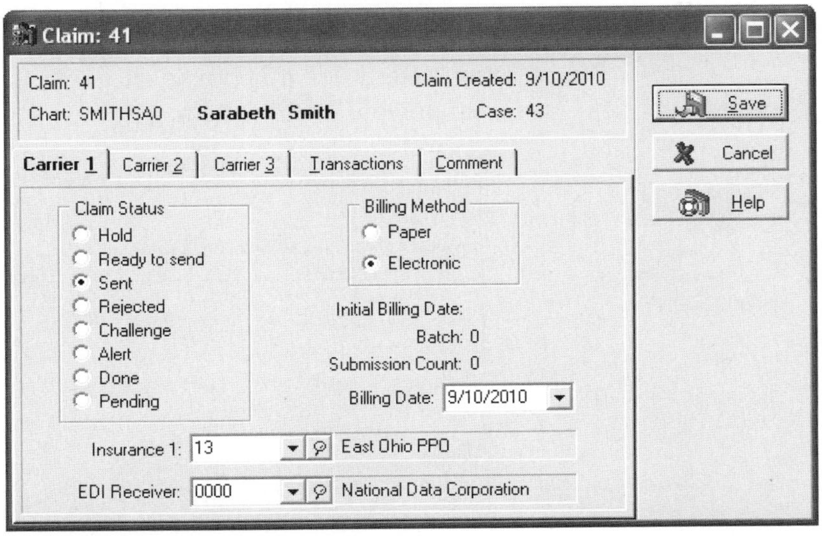

Figure 9-6 **Claim Dialog Box**

Batch   If the claim has been assigned to a batch, the batch number is displayed.

Submission Count   The Submission Count area lists the number of claims submitted.

Billing Date   The Billing Date box lists the date the bill was sent.

Insurance 1   The Insurance 1 box lists a patient's primary insurance carrier.

EDI Receiver   The EDI receiver is selected from the drop-down list.

CARRIER 2 AND CARRIER 3 TABS

The Carrier 2 and Carrier 3 tabs display information about claims being submitted to a patient's secondary (Carrier 2) and tertiary (Carrier 3) insurance carriers. The boxes in these tabs are the same as the boxes in the Carrier 1 tab, with the exception of the Claim Status box. In the Carrier 2 and Carrier 3 tabs, there is no Pending radio button in the Claim Status box. Otherwise the three tabs are the same.

TRANSACTIONS TAB

The Transactions tab lists information about the transactions included in a claim. The scroll bars can be used to view all the information in the Transactions tab (see Figure 9-7).

Diagnosis   The diagnosis for the listed transactions is displayed.

Date From   The Date From box lists the date on which service was provided.

Document   The Document box lists the document number of a transaction.

Procedure   The Procedure box displays the procedure code for a procedure performed.

Amount   In the Amount box, the dollar cost of a service is displayed.

Ins 1 Resp   If this box is checked, the primary insurance carrier is responsible for the claim.

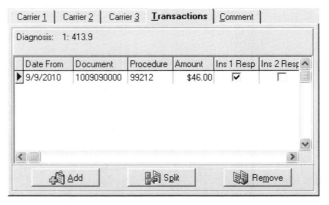

Figure 9-7 **Transactions Tab**

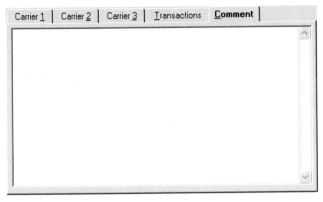

Figure 9-8 **Comment Tab**

Ins 2 Resp If this box is checked, the secondary insurance carrier is responsible for the claim.

Ins 3 Resp If this box is checked, the tertiary insurance carrier is responsible for the claim.

The Transactions tab also contains three buttons at the bottom of the dialog box: Add, Split, and Remove. The Add button is used to add a transaction to an existing claim. The Split button removes a single transaction from an existing claim and places it on a new claim. The Remove button deletes a transaction from the database.

COMMENT TAB The Comment tab provides a place to include any specific notes or comments about the claim (see Figure 9-8).

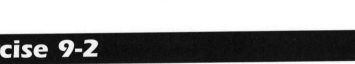

Review insurance claims for patients with East Ohio PPO as their insurance carrier.

Date: November 5, 2010

1. Open the Claim Management dialog box.

2. Click the List Only . . . button.

3. Click 13 East Ohio PPO on the drop-down list in the Insurance Carrier box.

4. Click the Apply button. You are returned to the Claim Management dialog box. Notice that only claims for patients who have East Ohio PPO as their insurance carrier are listed.

5. Click on the claim for Lawana Brooks (chart number BROOKLA∅).

6. Click the Edit button to review the claim. The Claim dialog box is displayed.

7. Review the information in the Carrier 1 tab.

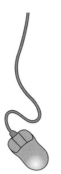

8. Review the information in the Transactions tab.

9. Click the Cancel button to exit the Claim dialog box without saving any changes. (The Cancel button does not cancel the claim; it just cancels any changes that may have been made.)

10. To restore the full list of claims in the Claim Management box, click the List Only . . . button and then click the Defaults button.

11. Click the Apply button.

12. Close the Claim Management dialog box.

ELECTRONIC CLAIMS

Before the implementaion of the HIPAA Transaction and Code Sets Standards in October of 2003, physician practices used many different electonic data interchange (EDI) systems to submit electronic claims. The HIPAA standards describe a particular electronic format that providers and payers must use to send and receive health care transactions. They also establish standard medical code sets, such as ICD and CPT-4, for use in health care transactions. Most of the setup requirements for creating and transmitting electronic claims are handled by the medical office's systems manager.

STEPS IN SUBMITTING ELECTRONIC CLAIMS

Because schools are not set up to transmit electronic claims, you will not be able to actually practice sending a claim electronically. However, here are the steps you would follow to send claims to a clearinghouse in an office setting.

1. Click Claim Management on the Activities menu. The Claim Management dialog box is displayed.

2. Click the Print/Send button.

3. The Print/Send Claims dialog box appears (see Figure 9-9). Click the Electronic button to change the billing method to electronic, if it is not already selected. Leave the Electronic Claim Receiver box set to NDC, which stands for National Data Corporation. Click the OK button.

Figure 9-9 **Print/Send Claims Dialog Box Set Up for Electronic Claims**

4. The Send Electronic Claims dialog box is displayed, with National Data Corporation displayed as the receiver (see Figure 9-10). Click the Send Claims Now button.

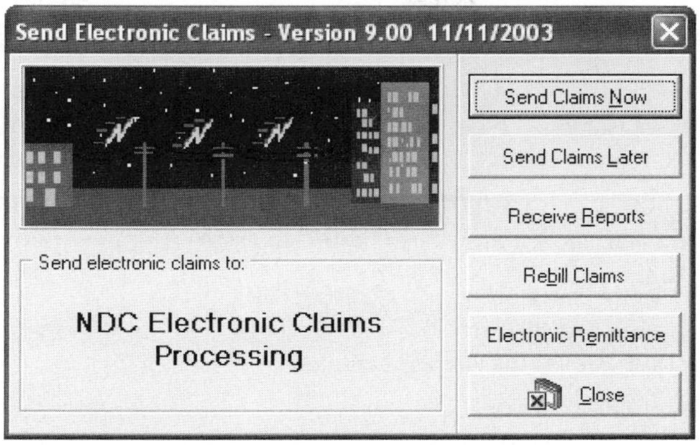

Figure 9-10 **Send Electronic Claims Dialog Box**

5. The Data Selection Questions dialog box appears. The various range boxes provide options for filtering the claims. Once these selections are made, click the OK button.

6. An Information dialog box appears, asking whether to display a Verification report. After clicking Yes, the Preview Report window appears with a copy of an EMC Verification report displayed (see Figure 9-11 on page 190). The report displays the details of each claim in the batch. Click the Close button when finished viewing the report. The Preview Report window closes, and an Information dialog box appears, asking you if you want to continue with the transmission.

7. If you were in a medical office, you would click the Yes button and the claim would be sent via cable lines, telephone lines, or satellite from your computer to a computer at the clearinghouse. However, because you are in a school setting and are not actually set up to submit electronic claims at this time, click the No button.

8. Click the Close button to close the Claim Management dialog box and return to the main NDCMedisoft window.

CHANGING THE STATUS OF CLAIMS

If claims were transmitted electronically, the Claim Status for each claim would automatically change from Ready to Send to Sent once the claims were sent. Since it is not possible to actually send electronic claims during these exercises, you will change the Claim Status manually from Ready to Send to Sent for the claims created earlier, as though the claims had actually been sent electronically.

Family Care Center
EMC Verification
EMC Batch Verification Report

Filename: c:\medidata\FCC8\EMC\ndcreq.dat
Chart Number Range: ALL
Date Created Range: ALL

Billing Code Range: ALL
Provider: ALL
Insurance Carrier Range: ALL

Claim#	Chart#	Patient Name	Policy#	Group#	Referring Provider	Facility
		Date From Proc. Code Modifiers Pos Tos		Units	Diagnoses	Amount

Provider: Katherine Yan (1)

49	JONESEL0 Elizabeth Jones	931001111B		Davis Marion	Not Found

Primary Carrier: Medicare (1)
Diagnoses: 1: 382.09 unspecified otitis media

| 10/28/2010 | 99212 | 11 | 1 | Diagnosis: 1 | $28.00 |

Claim 49 Total: $28.00

| 50 | JONESEL0 Elizabeth Jones | 931001111B | | Davis Marion | Not Found |

Primary Carrier: Medicare (1)
Diagnoses: 1: 427.9 Arrhythmia

| 11/05/2010 | 99214 | 11 | 1 | Diagnosis: 1 | $59.00 |
| 11/05/2010 | 93000 | 11 | 1 | Diagnosis: 1 | $29.00 |

Claim 50 Total: $88.00

Provider Katherine Yan (1) Total: $116.00

Provider: Patricia McGrath (4)

| 45 | BATTIAN0 Anthony Battistuta | 239550855 | | Davis Marion | Not Found |

Primary Carrier: Medicare (1)
Diagnoses: 1: 250.00 Diabetes mellitus

| 10/28/2010 | 99212 | 11 | 1 | Diagnosis: 1 | $28.00 |
| 10/28/2010 | 82947 | 11 | 1 | Diagnosis: 1 | $25.00 |

Claim 45 Total: $53.00

| 46 | BROOKLA0Lawana Brooks | 35068 | jd4800 | Davis Marion | Not Found |

Primary Carrier: East Ohio PPO (13)
Diagnoses: 1: 845.00 Ankle sprain

| 10/29/2010 | 99212 | 11 | 1 | Diagnosis: 1 | $46.00 |
| 10/29/2010 | 73600 | 11 | 1 | Diagnosis: 1 | $80.00 |

Claim 46 Total: $126.00

Figure 9-11 Sample Page from an Electronic Claims Verification Report

Exercise 9-3

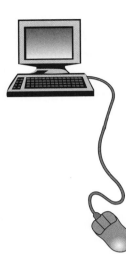

Change the Claim Status for the claims created on November 5, 2010, from Ready to Send to Sent.

Date: November 5, 2010

1. In the Claim Management dialog box, click the Change Status button. The Change Claim Status/Billing Method dialog box appears.

2. Click Batch and accept the default entry of 0.

3. Select Ready to Send in the Status From column.

4. Select Sent in the Status To column.

5. Click the OK button. The dialog box closes and the Claim Management dialog box reappears with the Claim Status column displaying Sent.

SENDING ELECTRONIC CLAIM ATTACHMENTS

When sending a claim electronically, an attachment that needs to accompany the claim, such as radiology films, must be referred to in the claim. In NDCMedisoft, the EDI Report area within the Diagnosis tab of the Case dialog box is used to indicate to the payer when an attachment will accompany the claim, and how the attachment will be transmitted (see Figure 9-12).

Figure 9-12 **Diagnosis Tab with EDI Report Fields**

The EDI Report section contains three boxes:

◆ Report Type Code box—This entry indicates the type of report that is to be attached (for example, a diagnostic report);

◆ Report Transmission Code—This indicates the means by which the report will be transmitted to the payer (for example, via mail, email, fax);

◆ Attachment Control Number—This box contains the attachment's reference number (up to seven digits, assigned by the practice).

Refer to the NDCMedisoft Help feature for a list of possible codes for the Report Type and Report Transmission boxes.

REVIEWING THE AUDIT/EDIT REPORT

When claims are transmitted to a clearinghouse, an audit/edit report is received immediately after claims are sent (see Figure 9-13). Options for viewing and printing the report are listed on-screen when the report is received. It is important to print a copy of the report, since some systems do not permit reports to be viewed online at a later time.

The audit/edit report marks each claim as accepted or rejected. Each claim is displayed on a separate line of the report. The Message column queries whether a claim will be sent to an insurance carrier. If a claim cannot be sent, the error is listed in the Message column. In the Flag column of the report, a "P" indicates that the claim will be sent on paper; an "R" indicates that the claim was rejected. A blank Flag column means that the claim has passed the audits and will be sent electronically. The report should be reviewed carefully. Any errors found by a clearinghouse must be corrected before a claim can be sent to an insurance carrier.

Exercise 9-4

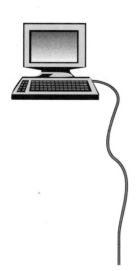

An audit/edit report has come back from the clearinghouse. A claim for James Smith has been rejected for submission to Blue Cross/Blue Shield. There are two reasons listed for rejection: "Missing Insured's ID no." and "Missing Insured's Group no." Locate the problem in NDCMedisoft, correct it, and prepare the claim for resubmission.

Date: November 5, 2010

1. Go to the Policy 1 tab in the Case dialog box to check whether Mr. Smith's insurance policy number and group number have been entered.

2. Notice that these boxes are blank. Someone forgot to enter data in them when creating the case for Mr. Smith.

3. Key *354691* in the Policy Number box.

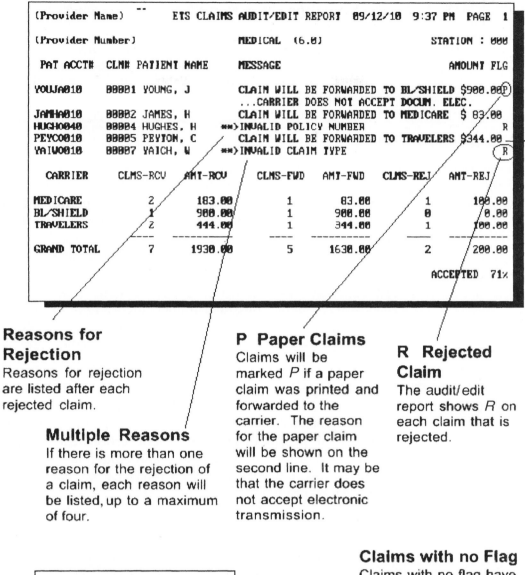

```
(Provider Name)  --        ETS CLAIMS AUDIT/EDIT REPORT  89/12/18  9:37 PM  PAGE  1

(Provider Number)          MEDICAL  (6.8)                    STATION : 888

  PAT ACCT#  CLM# PATIENT NAME    MESSAGE                      AMOUNT FLG

  YOUJA818   88881 YOUNG, J       CLAIM WILL BE FORWARDED TO BL/SHIELD $988.88 P
                                  ...CARRIER DOES NOT ACCEPT DOCUM. ELEC.
  JAMHA818   88882 JAMES, H       CLAIM WILL BE FORWARDED TO MEDICARE  $ 83.88
  HUGHO848   88884 HUGHES, H    **>INVALID POLICY NUMBER                      R
  PEYCO818   88885 PEYTON, C      CLAIM WILL BE FORWARDED TO TRAVELERS $344.88
  YAIVO818   88887 YAICH, W     **>INVALID CLAIM TYPE                        R

   CARRIER     CLMS-RCV   AMT-RCV    CLMS-FWD   AMT-FWD   CLMS-REJ   AMT-REJ

  MEDICARE        2        183.88       1        83.88        1       188.88
  BL/SHIELD       1        988.88       1       988.88        8         8.88
  TRAVELERS       2        444.88       1       344.88        1       188.88
                         ----------            ----------            ----------
  GRAND TOTAL     7       1938.88       5      1638.88        2       288.88

                                                            ACCEPTED  71%
```

Reasons for Rejection

Reasons for rejection are listed after each rejected claim.

Multiple Reasons

If there is more than one reason for the rejection of a claim, each reason will be listed, up to a maximum of four.

P Paper Claims

Claims will be marked *P* if a paper claim was printed and forwarded to the carrier. The reason for the paper claim will be shown on the second line. It may be that the carrier does not accept electronic transmission.

R Rejected Claim

The audit/edit report shows *R* on each claim that is rejected.

Claims with no Flag

Claims with no flag have passed the audits and will be forwarded electronically to the appropriate carrier.

T Test Claims Flag

Used during setup when testing claims with a carrier. Data will not be forwarded to the carrier.

Figure 9-13 Audit/Edit Report

4. Key *U339* in the Group Number box.

5. Click the Save button.

6. Close the Patient List dialog box.

7. In the Claim Management dialog box, double-click the claim for James Smith.

8. **Change the Claim Status from Sent to Ready to Send. Click the Save button.**

9. **Close the Claim Management dialog box. (Once again, because schools are not set up to transmit electronic media claims, this exercise ends without actually transmitting the claim.)**

CREATING STATEMENTS

patient statement *a list of the amount of money a patient owes.*

A **patient statement** lists the amount of money a patient owes, organized by the amount of time the money has been owed, the procedures performed, and the dates the procedures were performed. In earlier versions of NDCMedisoft, statements were created from the Reports menu. Beginning with Version 9, statements are created using the new Statement Management feature, which is listed on the Activities menu.

Just as Claim Management provides a range of options for billing insurance carriers, Statement Management offers multiple choices for billing patients. Within the Statement Management area of NDCMedisoft, statements are created and printed.

STATEMENT MANAGEMENT DIALOG BOX

The Statement Management dialog box is displayed by clicking Statement Management on the Activities menu or by clicking the Statement Management shortcut button on the toolbar (see Figure 9-14). The dialog box lists all statements that have already been created (see Figure 9-15). In this dialog box, several actions can be performed: existing statements can be reviewed and edited, new statements can be created, the status of existing statements can be changed, and statements can be printed.

Figure 9-14 Statement Management Shortcut Button

	Stmt #	Guarantor	Phone	Status	Initial Billing	Batch	Media	Type
	10	KLEINRA0	(614)022-2693	Ready to Send		0		Standard
	11	PATELRA0	(614)099-3624	Ready to Send		0		Standard
	12	PATTELE0	(614)666-0099	Ready to Send		0		Standard
	13	SIMMOJI0	(614)011-6767	Ready to Send		0		Standard
	14	SMITHJA0	(614)879-2222	Ready to Send		0		Standard
	15	SMITHSA0	(614)822-0000	Ready to Send		0		Standard
	16	SYZMAMI0	(614)086-4444	Ready to Send		0		Standard
	17	WONGJO10	(614)029-7777	Ready to Send		0		Standard
	18	WONGLIY0	(614)029-7777	Ready to Send		0		Standard

Search: _____ Sort By: Batch Number | List Only... | Change Status

Edit | Create Statements | Print/Send | Rebill Statement | Delete | Close

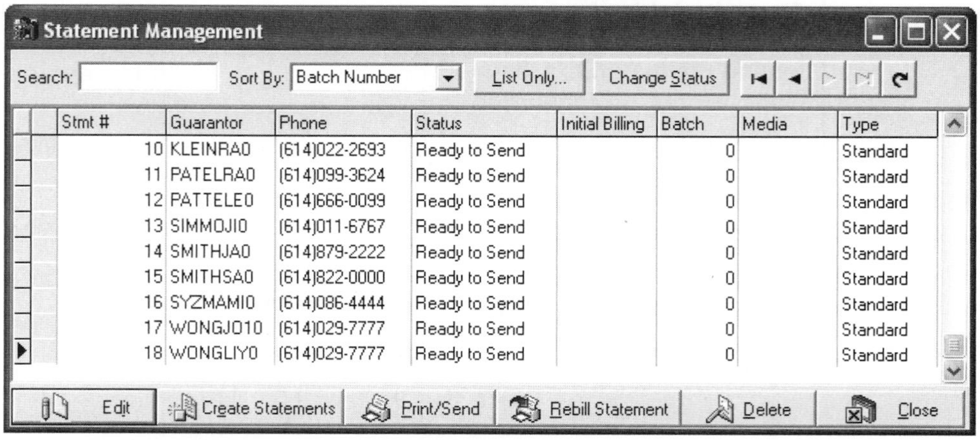

Figure 9-15 Statement Management Dialog Box

The following columns are listed in the Statement Management dialog box:

Stmt # The Stmt # column lists the statement number, which is generated by the program in sequential order

Guarantor In the Statement Management dialog box, guarantors rather than patients are listed, since statements are created only for those financially responsible for an account—the guarantor. For example, if a patient's father is the guarantor, a statement is created for the patient's father, not the patient. In the Statement Management dialog box, the statement is listed under the father's chart number. If the father is also guarantor on his wife's account, his chart number will appear twice in the Statement Management window. When statements are printed, however, all transactions for the guarantor's son and wife are billed on one statement.

Phone The Phone column lists the guarantors' phone numbers.

Status The status assigned to each statement depends on whether the statement has been billed, and on whether the account has a zero balance:

◆ Ready to Send—Transactions that have not been billed

◆ Sent—Transactions that have been billed but not fully paid

◆ Done—Transactions that have been billed and fully paid

Initial Billing The date the statement was initially sent appears in the Initial Billing column.

Batch The batch number assigned by NDCMedisoft is displayed.

Media The media format for the statement, either paper or electronic, is designated.

Type The type of statement, either Standard or Remainder, is listed.

CREATE STATEMENTS DIALOG BOX The Create Statements dialog box is where the information is entered that determines which statements are generated (see Figure 9-16 on page 196).

The following filters can be applied in the Create Statements dialog box:

Transaction Dates A range of dates is entered to select transactions that occur within those dates. The dates can be entered directly by keying in the boxes, or they can be selected from the calendar that is displayed

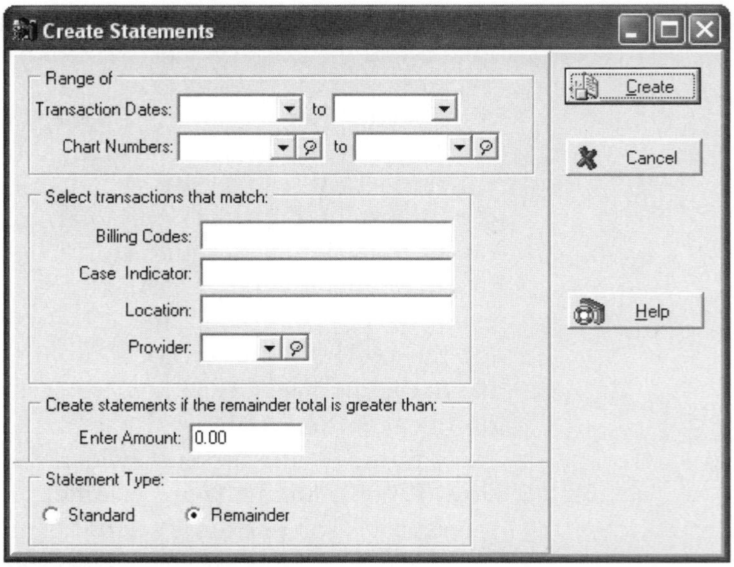

Figure 9-16 **Create Statements Dialog Box**

when the drop-down arrow is clicked. To create statements for all available transactions, leave both Transaction Dates boxes blank.

Chart Numbers In the Chart Numbers boxes, the starting and ending chart numbers for which statements will be created are entered. If the boxes are left blank, all chart numbers will be included.

Select Transactions That Match The options in this portion of the dialog box provide filters for creating statements for billing code(s), case indicator(s), location(s), and provider. In all instances, a comma must be placed between entries if more than one code is entered.

Create Statements if the Remainder Total Is Greater Than . . . Enter Amount The dollar amount entered in the Enter Amount field in this box is the minimum outstanding balance required for a statement to be created. For example, if 5.00 is entered in this field, the program would not create statements for accounts with a balance below 5.00. If this field is left blank, statements will be created for all accounts, regardless of the balance.

Statement Type The Statement Type box contains two options. **Standard statements** show all available charges regardless of whether the insurance has paid on the transactions. **Remainder statements** list only those charges that are not paid in full after all insurance carrier payments have been received. Once a statement type is selected, the setting remains in effect until a different type is selected.

After all selections are complete in the Create Statements dialog box, clicking the Create button instructs the program to generate state-

standard statements statement that list all available charges regardless of whether the insurance has paid on the transactions.

remainder statements statements that only list those charges that are not paid in full after all insurance carrier payments have been received.

ments. (*Note:* If you click the Create button and no statements can be created, the following message appears: "No new statements were created." Click OK to close the dialog box that contains the message.)

Exercise 9-5

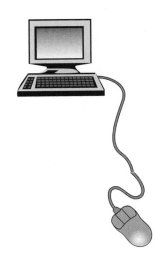

Create remainder statements for all patients with last names beginning with the letter "S" through the end of the alphabet. Date: September 30, 2010

1. Select Statement Management on the Activities menu.

2. Click the Create Statements button. The Create Statements dialog box is displayed.

3. Enter "S" in the first Chart Numbers box and WONGLI0 in the second.

4. Click the Create button.

5. An Information box appears, stating the number of statements that have been created. Click the OK button. The statements are listed in the Statement Management dialog box.

EDITING STATEMENTS

Statements can be edited by clicking the Edit button in the Statement Management dialog box. When the Edit button in the Statement Management dialog box is clicked, the statement dialog box is displayed (see Figure 9-17). The three tabs in the Statement dialog box contain important information about the statement.

Figure 9-17 The Statement Dialog Box

GENERAL TAB   The following information is located in the General tab:

Status The button in the Status box indicates the current status of the statement.

Billing Method The billing method can be either paper or electronic.

Type The Type field indicates whether the statement is a standard statement or a remainder statement.

Initial Billing Date This field lists the date the statement was first created.

Batch The batch number is assigned by the program.

Submission Count This field displays the number of times the statement has been sent to the guarantor. This information can be used when trying to collect on overdue accounts.

Billing Date If a statement has been sent more than once, the most recent date is shown in the Billing Date field located in the General Tab of the Edit Statement dialog box.

TRANSACTIONS TAB   The Transactions tab lists the transactions placed on the statement (see Figure 9-18). The buttons at the bottom of the tab are used to add, split, or remove transactions from the statement.

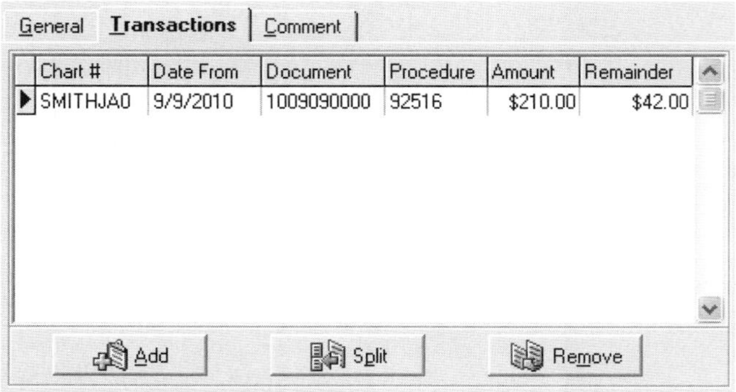

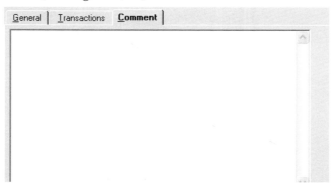

Figure 9-18 **Transactions Tab**

COMMENT TAB   The Comment tab provides a place to include notes about the statement (see Figure 9-19).

Figure 9-19 **Comment Tab**

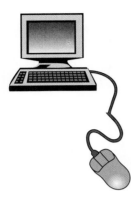

Exercise 9-6

Review one of the statements created in the Exercise 9-5.
Date: September 30, 2010

1. **Select a statement in the Statement Management dialog box by clicking on it.**

2. **Click the Edit button.**

3. **Review the information in the General tab.**

4. **Click on the Transactions tab to see the transactions that are on the statement.**

5. **Click the Cancel button to close the Statement dialog box.**

PRINTING STATEMENTS

Once statements have been created, the next step is to print the statements to a printer or to send them electronically. When the Print/Send button is clicked, the Print/Send Statements dialog box is displayed (see Figure 9-20). This dialog box is used to choose the type of statement that will be created—Paper or Electronic. Paper statements are printed and mailed by the practice. Electronic statements are sent electronically to a processing center where statements are printed and mailed. If the electronic format is indicated, the statement format is selected from a drop-down list in the Electronic Statement type box.

Figure 9-20 **Print/Send Statements Dialog Box**

The Exclude Billed Paid Entries box designates whether transactions that have been billed and paid are left out of the statement processing.

Once these selections are made, the OK button is clicked and the Open Report dialog box appears (see Figure 9-21 on page 200).

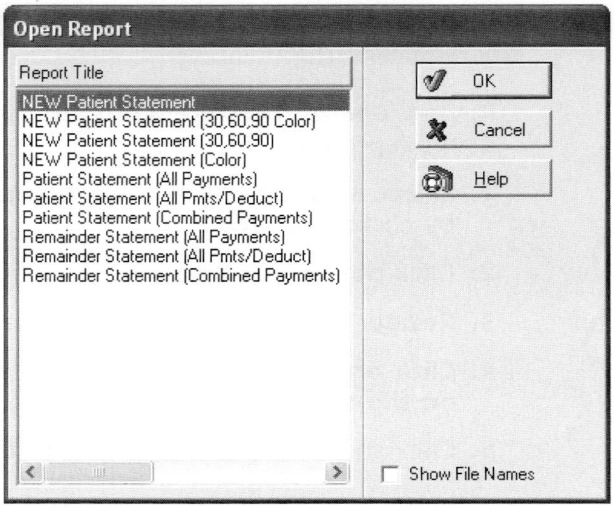

Figure 9-21 **Open Report dialog box**

SELECTING A REPORT FORMAT

The report selected in the Open Report dialog box must match the type of statement selected in the Statement Type field of the Create Statements dialog box—either Standard or Remainder. If Remainder was checked, statements will print only if one of the three Remainder Statement report formats is selected in the Open Report window:

◆ Remainder Statement (All Payments)

◆ Remainder Statement (All Pmts/Deduct)

◆ Remainder Statement (Combined Payments)

Likewise, for Standard statements to print, one of the seven other report formats must be chosen:

◆ NEW Patient Statement

◆ NEW Patient Statement (30,60,90 Color)

◆ NEW Patient Statement (30,60,90)

◆ NEW Patient Statement (Color)

◆ Patient Statement (All Payments)

◆ Patient Statement (All Pmts/Deduct)

◆ Patient Statement (Combined Payments)

After the report format is selected, click the OK button to display the Print Report Where? dialog box, which asks whether to preview the report on screen, send the report directly to the printer, or export the report to a file (see Figure 9-22).

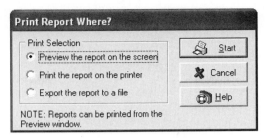

Figure 9-22 **Print Report Where? Dialog Box**

Once the Start button is clicked, the Data Selection Questions dialog box for the selected format appears (see Figure 9-23).

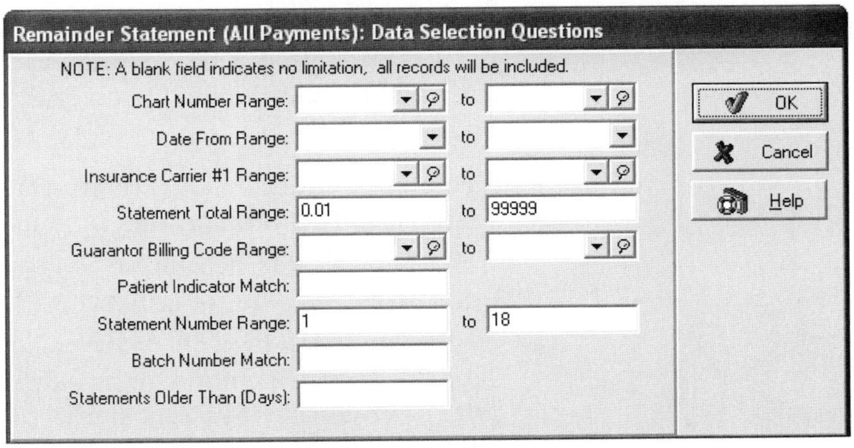

Figure 9-23 **Data Selection Questions Dialog Box**

SELECTING THE STATEMENT FILTERS AND PRINTING THE REPORT

once-a-month-billing A type of billing in which statements are mailed to all patients at the same time each month.

cycle billing A type of billing in which patients are divided into groups and statements are mailed on a staggered schedule throughout the month.

The fields in the Data Selection Questions dialog box are used to filter statement selections. For example, to print statements for a certain group of patients, entries are made in the Chart Number Range field. Many practices use cycle billing rather than **once-a-month billing,** in which all statements are printed and mailed at once. In a **cycle billing** system, patients are divided into groups and statement printing and mailing is staggered throughout the month. For example, statements for guarantors whose last names begin with the letters "A" to "F" are mailed on the first of the month, those with last names that begin with "G to "L" are mailed on the eighth of the month, and so on.

In addition to the Chart Number Range filter, other available filters include:

Date From Range—A range of dates is entered to print statements within a certain time frame.

Insurance Carrier #1 Range—A range of insurance carriers to be included is entered in the Insurance Carrier #1 Range boxes.

Statement Total Range—The Statement Total Range boxes are used to filter statements for guarantors with a balance within a specified range.

Guarantor Billing Code Range—The Guarantor Billing Code Range boxes are used to select statements for a range of guarantors assigned Billing Codes (from the Other Information tab in the Patient/Guarantor dialog box).

Patient Indicator Match—To print statements for patients assigned a particular patient indicator (from the Other Information tab in the Patient/Guarantor dialog box), an entry is made in the Patient Indicator Match box.

Statement Number Range—The Statement Number Range boxes are used to print a range of statements. Statement numbers (assigned by NDCMedisoft).

Batch Number Match—To print statements in a particular batch (assigned by NDCMedisoft), an entry is made in the Batch Number Match box.

Statements Older Than (Days)—statements that are older than a specified date can be printed by entering a date in the Statements Older Than (Days) box.

If no changes are made to the default entries in the Data Selection Questions dialog box, all statements that have a status of Ready to Send or Sent are included in the batch. If a practice does not want to print statements with a Sent status, a 0 (zero) is entered in the Batch Number Match field in the Data Selection Questions dialog box. All statements that are Ready to Send have a batch number of 0.

Once all selections are complete, clicking the Print/Send button sends the statements to a printer, to an electronic statement processor, or to a file. Figure 9-24 displays a sample patient remainder statement. (*Note:* If the Preview Report on the Screen option was selected in the Print Report Where? dialog box, the statements will be displayed in the Preview Report window, where they can also be printed.)

Exercise 9-7

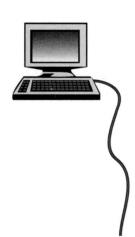

Print remainder statements for all patients with last names beginning with the letter "S" through the end of the alphabet.

Date: September 30, 2010

1. Click the Print/Send button in the Statement Management dialog box. The Print/Send Statements dialog box is displayed.

2. Select Paper as the statement method. Verify that the Exclude Billed Paid Entries box is checked. Click the OK button.

3. In the Open Report dialog box that appears, select Remainder Statement (All Payments). Click the OK button.

Family Care Center

285 Stephenson Boulevard

Stephenson, OH 60089

(614)555-0000

Statement Date	Chart Number	Page
09/30/2010	SMITHJA0	1

James L. Smith

17 Blacks Lane

Stephenson, OH 60089

Make Checks Payable To:
Family Care Center 285 Stephenson Boulevard Stephenson, OH 60089 (614)555-0000

Date of Last Payment: 9/10/2010	Amount: -168.00	Previous Balance:	0.00

Patient:	James L. Smith	Chart Number: SMITHJA0	Case:	Facial nerve paralysis

Dates	Procedure	Charge	Paid by Primary		Paid By Guarantor	Adjustments	Remainder
09/09/10	92516	210.00	-168.00			0.00	42.00

Amount Due
42.00

Figure 9-24 **Sample Patient Remainder Statement**

4. In the Print Report Where? dialog box, choose the option to preview the report on the screen. Click the Start button. The Data Selection Questions dialog box is displayed.

5. In the Chart Number Range boxes, enter the chart numbers that will select all patients with last names beginning with "S" through the end of the alphabet. Click the OK button.

6. Browse the statements in the Preview Report window. Click the Close button.

7. Notice that the status of the statements is still listed as Ready to Send. NDCMedisoft does not change the status until the statements are actually sent to the printer.

8. Close the Statement Management dialog box.

9. Create a backup of your work and exit NDCMedisoft by selecting Exit on the File menu or by clicking the Close button. The Backup Reminder dialog box is displayed.

10. Click the Back Up Data Now button. The Backup dialog box appears.

11. Enter the file path and file name in the Destination File Path and Name box or click the Find button and browse to the correct location. The file path will vary depending on your computer and network setup. Ask your instructor for the file path. The file should be named FCC8-9.mbk.

12. Click the Start Backup button. NDCMedisoft creates a backup file. When it is complete, and Information box is displayed, indicating that the backup is complete. Click OK. The Backup dialog box closes and the program shuts down.

CHAPTER REVIEW

USING TERMINOLOGY

Match the terms on the left with the definitions on the right.

_____ **1.** cycle billing

_____ **2.** filter

_____ **3.** navigator buttons

_____ **4.** once-a-month billing

_____ **5.** patient statement

_____ **6.** remainder statements

_____ **7.** standard statements

a. A list of the amount of money a patient owes, organized by the amount of time the money has been owed, the procedures performed, and the dates the procedures were performed.

b. A type of billing in which patients are divided into groups, and statement printing and mailing is staggered throughout the month.

c. Statements that show all available charges regardless of whether the insurance has paid on the transactions.

d. A condition that data must meet to be included in the selection.

e. Items that simplify the task of moving from one entry to another in a software program.

f. A type of billing in which statements are mailed to all patients at the same time each month.

g. Statements that list only those charges that are not paid in full after all insurance carrier payments have been received.

CHECKING YOUR UNDERSTANDING

Answer the questions below in the space provided.

8. A claim needs to be submitted for John Fitzwilliams. How would you select only those claims pertaining to John Fitzwilliams?

_____

_____

_____

9. On an audit/edit report, what does an "R" in the Flag column indicate?

_____

_____

_____

10. If an error is found on a claim, how is it corrected?

_____

_____

11. If a practice did not want to create statements for patients with an account balance below $5.00, how would this be done?

_____

_____

APPLYING KNOWLEDGE

Answer the questions below in the space provided.

12. You were asked to create claims for Samuel Bell. After entering his chart number in the Create Claims dialog box, you receive the message "No new claims were created." Why were no claims created for Samuel Bell?

_____

_____

13. Why do many practices send out remainder statements rather than standard statements?

_____

_____

AT THE COMPUTER

Answer the following questions at the computer.

14. How many claims were created on November 5, 2010?

_____

15. What transaction(s) were included on Sarabeth Smith's claim that was created on September 10, 2010?

_____

CHAPTER 10 Printing Reports

WHAT YOU NEED TO KNOW

To use this chapter, you need to know how to:
◆ Start NDCMedisoft, use menus, and enter and edit text.
◆ Work with chart numbers and codes.

WHAT YOU WILL LEARN

When you finish this chapter, you will be able to:
◆ Select the options available for different reports.
◆ Preview and print a variety of NDCMedisoft reports.
◆ Access NDCMedisoft's Report Designer.

KEY TERMS

aging report
day sheet
patient day sheet
patient ledger

payment day sheet
practice analysis report
procedure day sheet

REPORTS IN THE MEDICAL OFFICE

Reports are an important tool in managing a medical office. They provide useful information about a practice and its patients. Providers and office managers ask for different reports at different times. Some providers want to see a daily report of each day's transactions. Others want to see reports on particular patients' accounts on a weekly or bimonthly basis.

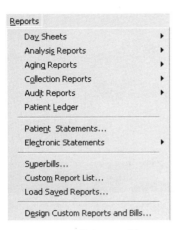

Reports
Day Sheets ▶
Analysis Reports ▶
Aging Reports ▶
Collection Reports ▶
Audit Reports ▶
Patient Ledger
Patient Statements...
Electronic Statements ▶
Superbills...
Custom Report List...
Load Saved Reports...
Design Custom Reports and Bills...

Figure 10-1 **Reports Menu**

NDCMedisoft provides a variety of standard reports, and has the ability to create custom reports using the Report Designer. Standard and custom reports are accessed through the Reports menu (see Figure 10-1). The Reports menu lists standard reports and also provides choices for designing custom reports using the Report Designer.

The standard reports are day sheets, analysis reports, aging reports, collection reports, audit reports, and patient ledger.

DAY SHEET REPORT

day sheet a report that provides information on practice activities for a twenty-four-hour period.

A **day sheet** is a report that provides information on practice activities for a twenty-four-hour period. In NDCMedisoft, there are three types of day sheet reports: patient day sheets, provider day sheets, and payment day sheets.

Patient Day Sheet

patient day sheet a summary of patient activity on a given day.

At the end of the day, many medical practices print a **patient day sheet,** which is a summary of the patient activity on that day (see Figures 10-2a, b, and c on pages 209–211). NDCMedisoft's version of this report lists the procedures for a particular day, grouped by patient, in alphabetical order by chart number. It includes:

◆ Procedures performed for a particular patient or group of patients

◆ Charges, receipts, adjustments, and balances for a particular patient or group of patients

◆ A summary of a practice's charges, payments, and adjustments

To print a patient day sheet, Day Sheets is clicked on the Reports menu and Patient Day Sheet on the submenu (see Figure 10-3 on page 211). Then, the Print Report Where? dialog box is displayed, asking whether the report should be previewed on the screen, sent directly to the printer, or exported to a file (see Figure 10-4 on page 211). Reports that are previewed on the screen can also be printed from the Preview Report window.

When the Preview the Report on the Screen radio button is selected and the Start button is clicked, the Data Selection Questions dialog box is displayed (see Figure 10-5 on page 212). This dialog box is

Patient Day Sheet

Entry	Date	Document	POS	Description	Provider	Code	Amount
ARLENSU0		**Susan Arlen**					
492	10/4/2010	1009060000		East Ohio PPO	5	EAPPAY	-46.00
		Patient's Charges		Patient's Receipts	Adjustments		Patient Balance
		$0.00		-$46.00	$0.00		$0.00
BELLHER0		**Herbert Bell**					
493	10/4/2010	1009060000		East Ohio PPO	2	EAPPAY	-30.00
		Patient's Charges		Patient's Receipts	Adjustments		Patient Balance
		$0.00		-$30.00	$0.00		$0.00
BELLJAN0		**Janine Bell**					
495	10/4/2010	1009060000		East Ohio PPO	3	EAPPAY	-103.00
494	10/4/2010	1009060000		East Ohio PPO	3	EAPPAY	-62.00
		Patient's Charges		Patient's Receipts	Adjustments		Patient Balance
		$0.00		-$165.00	$0.00		$0.00
BELLJON0		**Jonathan Bell**					
496	10/4/2010	1009060000		East Ohio PPO	3	EAPPAY	-177.60
		Patient's Charges		Patient's Receipts	Adjustments		Patient Balance
		$0.00		-$177.60	$0.00		$0.00
BELLSAM0		**Samuel Bell**					
497	10/4/2010	1009060000		East Ohio PPO	2	EAPPAY	-46.00
		Patient's Charges		Patient's Receipts	Adjustments		Patient Balance
		$0.00		-$46.00	$0.00		$0.00
BELLSAR0		**Sarina Bell**					
498	10/4/2010	1009060000		East Ohio PPO	3	EAPPAY	-62.00
		Patient's Charges		Patient's Receipts	Adjustments		Patient Balance
		$0.00		-$62.00	$0.00		$0.00
FITZWJO0		**John Fitzwilliams**					
474	10/4/2010	1010040000	11		2	99213	39.00
475	10/4/2010	1010040000	11		2	82270	8.00
476	10/4/2010	1010040000	11		2	CHVCOPAY	15.00
478	10/4/2010	1010040000	11		2	CHVCPAY	-15.00
479	10/4/2010	1009070000		#214778924 ChampVA	2	CHVPAY	-29.00
		Patient's Charges		Patient's Receipts	Adjustments		Patient Balance
		$62.00		-$44.00	$0.00		$47.00
FITZWSA0		**Sarah Fitzwilliams**					
480	10/4/2010	1009070000		#214778924 ChampVA	1	CHVPAY	-12.00
481	10/4/2010	1009070000		#214778924 ChampVA	1	CHVPAY	-29.00
		Patient's Charges		Patient's Receipts	Adjustments		Patient Balance
		$0.00		-$41.00	$0.00		$0.00
GARDIJO0		**John Gardiner**					
483	10/4/2010	1010040000	11		1	CAPADJ	-24.00

Figure 10-2a Page 1 of Patient Day Sheet Report

Patient Day Sheet

Entry	Date	Document	POS	Description	Provider	Code	Amount
		Patient's Charges $0.00		Patient's Receipts $0.00	Adjustments -$24.00		Patient Balance $0.00
JONESEL0		**Elizabeth Jones**					
473	10/4/2010	1010040000	11		1	99213	39.00
		Patient's Charges $39.00		Patient's Receipts $0.00	Adjustments $0.00		Patient Balance $155.00
PATTELE0		**Leila Patterson**					
484	10/4/2010	1010040000	11		2	CAPADJ	-24.00
		Patient's Charges $0.00		Patient's Receipts $0.00	Adjustments -$24.00		Patient Balance $0.00
TANAKHI0		**Hiro Tanaka**					
471	10/4/2010	0307140000	11		1	99202	62.00
472	10/4/2010	0307140000	11		1	OHCCOPAY	30.00
477	10/4/2010	1010040000	11		1	OHCCPAY	-30.00
		Patient's Charges $92.00		Patient's Receipts -$30.00	Adjustments $0.00		Patient Balance $62.00

Figure 10-2b **Page 2 of Patient Day Sheet Report**

used to select the patients, dates, and providers for whom a report is being generated. If any box is left blank, all values are included in the report. For example, if no chart numbers are entered, all patients will be included in the report. The selection options in the dialog box are as follows:

Chart Number Range In the Chart Number Range boxes, a range of chart numbers for patients is entered. If a report is needed for just one patient, that patient's chart number is entered in both boxes.

Date Created Range/Date From Range The Date Created Range refers to the actual date the charge was created. The Date From Range refers to the date of the transaction. The date created and the transaction date may or may not be the same. For example, suppose it is Monday morning, October 4, and transactions from the prior Friday, October 1, still need to be entered in NDCMedisoft. In this example, the Date Created is the date the transaction was entered—October 4. The Date From is the date on which the patient was in the office—October 1.

By default, NDCMedisoft enters the Windows System Date in both Date Created Range boxes. For the purposes of the exercises in this book, those dates must be deleted and the correct dates must be entered in the Date From Range boxes.

Family Care Center

Patient Day Sheet

Total # Patients	12
Total # Procedures	6
Total Procedure Charges	$193.00
Total Product Charges	$0.00
Total Inside Lab Charges	$0.00
Total Outside Lab Charges	$0.00
Total Billing Charges	$0.00
Total Tax Charges	$0.00
Total Charges	$193.00
Total Insurance Payments	-$596.60
Total Cash Copayments	$0.00
Total Check Copayments	-$45.00
Total Credit Card Copayments	$0.00
Total Patient Cash Payments	$0.00
Total Patient Check Payments	$0.00
Total Credit Card Payments	$0.00
Total Receipts	-$641.60
Total Credit Adjustments	$0.00
Total Debit Adjustments	$0.00
Total Insurance Debit Adjustments	$0.00
Total Insurance Credit Adjustments	-$48.00
Total Insurance Withholds	$0.00
Total Adjustments	-$48.00
Net Effect on Accounts Receivable	-$496.60

Figure 10-2c Page 3 of Patient Day Sheet Report

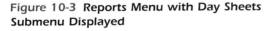

Figure 10-3 Reports Menu with Day Sheets Submenu Displayed

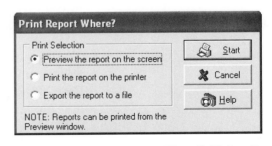

Figure 10-4 Print Report Where? Dialog Box

Day sheets can also be created for a range of dates. For example, if it were necessary to print patient day sheets for the period of May 1 to May 15, 2010, "05012010" would be entered in the first Date From Range box and "05152010" in the second Date From Range box.

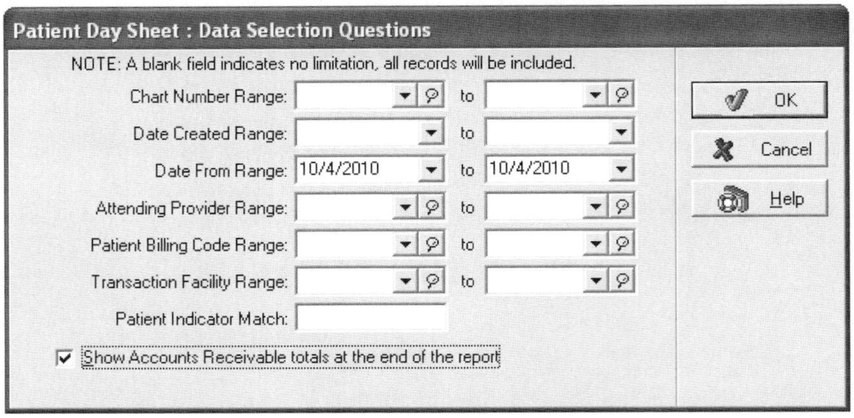

Figure 10-5 Data Selection Questions Dialog Box for Patient Day Sheet Report

Attending Provider Range A range of codes for the attending providers is entered in the Attending Provider Range boxes.

Patient Billing Code Range If the practice uses NDCMedisoft's Patient Billing Code feature, codes can be entered in this box to select only those patients with the designated billing code(s).

Transaction Facility Range A range of codes for the facility where the procedure was performed is entered.

Patient Indicator Match If the practice has assigned a Patient Indicator code to each patient, an entry can be made to select only those patients who match a specific code.

Show Accounts Receivable Totals at the End of the Report If this box is checked, accounts receivable totals will appear at the end of the patient day sheet report.

When these selection boxes have been completed, the OK button is clicked. NDCMedisoft begins creating the report. NDCMedisoft generates the report and displays it on-screen or sends it to a file or to the printer, depending on the selection made in the Print Report Where? dialog box.

The Preview Report window, common to all reports, provides options for viewing or printing a report (see Figure 10-6). The buttons on the Preview Report toolbar control how a report is displayed on-screen and movement from page to page within a report (see Figure 10-7).

The three zoom buttons at the left of the toolbar are used to affect the size of the report displayed on-screen. The zoom button farthest to the left reduces a report so that a full page fits on the screen. The middle zoom button displays a report at 100 percent of its size. This option acts like a magnifying glass, allowing a portion of a report to be viewed up close. The zoom button on the right displays the full width of a page on the screen.

Family Care Center
Patient Day Sheet

Entry	Date	Document	POS	Description	Provider	Code	Amount
ARLENSU0		**Susan Arlen**					
492	10/4/2010	1009060000		East Ohio PPO	5	EAPPAY	-46.00
		Patient's Charges $0.00		Patient's Receipts -$46.00	Adjustments $0.00		Patient Balance $0.00
BELLHER0		**Herbert Bell**					
493	10/4/2010	1009060000		East Ohio PPO	2	EAPPAY	-30.00
		Patient's Charges $0.00		Patient's Receipts -$30.00	Adjustments $0.00		Patient Balance $0.00
BELLJAN0		**Janine Bell**					
495	10/4/2010	1009060000		East Ohio PPO	3	EAPPAY	-103.00
494	10/4/2010	1009060000		East Ohio PPO	3	EAPPAY	-62.00
		Patient's Charges $0.00		Patient's Receipts -$165.00	Adjustments $0.00		Patient Balance $0.00
BELLJON0		**Jonathan Bell**					
496	10/4/2010	1009060000		East Ohio PPO	3	EAPPAY	-177.60
		Patient's Charges $0.00		Patient's Receipts -$177.60	Adjustments $0.00		Patient Balance $0.00
BELLSAM0		**Samuel Bell**					
497	10/4/2010	1009060000		East Ohio PPO	2	EAPPAY	-46.00
		Patient's Charges $0.00		Patient's Receipts -$46.00	Adjustments $0.00		Patient Balance $0.00
BELLSAR0		**Sarina Bell**					

Figure 10-6 **Preview Report Window**

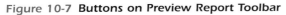

Figure 10-7 **Buttons on Preview Report Toolbar**

A series of four triangle buttons, two on the left and two on the right, are used to move through pages of a multipage report. The First Page button, farthest on the left, moves to the beginning of a report. The Previous Page button moves to the page that precedes the one currently displayed. The bar between the two sets of triangle buttons indicates how many pages are in a report and the number of the current page. To the right of the bar are the other two triangle buttons. The Next Page button moves to the page following the current one. The Last Page button moves to the end of a report.

The remaining buttons include the Print button, which is used to send a report to the printer, and the Disk button, which saves a report to disk. The Close button closes the Preview Report window, redisplaying the main NDCMedisoft window.

The Preview Report window also contains the Go to Page box, in which the number of a specific page to be displayed in the Preview Report window is entered.

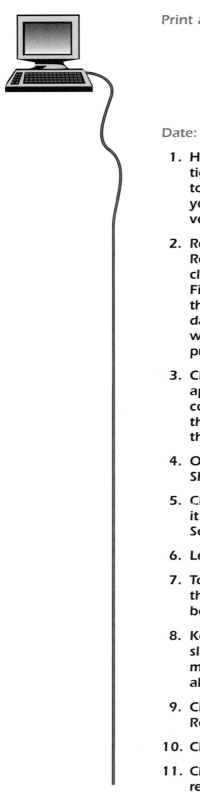

Exercise 10-1

Print a patient day sheet report for October 4, 2010.

> Note: Steps 1 through 3 are required at the beginning of each chapter. These steps start NDCMedisoft, set the path to the correct data location, and restore the data saved at the end of the last work session.

Date: October 4, 2010

1. Hold down the F7 key and start NDCMedisoft. Enter the location of the NDCMedisoft data in the Find NDCMedisoft Directory box and click OK. (If you are unsure what to enter, ask your instructor.) When the Open Practice dialog box appears, verify that Family Care Center is highlighted and click OK.

2. Restore the data from your last work session by selecting Restore Data on the File menu. When a Warning box appears, click OK. Enter the file path and file name in the Destination File Path and Name box or click the Find button and browse to the desired location. The file name should be FCC8-9.mbk (the database name followed by the chapter number that you last worked on). The file path will vary depending on your computer and network setup. Ask your instructor for the file path.

3. Click the Start Restore button. When a Confirm dialog box appears, click OK. NDCMedisoft restores the data. When it is complete, an Information box is displayed, indicating that the restore is complete. Click OK. the Restore box closes and the main NDCMedisoft window is displayed.

4. On the Reports menu, click Day Sheets and then Patient Day Sheet. The Print Report Where? dialog box is displayed.

5. Click the radio button for previewing the report on-screen if it is not already selected. Click the Start button. The Data Selection Questions dialog box is displayed.

6. Leave the Chart Number Range boxes blank.

7. Today's date—that is, the date on which you are working on this exercise—will likely appear in both Date Created Range boxes. Delete both entries.

8. Key *10042010* in both Date From Range boxes. Do not key any slashes between the numbers; NDCMedisoft does this automatically. Leave all other boxes blank. This will select data for all patients and attending providers for October 4, 2010.

9. Check the Show Accounts Receivable Totals at the End of the Report box.

10. Click the OK button. The patient day sheet report is displayed.

11. Click the appropriate zoom button on the toolbar to display the report the full width of the screen so that it is easier to read.

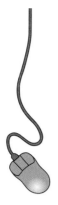

12. **Scroll down the page to view additional entries on the first page of the report.**

13. **Click the Next Page button to advance to the second page of the report.**

14. **Click the other zoom and triangle buttons on the toolbar to see their effects. Use the Go to Page box to move back to the first page of the report.**

15. **Click the Print button, and then click the OK button on the Print menu to print the report.**

16. **Click the Close button to exit the Preview Report window.**

Procedure Day Sheet

procedure day sheet *a report that lists all the procedures performed on a particular day, listed in numerical order.*

A **procedure day sheet** lists all procedures performed on a particular day, and gives the dates, patients, document numbers, places of service, debits, and credits relating to them (see Figures 10-8a and b on pages 216–217). Procedures are listed in numerical order. Procedure day sheets are printed by clicking Day Sheets on the Reports menu and then Procedure Day Sheet on the submenu. The same Print Report Where? dialog box used for a patient day sheet is displayed. Again, the report can be previewed on-screen, printed directly, or exported to a file.

Once the decision to preview, print, or export is made, the data selection criteria must be determined. The Data Selection Questions dialog box provides options to select by procedure codes, dates, and providers (see Figure 10-9 on page 217). A procedure day sheet will be generated only for data that meet the selection criteria. If any box is left blank, all values are included in the report.

The following boxes are listed in the Data Selection Questions dialog box.

Procedure Code Range   In the Procedure Code Range box, a range of procedure codes is entered. If a report is needed for a single code, it is entered in both boxes.

Date Created Range/Date From Range   These boxes have the same functionality as for the Patient Day Sheet report.

Attending Provider Range   Codes for attending providers are entered in the Attending Provider Range boxes.

Transaction Facility Range   A range of codes for the facility where the procedure was performed is entered.

Show Accounts Receivable Totals at the End of the Report   If this box is checked, accounts receivable totals will appear at the end of the report.

Procedure Code Day Sheet

Entry	Date	Chart	Name	Document	POS	Debits	Credits
82270			**Blood screening, occult; feces**				
475	10/4/2010	FITZWJO0	Fitzwilliams, John	1010040000	11	8.00	
		Total of 82270		Quantity:	1	$8.00	$0.00
99202			**OF –new patient, low**				
471	10/4/2010	TANAKHI0	Tanaka, Hiro	0307140000	11	62.00	
		Total of 99202		Quantity:	1	$62.00	$0.00
99213			**OF –established patient, detailed**				
473	10/4/2010	JONESEL0	Jones, Elizabeth	1010040000	11	39.00	
474	10/4/2010	FITZWJO0	Fitzwilliams, John	1010040000	11	39.00	
		Total of 99213		Quantity:	2	$78.00	$0.00
CAPADJ			**Capitation Adjustment**				
483	10/4/2010	GARDIJO0	Gardiner, John	1010040000	11		-24.00
484	10/4/2010	PATTELE0	Patterson, Leila	1010040000	11		-24.00
		Total of CAPADJ		Quantity:	2	$0.00	-$48.00
CHVCOPAY			**ChampVA Copayment Charge**				
476	10/4/2010	FITZWJO0	Fitzwilliams, John	1010040000	11	15.00	
		Total of CHVCOPAY		Quantity:	1	$15.00	$0.00
CHVCPAY			**ChampVA Copayment**				
478	10/4/2010	FITZWJO0	Fitzwilliams, John	1010040000	11		-15.00
		Total of CHVCPAY		Quantity:	1	$0.00	-$15.00
CHVPAY			**ChampVA Payment**				
479	10/4/2010	FITZWJO0	Fitzwilliams, John	1009070000			-29.00
480	10/4/2010	FITZWSA0	Fitzwilliams, Sarah	1009070000			-12.00
481	10/4/2010	FITZWSA0	Fitzwilliams, Sarah	1009070000			-29.00
		Total of CHVPAY		Quantity:	3	$0.00	-$70.00
EAPPAY			**East Ohio PPO Payment**				
498	10/4/2010	BELLSAR0	Bell, Sarina	1009060000			-62.00
497	10/4/2010	BELLSAM0	Bell, Samuel	1009060000			-46.00
495	10/4/2010	BELLJAN0	Bell, Janine	1009060000			-103.00
496	10/4/2010	BELLJON0	Bell, Jonathan	1009060000			-177.60
494	10/4/2010	BELLJAN0	Bell, Janine	1009060000			-62.00
493	10/4/2010	BELLHER0	Bell, Herbert	1009060000			-30.00
492	10/4/2010	ARLENSU0	Arlen, Susan	1009060000			-46.00
		Total of EAPPAY		Quantity:	7	$0.00	-$526.60
OHCCOPAY			**OhioCare HMO Copayment Charge**				
472	10/4/2010	TANAKHI0	Tanaka, Hiro	0307140000	11	30.00	
		Total of OHCCOPAY		Quantity:	1	$30.00	$0.00

Figure 10-8a Page 1 of Procedure Code Day Sheet

Family Care Center

Procedure Code Day Sheet

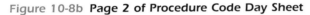

Entry	Date	Chart	Name	Document	POS	Debits	Credits
OHCCPAY			**OhioCare HMO Copayment**				
477	10/4/2010	TANAKHI0	Tanaka, Hiro	1010040000	11		-30.00
		Total of	OHCCPAY	Quantity:	1	$0.00	-$30.00

Total of Codes:	$193.00	-$689.60
Balance:	-$496.60	

Practice Totals

Total # Procedures	67
Total Charges	$2,911.60
Total Payments	-$1,948.40
Total Adjustments	-$48.00
Accounts Receivable	$915.20

Figure 10-8b **Page 2 of Procedure Code Day Sheet**

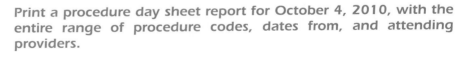

Figure 10-9 **Data Selection Questions Dialog Box for Procedure Code Day Sheet Report**

Exercise 10-2

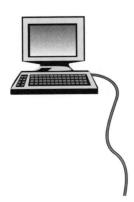

Print a procedure day sheet report for October 4, 2010, with the entire range of procedure codes, dates from, and attending providers.

Date: October 4, 2010

1. On the Reports menu, click Day Sheets and then Procedure Day Sheet. The Print Report Where? dialog box is displayed.

2. Click the radio button option for previewing the report on-screen. Click the Start button. The Data Selection Questions dialog box is displayed.

3. Leave the Procedure Code Range boxes blank.

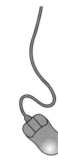

4. Delete the entries in both Date Created Range boxes.

5. Key *10042010* in both Date From Range boxes.

6. Check the Show Accounts Receivable Totals at the End of the Report box.

7. Click the OK button. The procedure day sheet report is displayed.

8. Send the report to the printer.

9. Exit the Preview Report window.

Payment Day Sheet

payment day sheet *a report that lists all payments received on a particular day, organized by provider.*

A **payment day sheet** lists all payments received on a particular day, organized by provider (see Figures 10-10a and b). It is printed by clicking Day Sheets on the Reports menu and then Payment Day Sheet on the submenu. The same Print Report Where? dialog box is

Family Care Center
Payment Day Sheet

Entry	Date	Document	Description	Chart	Code	Amount
1		**Yan, Katherine**				
477	10/4/2010	1010040000		TANAKHI0	OHCCPAY	-30.00
480	10/4/2010	1009070000	#214778924 Champ VA	FITZWSA0	CHVPAY	-12.00
481	10/4/2010	1009070000	#214778924 Champ VA	FITZWSA0	CHVPAY	-29.00
			Count: 3		**Provider Total**	-71.00
2		**Rudner, John**				
478	10/4/2010	1010040000		FITZWJO0	CHVCPAY	-15.00
479	10/4/2010	1009070000	#214778924 Champ VA	FITZWJO0	CHVPAY	-29.00
497	10/4/2010	1009060000	East Ohio PPO	BELLSAM0	EAPPAY	-46.00
493	10/4/2010	1009060000	East Ohio PPO	BELLHER0	EAPPAY	-30.00
			Count: 4		**Provider Total**	-120.00
3		**Rudner, Jessica**				
498	10/4/2010	1009060000	East Ohio PPO	BELLSAR0	EAPPAY	-62.00
495	10/4/2010	1009060000	East Ohio PPO	BELLJAN0	EAPPAY	-103.00
496	10/4/2010	1009060000	East Ohio PPO	BELLJON0	EAPPAY	-177.60
494	10/4/2010	1009060000	East Ohio PPO	BELLJAN0	EAPPAY	-62.00
			Count: 4		**Provider Total**	-404.60
5		**Beach, Robert**				
492	10/4/2010	1009060000	East Ohio PPO	ARLENSU0	EAPPAY	-46.00
			Count: 1		**Provider Total**	-46.00

Figure 10-10a Page 1 of Payment Day Sheet

Family Care Center
Payment Day Sheet

Report Totals

Total # Payments	12
Total Payments	-$641.60

Practice Totals

Total # Payments	49
Total Payments	-$1,948.40
Total Applied Payments	-$1,948.40
Total Unapplied Payments	$0.00

Accounts Receivable	$915.20

Figure 10-10b **Page 2 of Payment Day Sheet**

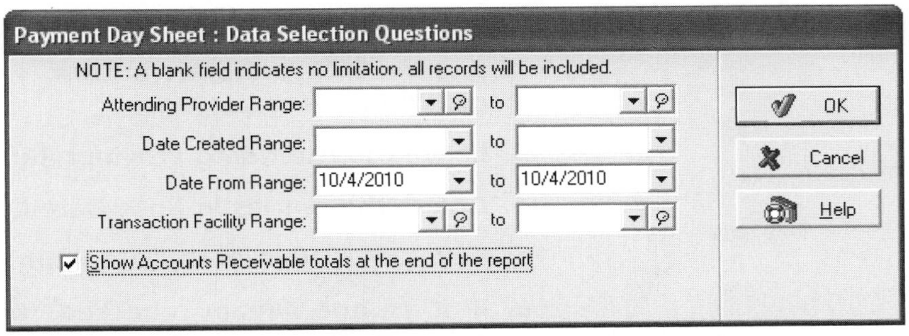

Figure 10-11 **Data Selection Questions Dialog Box for Payment Day Sheet Report**

displayed. Again, the report can be previewed on-screen, printed directly, or exported.

Once the decision to preview, print, or export is made, the data selection criteria must be determined. The Data Selection Questions dialog box provides options to select by attending provider and date (see Figure 10-11). A payment day sheet will be generated only for data that meet the selection criteria. If any box is left blank, all values for that box are included in the report.

The following boxes are listed in the Data Selection Questions dialog box.

Attending Provider Range Codes for attending providers are entered in the Attending Provider Range boxes.

Date Created Range A range of dates when transactions were entered in NDCMedisoft is entered in the two boxes. The Windows System Date is the default entry.

Date From Range A range of dates when each transaction occurred is entered in the Date From Range boxes.

Transaction Facility Range A range of codes for the facility where the procedure was performed is entered.

Show Accounts Receivable Totals at the End of the Report If this box is checked, accounts receivable totals will appear at the end of the report.

Exercise 10-3

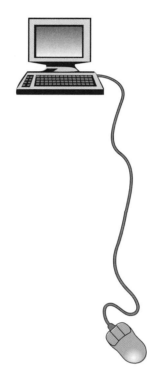

Print a payment day sheet report for October 4, 2010, with the entire range of attending providers.

Date: October 4, 2010

1. On the Reports menu, click Day Sheets and then Payment Day Sheet. The Print Report Where? dialog box is displayed.

2. Click the radio button option for previewing the report on-screen. Click the Start button. The Data Selection Questions dialog box is displayed.

3. Leave the Attending Provider Range boxes blank.

4. Delete the entries in both Date Created Range boxes.

5. Key *10042010* in both Date From Range boxes.

6. If it is not already checked, be sure to check the Show Accounts Receivable Totals at the End of the Report box.

7. Click the OK button. The payment day sheet report is displayed.

8. Send the report to the printer.

9. Exit the Preview Report window.

PRACTICE ANALYSIS REPORT

practice analysis report a report that analyzes the revenue of a practice for a specified period of time, usually a month or a year.

NDCMedisoft's **practice analysis report** analyzes the revenue of a practice for a specified period of time, usually a month or a year (see Figures 10-12a and b on pages 221–222). The report can be used to generate medical practice financial statements. It can also be used for profit analysis. The summary at the end of the report breaks down the information into total charges, total payments and copayments, and total adjustments.

The following boxes are listed in the Data Selection Questions dialog box (see Figure 10-13 on page 222).

Procedure Code Range A range of procedure codes is entered in the Procedure Code Range boxes.

Practice Analysis

From October 1, 2010 to October 31, 2010

Code	Modifier	Description	Amount	Units	Average	Cost	Net
71010		Chest x-ray, single view, frontal	91.00	1	91.00	0.00	91.00
73600		Ankle x-ray, AP and lateral views	80.00	1	80.00	0.00	80.00
80048		Basic metabolic panel	60.00	1	60.00	0.00	60.00
82270	90	Blood screening, occult; feces	8.00	1	8.00	0.00	8.00
82947		Glucose screening--quantitative	25.00	1	25.00	0.00	25.00
87086		Urine culture and colony count	51.00	1	51.00	0.00	51.00
87430		Strep test	58.00	1	58.00	0.00	58.00
99202		OF--new patient, low	62.00	1	62.00	0.00	62.00
99212		OF--established patient, low	248.00	6	41.33	0.00	248.00
99213		OF--established patient, detailed	212.00	4	53.00	0.00	212.00
CAPADJ		Capitation Adjustment	-48.00	2	-24.00	0.00	-48.00
CHVCOPAY		ChampVA Copayment Charge	15.00	1	15.00	0.00	15.00
CHVCPAY		ChampVA Copayment	-15.00	1	-15.00	0.00	-15.00
CHVPAY		ChampVA Payment	-70.00	3	-23.33	0.00	-70.00
EAPCOPAY		East Ohio PPO Copayment Charge	100.00	4	25.00	0.00	100.00
EAPCPAY		East Ohio PPO Copayment	-100.00	4	-25.00	0.00	-100.00
EAPPAY		East Ohio PPO Payment	-526.60	7	-75.23	0.00	-526.60
OHCCOPAY		OhioCare HMO Copayment Charge	30.00	1	30.00	0.00	30.00
OHCCPAY		OhioCare HMO Copayment	-30.00	1	-30.00	0.00	-30.00

Figure 10-12a **Page 1 of Practice Analysis Report**

Date Created Range A range of dates when transactions were entered in NDCMedisoft is entered in the two boxes. The Windows System Date is the default entry.

Date From Range A range of dates is entered in the Date From Range boxes. The system enters a default entry in the second of the two boxes. To change this date, highlight the default entry and enter the new date in MMDDCCYY format.

Attending Provider Range Codes for attending providers are entered in the Attending Provider Range boxes.

Place of Service Range Codes for place of service are entered if a report is required for a specific place of service.

Transaction Facility Range A range of codes for the facility where the procedure was performed is entered.

Show Accounts Receivable Totals at the End of the Report If this box is checked, accounts receivable totals will appear at the end of the report.

Family Care Center
Practice Analysis
From October 1, 2010 to October 31, 2010

Total Procedure Charges	$1,040.00
Total Product Charges	$0.00
Total Inside Lab Charges	$0.00
Total Outside Lab Charges	$0.00
Total Billing Charges	$0.00
Total Tax Charges	$0.00
Total Insurance Payments	-$596.60
Total Cash Copayments	$0.00
Total Check Copayments	-$145.00
Total Credit Card Copayments	$0.00
Total Patient Cash Payments	$0.00
Total Patient Check Payments	$0.00
Total Credit Card Payments	$0.00
Total Debit Adjustments	$0.00
Total Credit Adjustments	$0.00
Total Insurance Debit Adjustments	$0.00
Total Insurance Credit Adjustments	-$48.00
Total Insurance Withholds	$0.00
Net Effect on Accounts Receivable	$250.40

Practice Totals

Total # Procedures	67
Total Charges	$2,891.60
Total Payments	-$1,948.40
Total Adjustments	-$48.00
Accounts Receivable	$895.20

Figure 10-12b **Page 2 of Practice Analysis Report**

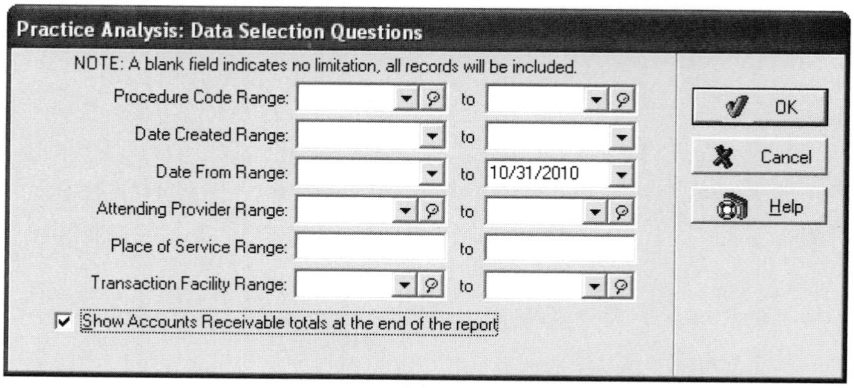

Figure 10-13 **Data Selection Questions dialog box for Practice Analysis Report**

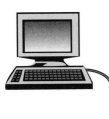

Exercise 10-4

Print a practice analysis report for October 2010.

Date: October 31, 2010

1. On the Reports menu, click Analysis Reports and then Practice Analysis.

2. Click the radio button for previewing the report on-screen. Click the Start button.

3. In the first Date From Range box, key *10012010*. In the second box, key *10312010*.

4. If it is not already checked, be sure to check the Show Accounts Receivable Totals at the End of the Report box.

5. Leave the rest of the boxes blank. Click the OK button.

6. View the report on-screen.

7. Go to the second page of the report.

8. Send the report to the printer.

9. Exit the Preview Report window.

PATIENT AGING REPORT

aging report a report that lists the amount of money owed to the practice, organized by the amount of time the money has been owed.

An **aging report** lists the amount of money owed to the practice, organized by the amount of time the money has been owed. A patient aging report lists a patient's balance by age, the date and amount of the last payment, and the telephone number. The columns display the amounts that are current and those that are 31–60, 61–90, and more than 90 days past due (see Figure 10-14). The aging begins on the date of the transaction. Patient aging reports are printed by clicking Aging Reports and then Patient Aging on the Reports menu. After making a selection in the Print Report Where? dialog box, the data must be selected.

Family Care Center
Patient Aging
As of September 30, 2010

Chart	Name	Birthdate	Current 0 - 30	Past 31 - 60	Past 61 - 90	Past 91 --->	Total Balance
WONGJO10	Jo Wong	9/6/1934	5.60		5.60		11.20
Last Pmt: -22.40	On: 9/14/2010	(614)029-7777					
	Report Aging Totals		$5.60	$0.00	$5.60	$0.00	11.20
	Percent of Aging Total		50.0%	0.0%	50.0%	0.0%	100.00%

Figure 10-14 **Patient Aging Report**

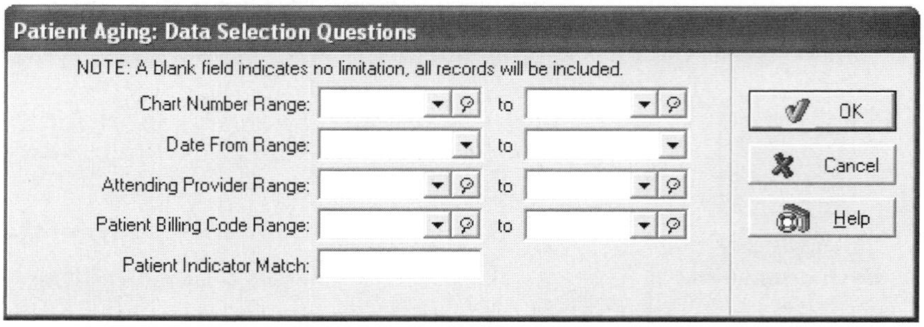

Figure 10-15 **Data Selection Questions dialog box for Patient Aging Report**

The boxes in the Data Selection Questions dialog box are as follows (see Figure 10-15).

Chart Number Range   In the Chart Number Range boxes, a range of chart numbers for patients is entered. If the report is needed for just one patient, that patient's chart number is entered in both boxes.

Date From Range   A range of dates is entered in the Date From Range boxes.

Attending Provider Range   A range of codes for the attending providers is entered in the Attending Provider Range boxes.

Patient Billing Code Range   If the practice uses NDCMedisoft's Billing Code feature, codes can be entered in this box to select only those patients with the designated billing code(s).

Patient Indicator Match   If the practice has assigned a Patient Indicator code to each patient, an entry can be made to select only those patients who match a specific code.

Exercise 10-5

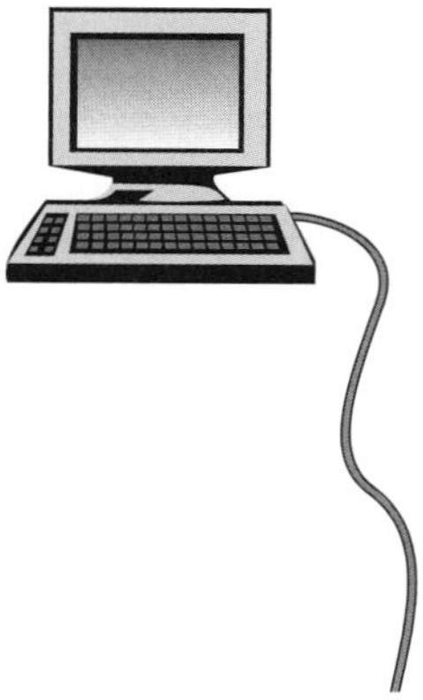

Print a patient aging report for Jo Wong.

Date: September 30, 2010

1. **On the Reports menu, click Aging Reports and then Patient Aging.**

2. **Click the radio button for previewing the report on-screen. Click the Start button.**

3. **Select Wong's chart number in both boxes of the Chart Number Range boxes.**

4. **Leave the starting date in the first of the Date From Range boxes blank, and key *09302010* in the second of the boxes.**

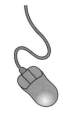

5. Leave the Attending Provider Range boxes blank. Click the OK button.

6. View the report on-screen.

7. Print the report.

8. Exit the Preview Report window.

INSURANCE AGING REPORT

An insurance aging report permits tracking of claims filed with insurance carriers. The report lists claims that have been on file 0–30 days, 31–60 days, 61–90 days, 91–120 days, and more than 120 days (see Figure 10-16). This information is used to follow up on overdue payments from insurance carriers. Printing the aging report and following up on overdue claims speeds the collection process. The aging begins on the date of billing. NDCMedisoft provides three insurance aging reports: primary, secondary, and tertiary.

Family Care Center

Primary Insurance Aging

Date of Service	Procedure	-- Past -- 0 - 30	-- Past -- 31 - 60	-- Past -- 61 - 90	-- Past -- 91 - 120	-- Past -- 121 ----->	Total Balance
Blue Cross Blue Shield (BLU01)							**(800)555-5555**
BORJO000	John Bordon		SS: 444556666		Policy: 740582	Group: 45k	
3/9/2010	99213					$60.00	60.00
3/9/2010	97260					$30.00	30.00
Claim: 7	Billed: 3/13/2010	0.00	0.00	0.00	0.00	90.00	90.00
3/15/2010	99213					$60.00	60.00
3/15/2010	97010					$10.00	10.00
Claim: 28	Billed: 9/7/2010	0.00	0.00	0.00	0.00	70.00	70.00
	Insurance Totals	$0.00	$0.00	$0.00	$0.00	$160.00	$160.00
Cigna (CIG00)							**(800)234-5678**
BRIJA000	Jay Brimley		SS:		Policy: 98547377	Group: 12d	
3/3/2010	99214					$65.00	65.00
3/3/2010	72052					$80.00	80.00
Claim: 2	Billed: 3/5/2010	0.00	0.00	0.00	0.00	145.00	145.00
BRISU000	Susan Brimley		SS:		Policy: 0394576	Group: 15c	
3/9/2010	99213					$60.00	60.00
3/9/2010	81000					$11.00	11.00
3/9/2010	99000					$8.00	8.00
Claim: 8	Billed: 3/13/2010	0.00	0.00	0.00	0.00	79.00	79.00
BRIJA000	Jay Brimley		SS:		Policy: 98547377	Group: 12d	
3/25/2010	99214					$65.00	65.00
Claim: 24	Billed: 4/21/2010	0.00	0.00	0.00	0.00	65.00	65.00
BRISU000	Susan Brimley		SS:		Policy: 0394576	Group: 15c	
3/15/2010	99213					$60.00	60.00
3/15/2010	DS					$40.00	40.00
Claim: 29	Billed: 9/7/2010	0.00	0.00	0.00	0.00	100.00	100.00
	Insurance Totals	$0.00	$0.00	$0.00	$0.00	$389.00	$389.00

Figure 10-16 **Primary Insurance Aging Report**

Primary Insurance Aging: Data Selection Questions

NOTE: A blank field indicates no limitation, all records will be included.

Insurance Carrier 1 Range:	▼ 🔎	to	▼ 🔎
Initial Billing Date 1 Range:	▼	to	▼
Attending Provider Range:	▼ 🔎	to	▼ 🔎
Transaction Facility Range:	▼ 🔎	to	▼ 🔎

✓ OK
✗ Cancel
🗃 Help

Figure 10-17 **Data Selection Questions dialog box for Primary Insurance Aging Report**

Boxes in the Data Selection Questions dialog box for the Primary Insurance Aging report is as follows (see Figure 10-17).

Insurance Carrier 1 Range   A range of codes for insurance carriers is entered in the Insurance Carrier 1 Range boxes.

Initial Billing Date 1 Range   A range of billing dates for the primary insurance carrier is entered in these boxes. The program displays the Windows System Date as the default entry in the second box.

Attending Provider Range   Codes for attending providers are entered in the Attending Provider Range boxes.

Transaction Facility Range   A range of codes for the facility where the procedure was performed is entered.

Boxes in the Data Selection Questions dialog box for the Secondary and Tertiary Insurance Aging report is the same except for the difference in the carrier number and billing date number.

COLLECTION REPORTS   NDCMedisoft provides a number of collection reports that can be used to locate overdue patient or insurance accounts (see Figure 10-18).

Patient Collection Report

The patient collection report uses information from the Statement Management feature to indicate the chart number, patient name,

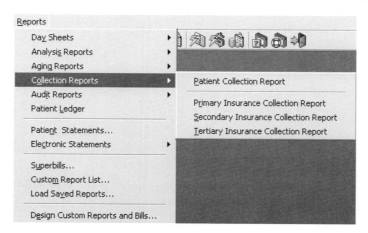

Figure 10-18 **Collection Reports Available in NDCMedisoft**

telephone number, Statement Number, Initial Bill Date, Last Bill Date, Last Patient Payment Date, Last Patient Payment Amount, Submission, Statement Type, and Statement Total of an account. A sample patient collection report is illustrated in Figure 10-19.

The selections for the report can be filtered by Chart Number Range, Date Created Range, Initial Billing Date Range, and Status Match.

Insurance Collection Reports

The insurance collection reports draw information from the Claim Management area of the program to provide details such as the Claim number, Chart number, Primary (Secondary, Tertiary) Bill Date, Batch 1 (2 or 3), Date Created, Submission Count, and Claim Total for each payer. Figure 10-20 on page 228 shows a sample insurance collection report.

Patient Collection Report
12/31/2010

Statement Number	Initial Bill Date	Last Bill Date	Last Patient Pay Date	Last Patient Pay Amount	Submission	Statement Type	Statement Total
BATTIAN0- Anthony Battistuta			Phone: (614)500-3619				
47					0	Remainder	$27.08
							$27.08
GILESSH0- Sheila Giles			Phone: (614)303-0579				
48					0	Remainder	$90.60
							$90.60
JONESEL0- Elizabeth Jones			Phone: (614)123-5555				
43	12/31/2010	12/31/2010			1	Remainder	$31.00
							$31.00
SIMMOJI0- Jill Simmons			Phone: (614)011-6767				
44	12/31/2010	12/31/2010			1	Remainder	$21.00
							$21.00
SMITHJA0- James L Smith			Phone: (614)879-2222				
45	12/31/2010	12/31/2010			1	Remainder	$42.00
							$42.00
WONGJO10- Jo Wong			Phone: (614)029-7777				
46	7/31/2010	7/31/2010			1	Remainder	$5.60
49					0	Remainder	$5.60
WONGLIY0- Li Y Wong			Phone: (614)029-7777				
50					0	Remainder	$2.80
							$2.80
						Total:	$225.68

Figure 10-19 **Sample Patient Collection Report**

Primary Insurance Collection Report

12/31/2010

Claim	Chart	Primary Bill Date	Batch 1	Date Created	Submission Count	Claim Total
1 - Medicare				Phone: (215)599-0000		
65	BATTIPA0		0	1/5/2011	0	$14.00
					Total:	$14.00
13 - East Ohio PPO				Phone: (419)444-1505		
58	BROOKLA0		0	11/30/2010	0	$210.00
70	SYZMADE0		0	1/5/2011	0	$337.60
					Total:	$547.60
15 - OhioCare HMO				Phone: (614)555-2229		
56	TANAKHI0		0	10/8/2003	0	$62.00
61	LOPEZCA0		0	11/30/2010	0	$38.00
67	JACKSLU0		0	1/5/2011	0	$113.00
69	STERNNA0		0	1/5/2011	0	$270.00
					Total:	$483.00
16 - Midwest Select HMO				Phone: (614)555-1211		
59	HSUDIAN0		0	11/30/2010	0	$67.00
60	HSUEDWI0		0	11/30/2010	0	$24.00
					Total:	$91.00
4 - Blue Cross/Blue Shield				Phone: (614)024-9000		
48	GILESSH0		0	10/8/2003	0	$221.00
54	SIMMOJI0		0	10/8/2003	0	$105.00
66	GILESSH0		0	1/5/2011	0	$85.00
68	SIMMOJI0		0	1/5/2011	0	$94.00
					Total:	$505.00
					Report Total:	$1,640.60

Figure 10-20 **Sample Insurance Collection Report**

The selections for the report can be filtered by Chart Number Range, Date Created Range, Initial Billing Date 1 Range (or 2 or 3 for secondary and tertiary claims), and Claim Status 1 Match (or 2 or 3 for secondary and tertiary claims).

PATIENT LEDGER

patient ledger a report that lists the financial activity in each patient's account, including charges, payments, and adjustments.

A **patient ledger** lists the financial activity in each patient's account, including charges, payments, and adjustments (see Figure 10-21). This information is especially useful if there is a question about a patient's account. A full set of patient ledgers details the status of every patient's account.

Patient Account Ledger
From July 1, 2010 to July 31, 2010

Entry	Date	POS	Description	Procedure	Document	Provider	Amount
SMITHSA0		**Sarabeth Smith**		(614)822-0000			
		Last Payment: -25.00	On: 6/9/2010				
404	7/12/2010			EAPCPAY	1007120000	3	-25.00
402	7/12/2010			99213	1007120000	3	62.00
403	7/12/2010			EAPCOPAY	1007120000	3	25.00
458	7/20/2010		#345687 East Ohio PPO	EAPPAY	1007120000	3	-62.00
		Patient Totals					0.00
WONGJO10		**Jo Wong**		(614)029-7777			
		Last Payment: -22.40	On: 6/14/2010				
405	7/12/2010			99212	1007120000	1	28.00
459	7/20/2010		#6457812 Medicare	MEDPAY	1007120000	1	-22.40
		Patient Totals					5.60
		Ledger Totals					5.60

Figure 10-21 Sample Patient Ledger Report

Patient ledgers are printed by clicking Patient Ledger on the Reports menu. The Print Report Where? dialog box is displayed. After the preview, print, or export selection is made, the Data Selection Questions dialog box is displayed, as it is with the other reports (see Figure 10-22). It provides options to select by chart numbers, patient reference balances, dates, and providers. A patient ledger is generated only for data that meet the selection criteria. If any selection box is left blank, all values are included in the report.

Chart Number Range In the Chart Number Range box, a range of chart numbers for patients is entered. If a report is needed for just one patient, that patient's chart number is entered in both boxes.

Patient Reference Balance Range Minimum and maximum dollar amounts are entered in the Patient Reference Balance Range boxes to delineate the dollar amount of an outstanding balance. The amounts are entered with decimal points.

Date From Range A range of dates is entered in the Date From Range boxes. For example, if it were necessary to print patient ledgers for the period of May 1 to May 15, 2010, "05012010" would be entered in the first box and "05152010" in the second box. If transactions were needed for the current date, that date would be entered in both boxes.

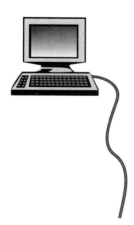

Patient Account Ledger : Data Selection Questions

NOTE: A blank field indicates no limitation, all records will be included.

Chart Number Range: [　　　▼ 🔍] to [　　　▼ 🔍]

Patient Reference Balance Range: [0.01] to [99999]

Date From Range: [7/1/2010 ▼] to [7/31/2010 ▼]

Attending Provider Range: [　　　▼ 🔍] to [　　　▼ 🔍]

Patient Billing Code Range: [　　　▼ 🔍] to [　　　▼ 🔍]

Patient Indicator Match: [　　　　　]

☐ Print one patient per page

☑ Show Accounts Receivable totals at the end of the report

✓ OK

✗ Cancel

🕮 Help

Figure 10-22 **Data Selection Questions dialog box for Patient Account Ledger Report**

Attending Provider Range   A range of codes for the attending providers is entered in the Attending Provider Range boxes.

Patient Billing Code Range   If the practice uses NDCMedisoft's Billing Code feature, codes can be entered in this box to select only those patients with the designated billing code(s).

Patient Indicator Match   If the practice has assigned a Patient Indicator code to each patient, an entry can be made to select only those patients who match a specific code.

Print One Patient Per Page   Clicking this box prints one report per page.

Show Accounts Receivable Totals at the End of the Report   If this box is checked, accounts receivable totals will appear at the end of the report.

Exercise 10-6

Print patient ledgers for July 2010 for patients whose last names begin with the letters *R* through *W*.

Date: July 31, 2010

1. On the Reports menu, click Patient Ledger.

2. If necessary, click the radio button for previewing the report on-screen. Click the Start button.

3. Key *R* in the first box of the Chart Number Range box and press Tab. Key *W* in the second box. Notice that the program stopped at the first patient with a last name beginning with *W*. To include all patients with last names beginning with *W*, key *WONGL* to select Li Wong, the last patient, and press Tab.

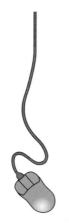

4. **In the first Date From Range box, enter July 1, 2010. In the second box, enter July 31, 2010.**

5. **Make certain that the Print One Patient Per Page box is not checked.**

6. **If it is not already checked, be sure to check the Show Accounts Receivable Totals at the End of the Report box.**

7. **Leave the remaining boxes blank.**

8. **Click the OK button.**

9. **Send the report to the printer.**

10. **Exit the Preview Report window.**

CUSTOM REPORTS

NDCMedisoft has already created a number of custom reports using the built-in Report Designer. These reports include:

◆ Lists of addresses, billing codes, EDI receivers, patients, patient recalls, procedure codes, providers, and referring providers

◆ The CMS(HCFA)-1500 and other claims in a variety of printer formats

◆ Patient statements and walkout receipts

◆ Superbills (encounter forms)

When Custom Report List is clicked on the Reports menu, the Open Report dialog box is displayed, listing a variety of custom reports already created in NDCMedisoft using the Report Designer (see Figure 10-23). Additional custom reports can be created using the Report Designer. When a new custom report is created, it is added to the list of custom reports that is displayed on-screen.

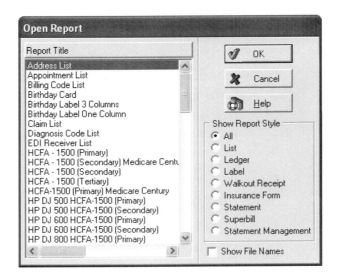

Figure 10-23 **Open Report Dialog Box**

The Open Report dialog box also contains nine radio buttons that are used to control the list of reports displayed in the dialog box. When the All radio button is clicked, all types of custom reports are listed in the dialog box. However, when one of the other radio buttons is clicked, only reports of that style are listed. For example, if the Insurance Form radio button is clicked, only reports that are insurance forms are listed.

To print a custom report, the title of the report is highlighted by clicking it, and then the OK button is clicked. The same options that are available with standard reports for previewing the report on-screen, sending it directly to the printer, or exporting it to a file are available with custom reports.

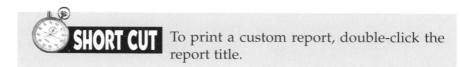 **SHORT CUT** To print a custom report, double-click the report title.

Exercise 10-7

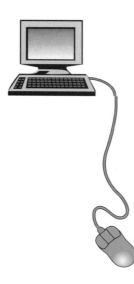

Print a list of all patients in the database.

Date: July 31, 2010

1. On the Reports menu, click Custom Report List.

2. Select Patient List. Click the OK button.

3. Click the radio button to preview the report on-screen. Click the Start button.

4. Leave the Chart Number Range boxes blank to select all patients.

5. Click the OK button.

6. View the report on-screen.

7. Send the report to the printer.

8. Exit the Preview Report window.

Exercise 10-8

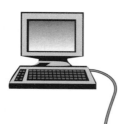

Print a list of all procedure codes in the database.

Date: July 31, 2010

1. On the Reports menu, click Custom Report List.

2. In the Show Report Style section of the dialog box, click the List radio button.

3. Select Procedure Code List. Click the OK button.

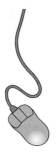

4. Click the radio button to preview the report on-screen. Click the Start button.

5. Leave the Code 1 Range boxes blank to select all procedure codes. Click the OK button.

6. View the report on-screen.

7. Send the report to the printer.

8. Exit the Preview Report window.

USING REPORT DESIGNER

NDCMedisoft's Report Designer provides maximum flexibility and control over data in the report and how they are displayed. Formatting styles include list, ledger, statement, and insurance. Reports can be created from scratch, or an existing report can be used as a starting point. The details of how to create new custom reports with the Report Designer is beyond the coverage of this book, but Exercise 10-9 offers practice working with the Report Designer to modify an existing report. The Report Designer is accessed by clicking Design Custom Reports and Bills on the Reports menu. This action causes the Report Designer window to be displayed (see Figure 10-24).

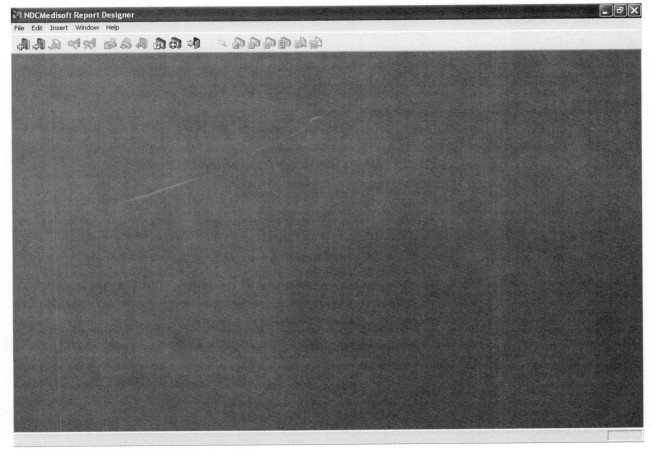

Figure 10-24 **The Report Designer Window**

Exercise 10-9

Modify the Patient List report so that a work telephone number replaces a home telephone number in the report.

Date: July 31, 2010

1. On the Reports menu, click Design Custom Reports and Bills. The Report Designer window is displayed.

2. Click Open Report on the File menu. The Open Report dialog box is displayed.

3. Double-click Patient List in the list. The Patient List report is displayed (see Figure 10-25).

4. Double-click on Phone that appears between the two horizontal black lines near the top of the report to select it. Then, double-click Phone again to edit it. The Text Properties dialog box is displayed (see Figure 10-26).

5. Enter *Work Phone* in the Text box that currently reads Phone.

6. Since Work Phone contains more letters than Phone, it is necessary to lengthen the space allotted for the label on the report so all the letters can be displayed. This is done in the section of the dialog box labeled Size. Click in the Auto Size box to deselect that option. In the Width box, delete the existing entry by using the Backspace key and enter *120*.

7. Click the OK button. Work Phone is displayed in the band where Phone used to be.

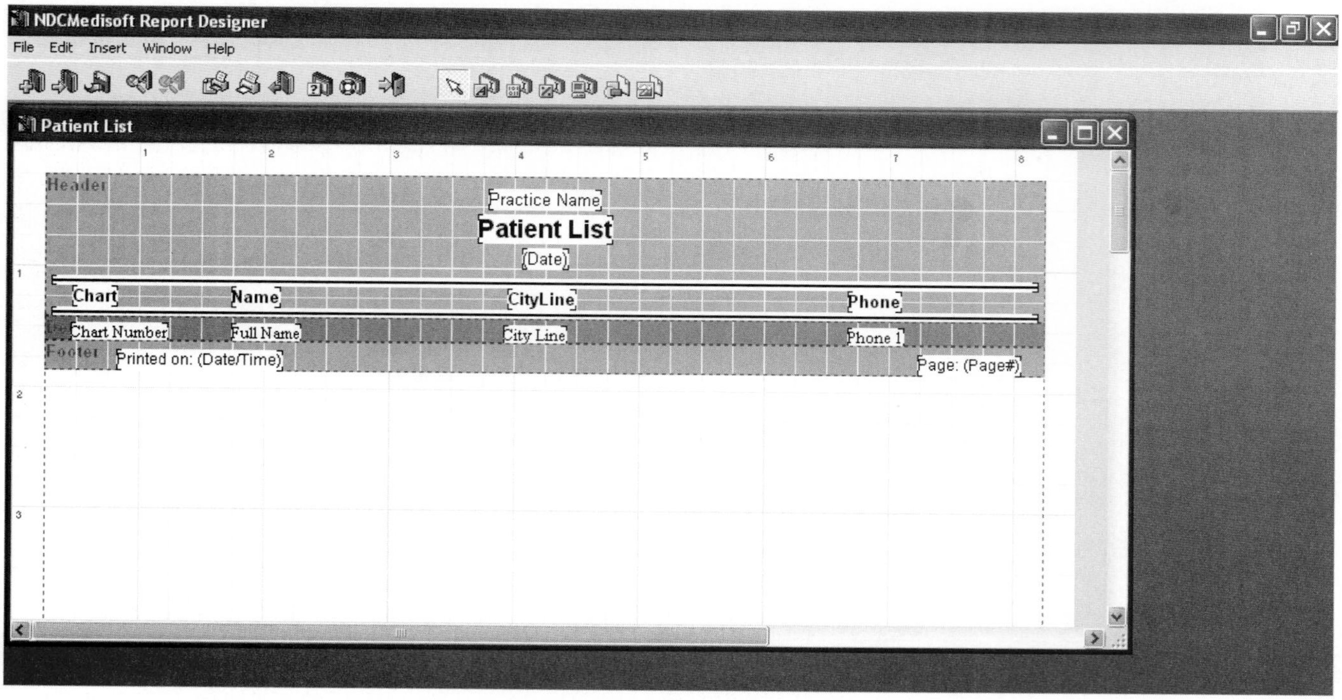

Figure 10-25 **Patient List Report Open in NDCMedisoft Report Designer**

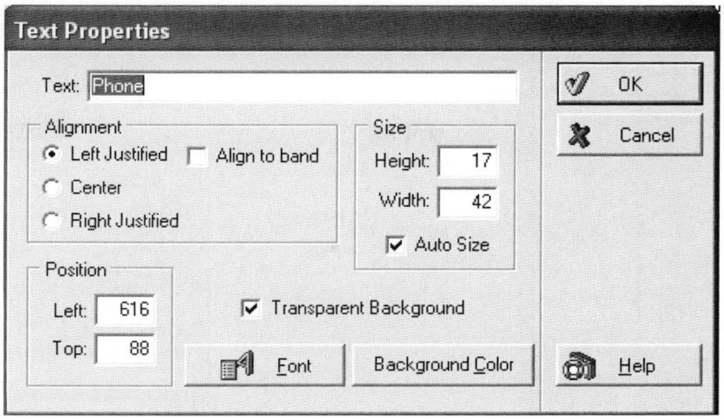

Figure 10-26 **Text Properties Dialog Box**

8. **In the green band below the band in which Work Phone appears, click the Phone 1 box to select it. Then double-click the Phone 1 box again to edit its contents. The Data Field Properties dialog box is displayed (see Figure 10-27).**

9. **The current data box, Print Patient Phone 1, is active in the Data Field and Expressions box. Click the Edit button to change this box. The Select Data Field dialog box is displayed (see Figure 10-28 on page 236).**

10. **In the Fields column, scroll down and highlight Work Phone and click OK. The Data Field and Expressions box now lists Print Patient Work Phone.**

11. **To increase the space allotted in the report for this new value, click the Auto Size box to deselect it. Then go to the Width box, delete the existing entry, and key *120.* Click the OK button. Work Phone is displayed where Phone 1 used to be.**

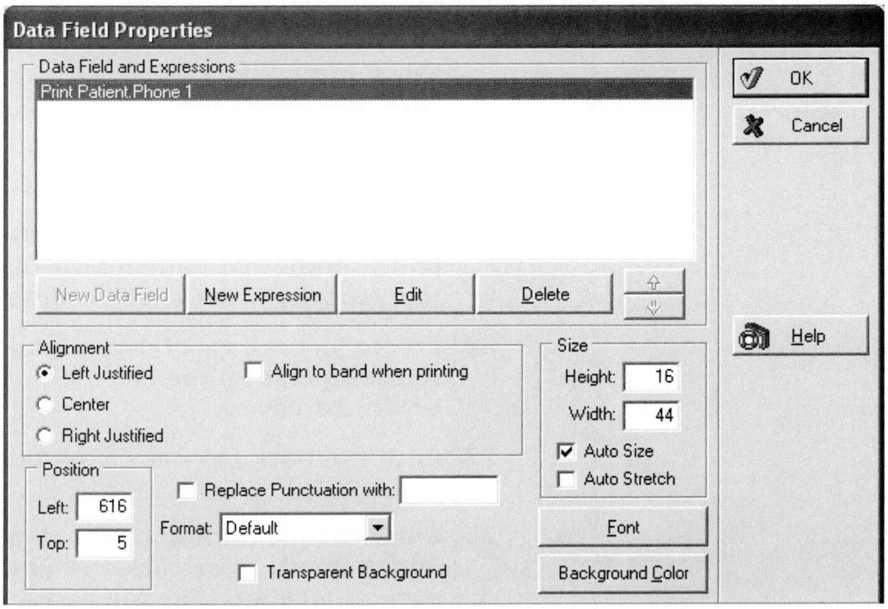

Figure 10-27 **Data Field Properties Dialog Box**

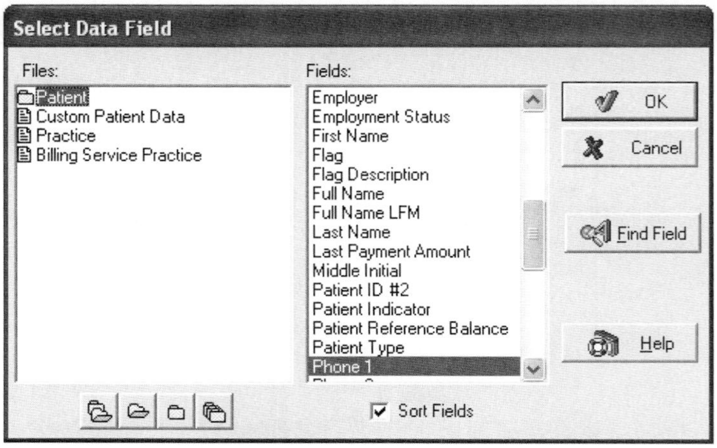

Figure 10-28 **Select Data Field Dialog Box**

12. On the Report Designer File menu, click Preview Report to see how the report will look when printed. The Save Report As. . . dialog box is displayed.

13. Key *Patient List—Work* in the Report Title box. Click the OK button. The Data Selection Questions dialog box is displayed.

14. Leave the Chart Number Range boxes blank to select all patients for the report.

15. Click the OK button.

16. The Preview Report dialog box is displayed, showing the report.

17. Click the Print button to print the report.

18. Exit the Preview Report window.

19. Click Close on the Report Designer File menu, or click the Close button in the top-right corner of the dialog box, to close the report file.

20. Click Exit on the File menu, or click the Exit button on the toolbar, to leave NDCMedisoft's Report Designer.

21. Select Custom Report List on the Reports menu. Scroll down and confirm that Patient List—Work appears in the list of custom reports. Click Cancel to close the Open Report dialog box.

22. Create a backup of your work and exit NDCMedisoft by selecting Exit on the File menu. The Backup Reminder dialog box is displayed.

23. Click the Back Up Data Now button. The Backup dialog box appears.

24. Enter the file path and file name in the Destination File Path and Name box or click the Find button and browse to the desired location. The file name should be FCC8-10.mbk (the database name followed by the chapter number). The file

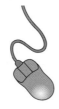

path will vary depending on your computer and network setup. Ask your instructor for the file path.

25. Click the Start Backup button. NDCMedisoft creates a backup file. When it is complete, an Information box is displayed, indicating that the backup is complete. Click OK. The Backup dialog box closes and the program is shut down.

CHAPTER REVIEW

USING TERMINOLOGY

Match the terms on the left with the definitions on the right.

_____ **1.** aging report

_____ **2.** day sheet

_____ **3.** patient day sheet

_____ **4.** patient ledger

_____ **5.** payment day sheet

_____ **6.** practice analysis report

_____ **7.** procedure day sheet

a. A summary of the activity of a patient on a given day.

b. A report that lists the amount of money owed the practice, organized by the length of time the money has been owed.

c. A report that provides information on practice activities for a twenty-four-hour period.

d. A report that lists the financial activity in each patient's account, including charges, payments, and adjustments.

e. A report that lists payments received on a given day, organized by provider.

f. A report that analyzes the revenue of a practice for a specified period of time, usually a month or a year.

g. A report that lists the procedures performed on a given day, listed in numerical order.

CHECKING YOUR UNDERSTANDING

Answer the questions below in the space provided.

8. What is the difference between a patient day sheet and a procedure day sheet? Which report is printed and mailed to patients with an outstanding balance?

_____

_____

9. What is the name of the dialog box that provides options for filtering data included on a report?

_____

_____

10. Which report indicates how far past due a patient's account is?

_____

_____

11. Which entries print in a report if the boxes in the Data Selection Questions dialog box are left blank?

_____

_____

APPLYING KNOWLEDGE

Answer the questions below in the space provided.

12. One of the providers in a practice asks for a report of yesterday's transactions. How would this report be created?

_____

_____

_____

13. A patient is unsure of whether she mailed a check last month for an outstanding balance on her account. How could you use NDCMedisoft's Reports feature to help answer the question?

_____

_____

_____

CHAPTER 11

Using Utilities

To use this chapter, you need to know how to:
◆ Start NDCMedisoft and use menus.
◆ Enter and edit text.

WHAT YOU WILL LEARN

When you finish this chapter, you will be able to:
◆ Make backup copies of data.
◆ View and restore backed up data.
◆ Use NDCMedisoft's file maintenance features.

KEY TERMS

packing data
purging data

rebuilding indexes
restoring data

NDCMEDISOFT'S UTILITY FEATURES

NDCMedisoft provides a number of built-in utilities to manage and maintain the data stored in the system. The utilities in NDCMedisoft are used for saving and storing data, retrieving data, maintaining data files, and deleting data that are no longer needed. All of NDCMedisoft's utilities are accessed through the File menu.

Whenever information is stored on a computer, it is possible to lose it. The cause can be a machine failure, sometimes called a hard disk crash, or the cause can be human error, such as when data are erased by accidentally pressing the wrong key. NDCMedisoft's backup utility can minimize the amount of data that have to be reentered should a loss occur. If copies of computer data files, called backups (see Chapter 3), are created on a regular basis, the amount of actual data gone from a system when a data loss occurs is minimal. It is limited to the amount entered between the time of the loss and the time the last backup was performed.

BACKING UP DATA

Medical offices generally have a regular schedule for backing up data. Depending on the volume of information, backups may be done as often as once a day or as infrequently as once a week. When data are backed up, they are stored on a removable media device. A removable media device stores data but is not a permanent part of a computer. Examples of removable media devices include disks, cartridges, tapes, and CD-ROMs. Removable media devices may be stored at a location other than the office to protect them from fire or theft.

To perform a data backup in an office situation, you would complete the following steps.

1. Click Backup Data on the File menu. The NDCMedisoft Backup dialog box is displayed (see Figure 11-1).

2. Insert the removable media device in the drive.

3. In the Destination File Path and Name box at the top of the NDCMedisoft Backup dialog box, key the drive, directory, and filename of the location where the backup copy of the data is to be stored. This should correspond to the drive that contains the removable media device, and should include a name for the backup file, such as A:\FCC8.mbk.

4. After the Destination File Path and Name box is complete, click the Start Backup button. The program copies the data from the source (indicated in the Source Path box in the lower half of the NDCMedisoft Backup dialog box) to the location indicated in the

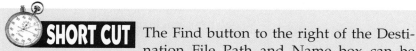

SHORT CUT The Find button to the right of the Destination File Path and Name box can be used to browse through and locate a destination drive and directory on your system. When you click Find, the Browse for Folder dialog box appears. Locate the appropriate destination drive and directory name in the dialog box and then click the OK button. The Browse for Folder dialog box closes, and the selected drive and directory name are copied to the Destination File Path and Name box for you. The name of the backup file is added to the drive and directory name to complete the entry in the Destination File Path and Name box.

Destination File Path and Name box. In the backup process, the source path is the drive and directory of the file that is being backed up.

5. When the backup is complete, an Information dialog box appears with the message "Backup complete." Click the OK button to continue.

6. The NDCMedisoft Backup dialog box disappears. Eject the removable media device, and label it with the date and time of the backup and with any other information required by the medical office.

As a security feature for protecting data, the NDCMedisoft Backup dialog box also contains a Password box. If a password is assigned

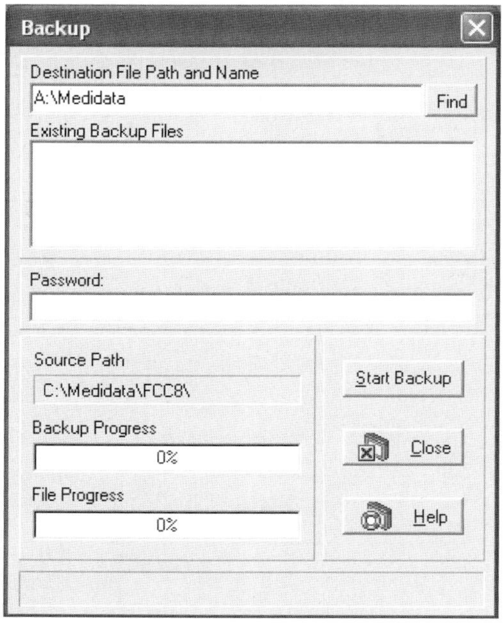

Figure 11-1 **Backup Dialog Box**

to a backup file, the password must be used to restore the data to the system. Each backup file can be assigned a different password.

Viewing Backup Data

NDCMedisoft provides a feature that allows a list of files on a backup device to be viewed on-screen or in a printed format. Information about the backup files is listed in the Backup View dialog box. In the top section of the dialog box, the following information is displayed: the name of the backup file and its location, the time and date it was created, the original data path, and the total number of files. The middle of the dialog box contains information about each file in the backup. File names, dates, times, original and compressed sizes, and the percentage of disk space saved by compression are listed.

To view backup data in an office situation, you would complete the following steps.

1. Click View Backup Disks on the File menu. The View Backup dialog box is displayed (see Figure 11-2).

2. Enter the data path for the backup files in the Source Path box, or use the Find button to locate the disk or the device with the backup files.

3. Click the View Backup button. The Backup View dialog box is displayed (see Figure 11-3).

4. Review the information on-screen, or print it by clicking the Print button.

5. Click the Close button to exit the Backup View dialog box.

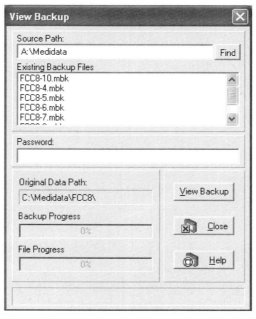

Figure 11-2 **View Backup Dialog Box**

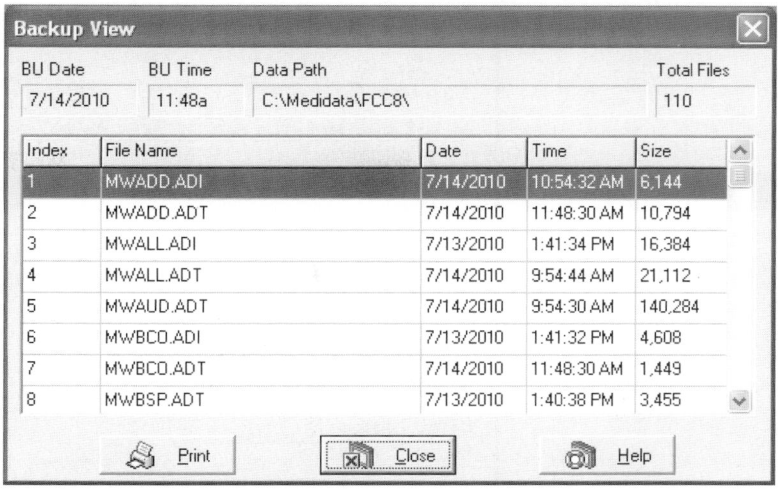

Figure 11-3 **Backup View Dialog Box**

RESTORING DATA

restoring data the process of retrieving data from backup storage devices.

The process of retrieving data from backup storage devices is called **restoring data.** Restoring data replaces all other data in the database. Since backup data are typically at least one day old, all the transactions, patient data, and appointments that were entered since the backup was made need to be reentered. This is one reason why it is important to print daily reports of activity in the practice. These reports can be used to reenter data when data need to be restored.

Under normal working conditions, data are not restored very often. In an office, only if there were serious problems with the current data would it be necessary to use NDCMedisoft's restore feature. However, in an instructional environment where computers are shared by many people, a program's restore feature is often used in combination with a backup feature to save students' work. In this text, data are restored from the Student Data Disk to the hard drive at the beginning of each session and then backed up again to the Student Data Disk at the end of each session. By restoring their files before each session, students are certain to be working on their own data.

To restore data, you would complete the following steps.

1. Click Restore Data on the File menu. A Warning box is displayed, stating that the current files are about to be overwritten. The options in this box are OK and Cancel. If the OK button is clicked, the Restore dialog box is displayed (see Figure 11-4 on page 246).

2. Insert the removable media device that contains the backup data in the drive.

3. The Restore dialog box is displayed (Figure 11-4).

4. In the Backup File Path and Name box at the top of the dialog box, key the drive, directory, and file name of the disk or the device containing the backup file that is to be restored, for example, *A:\FCC8.mbk*.

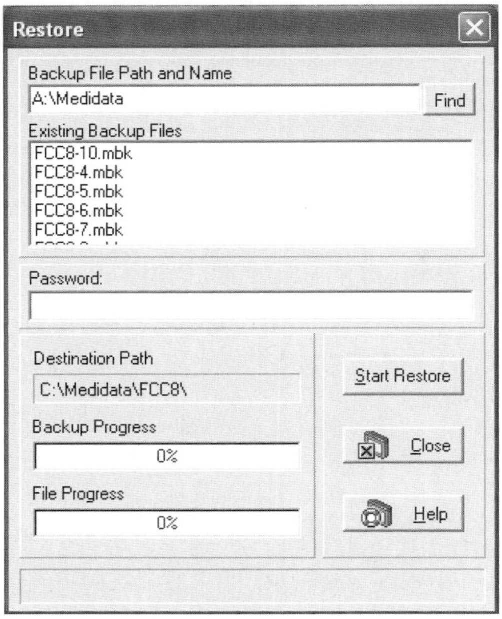

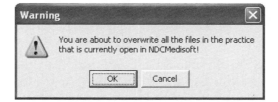

Figure 11-4 **Restore Dialog Box**

> **TIP>** The Find button to the right of the Backup File Path and Name box can be used to browse and locate the source drive and directory.

5. Click the Start Restore button. A Warning dialog box is displayed (see Figure 11-5). Click the OK button to continue. (Clicking the Cancel button cancels the restore process.)

6. After the program restores the data to the system, an information dialog box is displayed, indicating that the restore is complete. Click OK.

7. The Restore dialog box disappears.

FILE MAINTENANCE UTILITIES

NDCMedisoft provides four features to assist in maintaining data files stored in a system. These four features are found on tabs in the File Maintenance dialog box (see Figure 11-6).

1. Rebuild indexes

2. Pack data

Figure 11-5 **Restore Warning Dialog Box**

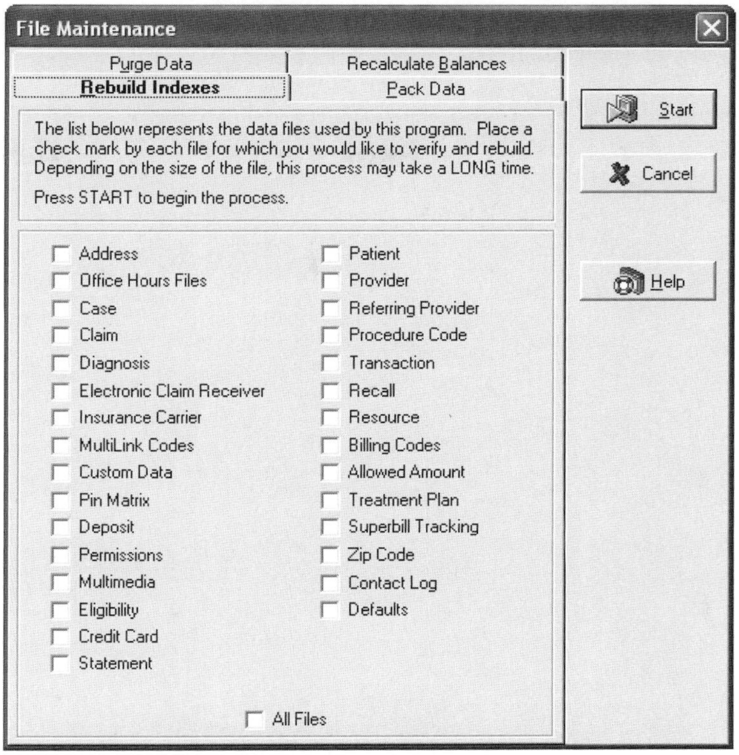

Figure 11-6 **File Maintenance Dialog Box**

3. Purge data

4. Recalculate balances

The dialog box is accessed by clicking File Maintenance on the File menu.

If the medical office's database is large, NDCMedisoft's utilities may take a long time to finish. For this reason, it is usually a good idea to use the utility functions at the end of the day or when the system will not be needed for a while.

Rebuilding Indexes

rebuilding indexes a process that checks and verifies data and corrects any internal problems with the data.

Rebuilding indexes is a process that checks and verifies data and corrects any internal problems with the data. The rebuild process does not check or verify the content of the data. For example, the system will not check whether John Fitzwilliams paid $50 on his last visit. Rebuilding does not change the content of any data files. To keep files working efficiently, files should be rebuilt about once a month. Files to be rebuilt are selected from the list of files in the Rebuild Indexes tab (see Figure 11-7 on page 248). If the database is large, rebuilding indexes could take a long time.

To rebuild files in NDCMedisoft in an office, you would complete the following steps.

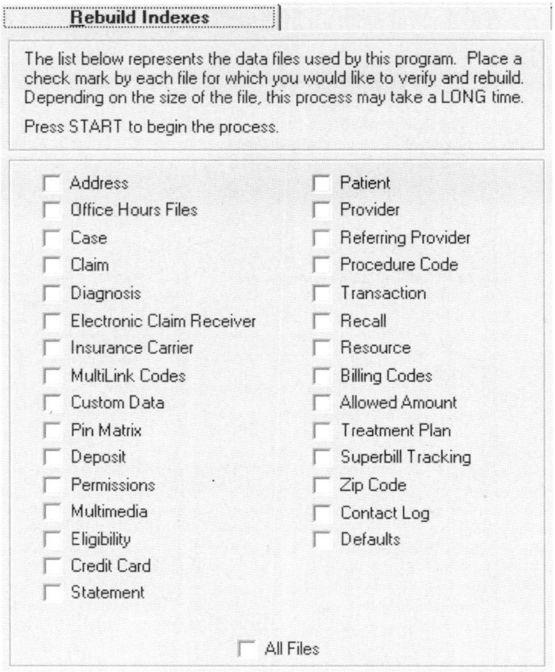

Rebuild Indexes

The list below represents the data files used by this program. Place a check mark by each file for which you would like to verify and rebuild. Depending on the size of the file, this process may take a LONG time.

Press START to begin the process.

☐ Address   ☐ Patient
☐ Office Hours Files   ☐ Provider
☐ Case   ☐ Referring Provider
☐ Claim   ☐ Procedure Code
☐ Diagnosis   ☐ Transaction
☐ Electronic Claim Receiver ☐ Recall
☐ Insurance Carrier   ☐ Resource
☐ MultiLink Codes   ☐ Billing Codes
☐ Custom Data   ☐ Allowed Amount
☐ Pin Matrix   ☐ Treatment Plan
☐ Deposit   ☐ Superbill Tracking
☐ Permissions   ☐ Zip Code
☐ Multimedia   ☐ Contact Log
☐ Eligibility   ☐ Defaults
☐ Credit Card
☐ Statement

                    ☐ All Files

Figure 11-7 Rebuild Indexes Tab

1. Click File Maintenance on the File menu. The File Maintenance dialog box is displayed with the Rebuild Indexes tab active.

2. Click in each check box next to the files that are to be verified and rebuilt. If all files are to be rebuilt, click the All Files box at the bottom of the list of files. This saves the time it would take to click a box for every NDCMedisoft file.

3. Click the Start button. The Confirm dialog box is displayed with the message "All of the checked file processes will be performed. Do you want to continue?" Click the OK button to continue. (Clicking the Cancel button aborts the process.)

4. The rebuild process is performed automatically. When the process is complete, an Information dialog box displays the message "All checked file processes are complete." Click the OK button.

Packing Data

When data are deleted in NDCMedisoft, the system empties the data from the record but keeps the empty slot in the database so it is available when new data need to be entered in the system. For example, if a patient was deleted in the Patient List dialog box, the system would delete all the records pertaining to that patient but would maintain an empty slot in the patient database. Then, the next time a new patient is entered, the data for the new patient occupies the vacant slot. When there is not much space available on the hard disk, it is sometimes desirable to delete the vacant slots to make more disk space available. The deletion of vacant slots from the

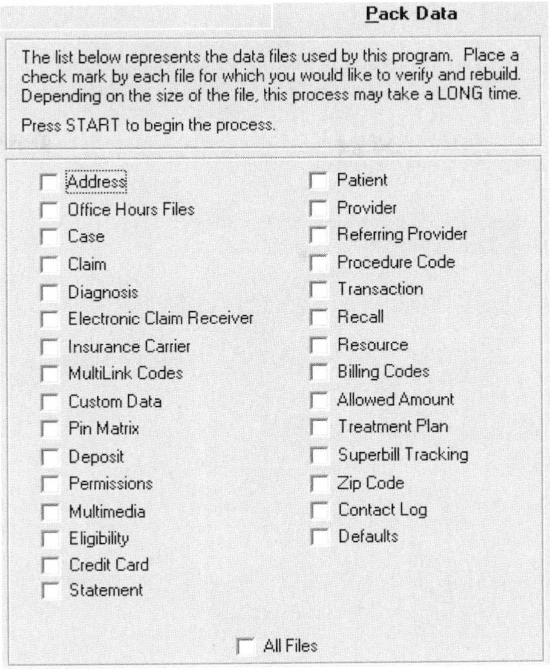

Pack Data	
The list below represents the data files used by this program. Place a check mark by each file for which you would like to verify and rebuild. Depending on the size of the file, this process may take a LONG time. Press START to begin the process.	

☐ Address   ☐ Patient
☐ Office Hours Files ☐ Provider
☐ Case   ☐ Referring Provider
☐ Claim   ☐ Procedure Code
☐ Diagnosis   ☐ Transaction
☐ Electronic Claim Receiver ☐ Recall
☐ Insurance Carrier ☐ Resource
☐ MultiLink Codes   ☐ Billing Codes
☐ Custom Data   ☐ Allowed Amount
☐ Pin Matrix   ☐ Treatment Plan
☐ Deposit   ☐ Superbill Tracking
☐ Permissions   ☐ Zip Code
☐ Multimedia   ☐ Contact Log
☐ Eligibility   ☐ Defaults
☐ Credit Card
☐ Statement

☐ All Files

Figure 11-8 **Pack Data Tab**

packing data *the deletion of vacant slots from the database.*

database is known as **packing data.** Data for packing can be selected from the list of files in the Pack Data tab (see Figure 11-8). (Only transaction files with a zero balance can be deleted.) If the database is large, packing data can take a long time.

To pack files in an office situation, you would complete the following steps.

1. Click File Maintenance on the File menu. The File Maintenance dialog box is displayed with the Rebuild Indexes tab active. Make the Pack Data tab active.

2. Click in each check box next to the files that are to have deleted data removed. If all files are to be checked for deleted data, click the All Files box at the bottom of the list of files.

3. Click the Start button. The Confirm dialog box is displayed with the message "All of the checked file processes will be performed. Do you want to continue?" Click the OK button to continue. (Clicking the Cancel button aborts the process.)

4. The pack process is performed automatically. When the process is complete, an Information dialog box displays the message "All checked file processes are complete." Click the OK button.

purging data *the process of deleting files of patients who are no longer seen by a provider in a practice.*

Purging Data

The process of deleting files of patients who are no longer seen by a provider in a practice is called **purging data.** Purging data frees space

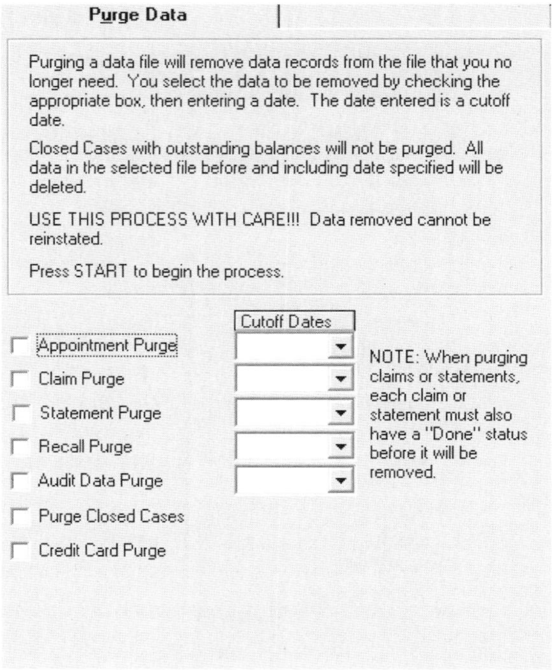

Figure 11-9 **Purge Data Tab**

on the computer and permits the system to run more efficiently. However, purging should be done with great caution. Once data are purged from the system, they cannot be retrieved, except from a backup file. As a safety precaution, always perform a backup before purging.

The Purge Data tab offers several options (see Figure 11-9). Data can be purged for appointments, claims, statements, appointment recalls, audit data, closed cases, or credit card information. All options except Purge Closed Cases are purged by date. A cutoff date is entered, and NDCMedisoft deletes all data up to that date. For example, if all the data entered prior to December 31, 2000, are to be purged, that date would be entered as the cutoff date. Data entered in cases that have been closed are purged by clicking the check box labeled "Purge Closed Cases."

To purge data in an office situation, you would complete the following steps.

1. Click File Maintenance on the File menu. The File Maintenance dialog box is displayed with the Rebuild Indexes tab active. Make the Purge Data tab active.

2. Click in each check box next to the files that are to be purged. Enter a cutoff date in the Cutoff Dates box.

3. Click the Start button. The Confirm dialog box is displayed with the message "All of the checked file processes will be performed.

Do you want to continue?" Click the OK button to continue. (Clicking the Cancel button aborts the process.)

4. The purge process is performed automatically. When the process is complete, an Information dialog box displays the message "All checked file processes are complete." Click the OK button.

Recalculating Patient Balances

As transaction entries are changed or deleted, there are times when the balance listed on-screen is not accurate. To update balances to reflect the most recent changes made to the data, the Recalculate Balances feature is used. This feature is accessed through the Recalculate Balances tab on the File Maintenance dialog box (see Figure 11-10).

When balances are recalculated, the system reviews every patient's data and recalculates the balances. The process of recalculating balances can be time-consuming. Individual patient balances can be recalculated in the Transaction Entry dialog box by clicking the Account Total column.

To recalculate balances in an office situation, you would complete the following steps.

1. Click File Maintenance on the File menu. The File Maintenance dialog box is displayed with the Rebuild Indexes tab active. Make the Recalculate Balances tab active.

2. Click to place a check mark in the Recalculate Balances box.

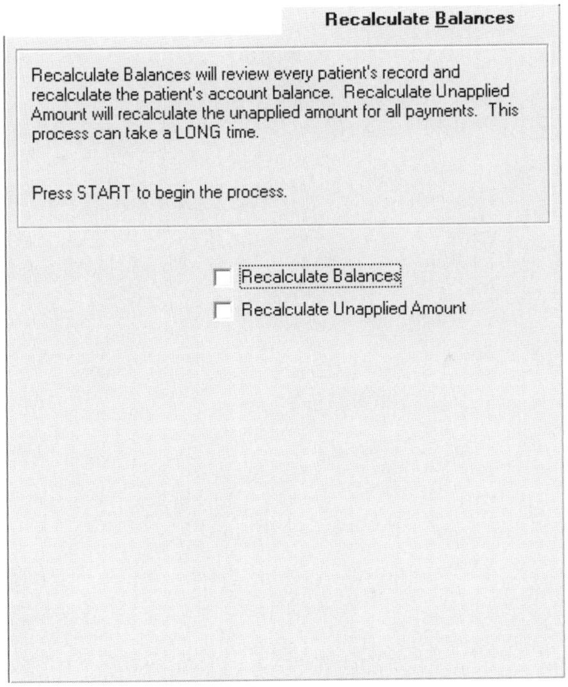

Figure 11-10 **Recalculate Balances Tab**

3. Click the Start button. The Confirm dialog box is displayed with the message "All of the checked file processes will be performed. Do you want to continue?" Click the OK button to continue. (Clicking the Cancel button aborts the process.)

4. The recalculate process is performed automatically. When the process is complete, an Information dialog box displays the message "All checked file processes are complete." Click the OK button.

CHAPTER REVIEW

USING TERMINOLOGY

Match the terms on the left with the definitions on the right.

_____ 1. packing data

_____ 2. purging data

_____ 3. rebuilding indexes

_____ 4. restoring data

a. the process of retrieving data from backup storage devices.

b. the process of deleting files of patients who are no longer seen by a provider in a practice.

c. a process that checks and verifies data and corrects any internal problems with the data.

d. the deletion of vacant slots from the database.

CHECKING YOUR UNDERSTANDING

Answer the questions below in the space provided.

5. Why is it important to back up data regularly?

_____

_____

6. Why is extra caution required when purging data?

_____

_____

7. When is a data restore performed in an office setting?

_____

_____

8. In NDCMedisoft, where are the two places a patient's balance can be recalculated?

_____

_____

APPLYING KNOWLEDGE

Answer the question below in the space provided.

9. You come to work on a Monday morning and find that the office computer is not working. The systems manager informs everyone that the computer's hard disk crashed, and that all data that were not backed up are lost. What do you do?

_____

_____

_____

Applying
Your
Knowledge

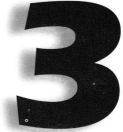

CHAPTER 12

Handling Patient Records and Transactions

WHAT YOU NEED TO KNOW

To complete the exercises in this chapter, you need to know how to:

◆ Locate patient information.

◆ Change the NDCMedisoft Program Date.

◆ Assign a new chart number and enter information on a new patient.

◆ Create a new case for a patient.

◆ Change information on an established patient.

◆ Add an insurance company to the database.

◆ Enter procedures, charges, and diagnoses.

◆ Record payments from patients and insurance carriers.

◆ Print walkout statements.

All office personnel at the Family Care Center (FCC) know how to input patient information in the Patient/Guarantor dialog box and in the Case dialog box. Whenever possible, all information for both dialog boxes is entered into the computer as soon as patients complete the handwritten information sheet and return it to the receptionist. On busy days, however, or when the office is understaffed because one of the medical assistants is sick or on vacation, input operations may be delayed.

EXERCISE 12-1: INPUTTING PATIENT INFORMATION

Note: Steps 1 through 3 are required at the beginning of each chapter. These steps start NDCMedisoft, set the path to the correct data location, and restore the data saved at the end of the last work session.

1. Hold down the F7 key and start NDCMedisoft. Enter the location of the NDCMedisoft data in the Find NDCMedisoft Directory box and click OK. (If you are unsure what to enter, ask your instructor.) When the Open Practice dialog box appears, verify that Family Care Center is highlighted and click OK.

2. Restore the data from your last work session by selecting Restore Data on the File menu. When a Warning box appears, click OK. Enter the file path and file name in the Destination File Path and Name or click the Find button and browse to the desired location. The file name should be FCC8-10.mbk (since no exercises were completed in Chapter 11). The file path will vary depending on your computer and network set up. Ask your instructor for the file path.

3. Click the Start Restore button. When a Confirm dialog box appears, click OK. NDCMedisoft restores the data. When it is complete, an Information box is displayed, indicating that the restore is complete. Click OK. The Restore box closes and the main NDCMedisoft window is displayed.

For this exercise, you need Source Documents 10–16.

It is Monday, November 15, 2010. You are a records/billing clerk at the Family Care Center. On your desk is a small pile of information sheets and encounter forms from Friday afternoon, November 12. You decide to input all patient information first, and then go back and record the transactions. First, you arrange the papers alphabetically:

    Battistuta

    Brooks

    Hsu

    Syzmanski

Then you begin. (Remember to change the NDCMedisoft Program Date to November 12, 2010.)

Patient 1: Anthony Battistuta

Record the address change that is written on Mr. Battistuta's encounter form (Source Document 10).

1. Click Patients/Guarantors and Cases on the Lists menu. The Patient List dialog box is displayed.

2. Select Anthony Battistuta from the list of patients.

3. Click the Edit Patient button. The Patient/Guarantor dialog box is displayed, with the Name, Address tab active.

4. Enter the new address.

5. Click the Save button.

Patient 2: Lawana Brooks

You can see from the encounter form (Source Document 11) that Ms. Brooks is an established patient. There are no changes to be made for her in the Patient/Guarantor dialog box. The work you need to do must take place in the Case dialog box. Ms. Brooks has had an accident at work, so a new case must be created.

1. After saving the changes for Mr. Battistuta in the Patient/ Guarantor dialog box, the Patient List dialog box is redisplayed.

2. In the list of patients, click the listing for Brooks to select her as the patient. In the list of cases, click the ankle sprain case. (You will not enter new information in the ankle sprain case; instead, you will copy information from the ankle sprain case to create a new case.)

3. Click the Copy Case button to copy the information from the existing case into a new case. A duplicate case is displayed.

4. Using Source Documents 11 and 12, edit the information in the case to reflect the information relevant to the new case by changing the information in the NDCMedisoft boxes listed below. If a box is not listed, either the information in that box does not need to be changed, or the box is to remain blank.

Personal Tab

Description

Diagnosis Tab

Default Diagnosis 1

Default Diagnosis 2

Default Diagnosis 3

Condition Tab

Injury/Illness/LMP Date

Illness Indicator

First Consultation Date (when a message about the date entry appears, click the No button)

Employment Related

Emergency

Accident Related to

Nature of

5. Save your work.

> **TIP** When entering information on different tabs within a dialog box, it is not necessary to click the Save button after completing work on each tab. However, the Save button must be clicked once all the tabs are complete, before exiting the dialog box.

Patient 3: Edwin Hsu

1. The information you need to make the necessary changes to the Patient/Guarantor dialog box for Edwin Hsu is on Source Documents 13 and 14. The new insurance company, Midwest Select, is not on the patient information form, nor is it in FCC's database. Edwin Hsu does not have his insurance card. You look up Midwest Select in the phone book, find the correct ZIP code on the map in the front of the phone book, and call the insurance company to find out what percentage of charges are covered by the plan. Midwest pays 100 percent after a $30 copayment.

2. After saving the new case for Brooks, you are in the Patient List dialog box. Select Edwin Hsu, and click the Edit Patient button.

3. Move to the Street box, and enter the new address.

4. Move to the home phone box and enter the new phone number.

5. Save the information you just entered.

6. Now the new insurance carrier must be added to the database. From the Lists menu, click Insurance Carriers.

> **TIP** If the entire dialog box is not visible on your monitor, resize the dialog box or use the scroll bars to see the additional entries.

7. The Insurance Carrier List dialog box is displayed.

8. Click the New Button to add information for Midwest Select.

9. Using the information on Source Document 14, enter the information in the following boxes.

Address Tab

Code

Name

Street

City

State

Zip Code

Phone

Practice ID

Options Tab

Plan Name

Type

Procedure Code Set

Diagnosis Code Set

Patient Signature on File

Insured Signature on File

Physician Signature on File

Print PINs on Forms

Default Billing Method

EDI, Codes Tab

EDI Receiver

EDI Payor Number

EDI Sub ID

NDC Record Code

EDI Max Transactions

Payment*

Adjustment

Withhold

Deductible

Take Back

* Notice that there are no Payment, Adjustment, Withhold, Deductible, or Take Back codes for Midwest Select, so they must be created.

Codes can be created from within the EDI, Codes tab by clicking in each box and pressing the F8 key. For example, to create a new Payment code, click in the Payment box and press F8. The Procedure/Payment/ Adjustment (new) dialog box opens. In the Code 1 box, key *MID-PAY*. Press Tab.

Key *Midwest Select Payment* in the Description box. Press the Tab key.

Click the Save button. The Procedure/Payment/Adjustment dialog box closes and MIDPAY is displayed in the Payment box on the EDI, Codes tab for Midwest Select.

Follow the same procedure to create Adjustment, Withhold, Take Back, and Deductible codes.

10. Click the Save button. Midwest Select is now displayed on the list of insurance carriers.

11. With Midwest Select HMO highlighted, click the Edit button. Continuing to use Source Document 14, complete the following boxes in the PINs tab.

Provider   PIN   Group ID

McGrath

Beach

Banu

12. Click the Save button.

13. Close the Insurance Carrier List dialog box. The Patient List dialog box is still displayed. Edwin Hsu is still the selected patient.

Create a charge code for the $30 copayment. This is the procedure code that is used to enter the charge for the $30 copayment.

14. Create a $30 copayment charge code for Midwest Select HMO, using the Procedure/Payment/Adjustment Codes option on the Lists menu.

15. Click the New button.

16. Key *MIDCOPAY* in the Code 1 box.

17. Enter *Midwest Select Copayment Charge* in the Description box.

18. Enter *16* in the Don't Bill to Insurance field, since the copayment charge should not be billed to the insurance carrier (16—Midwest Select).

19. Click on the Amounts tab. Enter *30* in the A field, since Midwest Select uses Price Code A.

20. Click the Save button.

Create a payment code for the $30 copayment. This is the procedure code that is used to enter the payment of the copayment.

21. Create a $30 copayment payment code for Midwest Select HMO.

22. The Procedure/Payment/Adjustment List dialog box should still be displayed.

23. Click the New button.

24. Key *MIDCPAY* in the Code 1 box.

25. Enter *Midwest Select Copayment* in the Description box.

26. Select Check copayment in the Code Type box.

27. Click on the Amounts tab. Enter *30* in the A field, since Midwest Select uses Price Code A.

28. Click the Save button. Close the Procedure/Payment/Adjustment List dialog box.

Create a new case.

29. Create a new case for Edwin Hsu by copying his existing case.

30. Using Source Documents 13 and 14, edit the information in the copied case to reflect the information relevant to the new case. Change information in the following boxes:

Personal Tab

Description

Account Tab

Price Code

Diagnosis Tab

Default Diagnosis 1

Policy 1 Tab

Insurance 1

Policy Holder 1

Relationship to Insured

Policy Number

Group Number

Accept Assignment

Capitated Plan

Copayment Amount

Insurance Coverage Percents by Service Classification: Enter 100 in all boxes if not already entered.

31. Click the Save button to save the new case.

> **TIP**> Do not change the insurance carrier in the urinary tract infection case for Edwin Hsu, because at the time he was treated for that condition, Hsu was covered by East Ohio PPO, not Midwest Select.

Patient 4: Hannah Syzmanski

Use Source Documents 15 and 16 to enter information on a new patient, Hannah Syzmanski. Hannah is the daughter of Michael and Debra Syzmanski, who are patients of Dr. Dana Banu. Hannah has been seeing her own doctor, a pediatrician, but is now switching to the Family Care Center.

1. Go to the Patient List dialog box, and click the New Patient button.

2. Key *SYZMAHAØ* in the Chart Number box.

3. Complete the Last Name and First Name boxes.

4. Click the Copy Address button. Select Hannah's father, Michael Syzmanski, on the list of patients, and then click the OK button. The program completes the address and phone number fields for you.

5. Complete the boxes for birth date, sex, and Social Security number.

6. Complete the following boxes in the Other Information tab.

   Type

   Assigned Provider

   Signature on File

   Signature Date

7. Save your work.

8. Click the Case radio button to make the Case portion of the Patient List dialog box active.

9. Click the New Case button to open a new Case dialog box.

10. Complete the following tabs in the Case dialog box.

    Personal Tab

    Description

    Guarantor

    Marital Status

    Student Status

    Account Tab

    Referring Provider

    Price Code*

* You will need to look up this information—Hannah is covered by her father's insurance policy. Because you can only have one case open at a time, click the Save button to save your work and close Hannah's case. Look up the information by opening Michael Syzmanski's acne case and checking the Account tab. Then return to Hannah's case.

Diagnosis Tab

Default Diagnosis 1

Allergies and Notes

Policy 1 Tab

When you attempt to complete the Policy 1 tab, you notice that Hannah has not filled in her insurance information. Since she is covered under her father's policy, it is easy to locate the information required to complete the Policy 1 tab.

First save your work on Hannah's case. As before, open the Case dialog box for the acne case for Michael Syzmanski. This time go to the Policy 1 tab. Use the information on that tab to fill in the missing insurance data for Hannah Syzmanski.

When completing the Policy 1 tab for Hannah, remember to list Michael Syzmanski in the Policy Holder 1 box and to click Child in the Relationship to Insured field.

11. Save your work.

EXERCISE 12-2: AN EMERGENCY VISIT

You will need Source Document 17 for this exercise.

It is still Monday morning, November 15, 2010. Carlos Lopez has just seen Dr. McGrath on an emergency basis. Mr. Lopez thought he was having a heart attack. Fortunately, Dr. McGrath has determined that he was just suffering from heart palpitations. You need to enter the procedure charges, accept his payment, and print a walkout receipt. Make sure all transaction information is properly recorded in the database.

1. Verify that the NDCMedisoft Program Date is November 15, 2010.

2. From the Patient List dialog box, create a new case for Carlos Lopez by copying the information in the case that already exists.

3. Using Source Document 17, complete the following boxes.

Personal Tab

Description

Diagnosis Tab

Default Diagnosis 1

Condition Tab

Injury/Illness/LMP Date

Illness Indicator

First Consultation Date

Emergency

4. Save your work. Close the Patient List dialog box.

5. Click Enter Transactions on the Activities menu.

6. Select Mr. Lopez in the Chart box.

7. Select Palpitations in the Case box.

8. Click the New button in the Charges section to create a new transaction.

9. Verify that the entry in the Date box is 11152010.

10. Enter the procedures marked on the encounter form. A reminder appears stating that the case requires a $30 copayment. Enter a charge for this copayment.

11. Now enter Lopez's $30 payment. Remember to enter a check number in the Check Number box. Then click the Apply button and apply the payment to the $30 copayment charge.

12. Click the Save Transactions button to save your work. When the Date of Service Validation boxes appear, click Yes to save the transactions. (*Note:* The box will appear once for each transaction entered that has a date in the future.)

13. Click the Quick Receipt button to print a walkout statement.

14. Close the Transaction Entry dialog box.

EXERCISE 12-3: INPUTTING TRANSACTION DATA

For this exercise, you need Source Documents 10, 11, 13, and 16.

You are now ready to record the transactions from Friday's four encounter forms. Before you begin, set the NDCMedisoft Program Date to November 12, 2010.

Anthony Battistuta

1. Click Enter Transactions on the Activities menu.

2. Select Anthony Battistuta in the Chart box.

3. Verify that Diabetes is displayed to the right of the Case box.

4. Record the procedures, one at a time.

5. Save your work.

Lawana Brooks

Follow essentially the same procedures to enter the transaction data. Remember to save your work.

Edwin Hsu

Follow essentially the same procedures to enter the transaction data. You need to record the code for the procedure as well as for the copayment charge. Then enter Hsu's payment, apply the payment to the charges, and save your work.

Hannah Syzmanski

Follow essentially the same procedures to enter the transaction data. You need to record the date and procedure, and Syzmanski's payment. Apply the payment to the charges, and save your work.

EXERCISE 12-4: ENTERING A NEW PATIENT AND TRANSACTIONS

For this exercise, you need Source Documents 18 and 19.

The date is November 12, 2010. Enter patient information and all transactions for Christopher Palmer, a new patient of Dr. Beach.

EXERCISE 12-5: ENTERING AND APPLYING AN INSURANCE CARRIER PAYMENT

For this exercise, you need Source Document 20.

The date is November 12, 2010. A remittance advice has just been received from East Ohio PPO with an Electronic Funds Transfer (EFT). Enter the deposit in NDCMedisoft and apply the payment to the appropriate patient accounts.

1. Open the Deposit List dialog box.

2. If necessary, change the date in the Deposit Date box to November 12, 2010.

3. Enter the deposit.

4. Apply the payment to the patient charges. Be sure to click the Save Payments/Adjustments button after each patient. Notice that as you enter and save payments, the amount listed in the Unapplied box decreases.

5. When you are finished, click the Detail button in the Deposit List dialog box to verify that the amount in the Unapplied column for each patient is 0.00.

6. Payments entered in the Deposit List dialog box are automatically linked to data in the Transaction Entry dialog box. Open the Transaction Entry dialog box and confirm that the insurance company payments and adjustments appear in the transaction list at the bottom of the window for each patient in this exercise. Close the Transaction Entry dialog box.

7. Create a backup of your work, and then exit NDCMedisoft. (Save the backup file as FCC8-12.mbk.)

CHAPTER 13

Setting Up Appointments

WHAT YOU NEED TO KNOW

To complete the exercises in this chapter, you need to know how to:

◆ Start Office Hours.
◆ Move around in the schedule.
◆ Enter appointments.
◆ Change appointment information.
◆ Move or copy an appointment.
◆ Schedule a recall appointment.
◆ Create a new case record for a patient.
◆ Change a transaction record.

The Family Care Center uses Office Hours as the primary tool for recording appointments. For the simulations in this chapter, assume that you are the front-desk receptionist and are responsible for most of the Center's scheduling tasks. Remember, you can access Office Hours at any time, no matter what you are working on. For example, suppose you are typing a letter for one of the doctors, and you get a phone call from a patient who wants to make an appointment. All you have to do is click the Start button on the task bar; select Programs—NDCMedisoft, and then Office Hours; enter the appointment; exit Office Hours; and return to your word-processing program. Office Hours can also be accessed from within NDCMedisoft, either by clicking the shortcut button or by clicking Appointment Book on the Activities menu.

EXERCISE 13-1: SCHEDULING APPOINTMENTS

Note: Steps 1 through 3 are required at the beginning of each chapter. These steps start NDCMedisoft, set the path to the correct data location, and restore the data saved at the end of the last work session.

1. Hold down the F7 key and start NDCMedisoft. Enter the location of the NDCMedisoft data in the Find NDCMedisoft Directory box and click OK. (If you are unsure what to enter, ask your instructor.) When the Open Practice dialog box appears, verify that Family Care Center is highlighted and click OK.

2. Restore the data from your last work session by selecting Restore Data on the File menu. When a Warning box appears, click OK. Enter the file path and file name in the Destination File Path and Name box or click the Find button and browse to the desired location. The file name should be FCC8-12.mbk. The file path will vary depending on your computer and network set up. Ask your instructor for the file path.

3. Click the Start Restore button. When a Confirm dialog box appears, click OK. NDCMedisoft restores the data. When it is complete, an Information box is displayed, indicating that the restore is complete. Click OK. The Restore box closes and the main NDCMedisoft window is displayed.

It is Monday, November 15, 2010. In Office Hours, schedule the following patient appointments on December 10, 2010:

Patient	Provider	Time	Length
Nancy Stern	P. McGrath	9:30	30 minutes
Sheila Giles	R. Beach	10:00	45 minutes
Raji Patel	D. Banu	2:45	30 minutes

4. Open Office Hours.

5. Go to December 10, 2010.

6. Select each patient's provider from the Provider drop-down list and enter the appointments.

EXERCISE 13-2: MAKING AN APPOINTMENT CHANGE

Carlos Lopez has just called to say that he lost his appointment card and cannot remember what time his appointment is on December 1. He thinks there may be a scheduling conflict with a meeting he has that day. If the appointment is in the morning, he wants you to change it to 2:00 that same day. If the 2:00 slot is not available, he needs to make the appointment for the next day at the earliest possible time.

1. Open Office Hours if it is not already open.

2. Go to December 1, 2010.

3. Find out who Lopez's doctor is by calling up the Patient/Guarantor dialog box in NDCMedisoft. Select the Other Information tab, and check the Assigned Provider box. Then select Lopez's provider from the Provider drop-down list in Office Hours.

4. Locate Mr. Lopez's appointment.

5. Check to see whether 2:00 P.M., the time he wanted to change the appointment to, is available.

6. Since 2:00 is not available, move to December 2 on the calendar and see if 8:00 A.M. is available.

7. Go back to December 1. Move Mr. Lopez's appointment from December 1 to December 2. (If you do not remember how to move an appointment, see Chapter 8.)

EXERCISE 13-3: JUGGLING SCHEDULES

Mrs. Jackson's sister is on the phone. She will be taking care of the Jackson twins, Darnell and Tyrone, on Saturday, December 11, 2010, and she needs to make an appointment for both of them for physicals and tetanus shots some time after 9:00 A.M. That is the only day they can come in, so she hopes you can accommodate her. She does not remember the name of their doctor.

1. Find out who the twins' doctor is by looking up the information in NDCMedisoft.

2. Go into Office Hours, and check the twins' provider's schedule for December 11. The doctor is booked solid from 8:00 A.M. until she leaves at 1:00 P.M.

3. Check the schedules of Dr. McGrath and Dr. Beach. Since Dr. McGrath is unavailable, book Darnell in the 10:30 A.M. time slot and Tyrone in the 10:45 A.M. slot with Dr. Beach.

EXERCISE 13-4: ADDING PATIENTS TO THE RECALL LIST

Darnell and Tyrone Jackson need to be called back for follow-up appointments in six months. Add both names to the Recall list for six months from December 11, 2010.

1. Click Patient Recall on the Lists menu in NDCMedisoft. The Patient Recall List dialog box is displayed.

2. Click the New button.

3. Enter June 11, 2011, in the Recall Date box.

4. Select Dr. Dana Banu in the Provider box.

5. Select Darnell Jackson's chart number from the drop-down list in the Chart box. Press the Tab key.

6. In the Message box, key *Six month follow-up appointment needed.*

7. Verify that the Call radio button in the Recall Status box is selected.

8. Click the Save button to save the entry.

9. Repeat the steps to add Tyrone Jackson to the Patient Recall List.

10. Close the Patient Recall List dialog box.

EXERCISE 13-5: DIANE HSU AND MICHAEL SYZMANSKI

For this simulation, you will need Source Documents 21 and 22.

It is Monday, November 15, 2010. Diane Hsu and Michael Syzmanski are leaving the office after their appointments. Use the information on Source Documents 21 and 22 to perform the following tasks:

1. Create new cases for both patients by copying existing cases.

For Hsu, complete the boxes listed below in the Personal, Account, Diagnosis, and Policy 1 tabs. When completing the Account and Policy 1 tabs for Hsu, remember that her husband changed insurance carriers to Midwest Select, and since she is covered under her husband's policy, the new insurance company information must be used. This information can be found in Edwin Hsu's acute sinusitis case (see also Source Document 14).

Personal Tab

Description

Account Tab

Price Code

Diagnosis Tab

Diagnosis 1

Policy 1 Tab

Insurance 1

Policy Number

Group Number

Policy Dates Start

Capitated Plan

Copayment Amount

For Syzmanski, complete the following boxes in the Personal and Diagnosis tabs.

Personal Tab

Description

Diagnosis Tab

Diagnosis 1

2. Record the charges in the Transaction Entry dialog box.

3. Record the payments and apply the payments to the charges.

4. Make the appointment indicated on Mrs. Hsu's encounter form, using Office Hours. Do not exit NDCMedisoft.

EXERCISE 13-6: CHANGING A TRANSACTION RECORD

Just as you finish making Mrs. Hsu's appointment, Dr. Robert Beach comes to the desk to say that he thinks he forgot to mark the encounter form for the strep test he performed on Christopher Palmer on November 12, 2010. He asks you to check and add the charge if necessary.

1. Go to the Transaction Entry dialog box. Check through the entries to find out whether the charge was entered. (It was not.)

2. Enter the new charge. (*Hint:* Remember to change the default date entry in the Date box to November 12, 2010.)

3. Create a backup of your work, and then exit NDCMedisoft. (Save the backup file as FCC8-13.mbk).

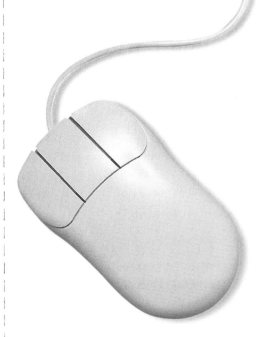

CHAPTER
14

Printing Lists and Reports

To complete the exercises in this chapter, you need to know how to:

- ◆ Create a patient ledger.
- ◆ Create a day sheet report.
- ◆ Understand what aging means, in an accounting sense.
- ◆ Create a patient aging report.
- ◆ Enter transactions.
- ◆ Print an appointment list.
- ◆ Print a patient ledger report.

Because NDCMedisoft is an accounting package, its most powerful features involve computerized manipulation of account data for patients. NDCMedisoft uses information in the system to produce reports on any facet of patients' or insurers' accounts and to generate bills for patients and insurance companies. For example, as long as the office personnel in the Family Care Center have entered transactions correctly and have performed basic accounting procedures, the NDCMedisoft program can be used to print current reports on the center's finances. You can print a report showing details of a day's transactions for any one of the center's physicians or for all physicians. You can print a report of late accounts for a particular patient or for all patients, for one insurance company or for all insurance companies.

Before starting the exercises in this chapter, you should understand some basic aspects of medical office accounting procedures.

Every medical office must keep a daily record of charges and payments made for every patient of every doctor. For charges, the record usually includes the name of the patient, the type of service provided, and the amount of the charge. For payments, the record usually includes the name of the patient whose account is being credited and the amount of the payment. Whereas day sheets record information on charges and payments for a single day, ledgers show all current information up to and including the date shown on the ledger.

As the name suggests, aging reports show clearly how long unpaid charges have been due. In NDCMedisoft, aging reports are divided into four columns, showing, in order, accounts that are currently due, accounts that have been due for 31–60 days, 61–90 days, 91–120 days, and accounts that have been due for more than 120 days.

EXERCISE 14-1: FINDING A PATIENT'S BALANCE

Note: Steps 1 through 3 are required at the beginning of each chapter. These steps start NDCMedisoft, set the path to the correct data location, and restore the data saved at the end of the last work session.

1. Hold down the F7 key and start NDCMedisoft. Enter the location of the NDCMedisoft data in the Find NDCMedisoft Directory box and click OK. (If you are unsure what to enter, ask your instructor.) When the Open Practice dialog box appears, verify that Family Care Center is highlighted and click OK.

2. Restore the data from your last work session by selecting Restore Data on the File menu. When a Warning box appears, click OK. Enter the file path and file name in the Destination File Path and Name box or click the Find button and browse to the desired location. The file name should be FCC8-13.mbk. The file path will vary depending on your computer and network set up. Ask your instructor for the file path.

3. Click the Start Restore button. When a Confirm dialog box appears, click OK. NDCMedisoft restores the data. When it is complete, an Information box is displayed, indicating that the restore is complete. Click OK. The Restore box closes and the main NDCMedisoft window is displayed.

It is still Monday, November 15, 2010. Anthony Battistuta calls. He would like to know the amount of the charges from November 12 that he is responsible for, assuming that Medicare pays its portion of the total charges. How can you find the amount he is responsible for?

4. On the Activities menu, click Enter Transactions.

5. In the Chart box, select Anthony Battistuta's chart number.

6. Verify that the Diabetes case is active in the Case box.

7. Look at the top section of the dialog box, where the information about estimated financial responsibility is listed. Determine the insurance carrier's portion of the charges, and then determine what amount of the charges is the guarantor's responsibility.

EXERCISE 14-2: PRINTING A SCHEDULE

Print the appointment schedule for Dr. Dana Banu for Saturday, December 11, 2010.

1. Open Office Hours.

2. Click Appointment List on the Office Hours Reports menu.

3. Select the option to print the report on the printer.

4. Click the Start button. The Data Selection dialog box appears.

5. Enter *12112010* in both Dates boxes.

6. Enter *6* in both Providers boxes.

7. Click the OK button.

8. When the Print dialog box is displayed, click the OK button.

9. Exit Office Hours.

EXERCISE 14-3: PRINTING DAY SHEET REPORTS

Patient day sheets and procedure day sheets can be viewed and/or printed using options on the Reports menu.

NDCMedisoft Program Date: November 12, 2010

Creating a Patient Day Sheet Report

1. On the Reports menu, click Day Sheets and then Patient Day Sheet.

2. Select the option to preview the report on-screen. Click the Start button.

3. Leave the Chart Number Range boxes blank, to include all patients.

4. Delete the entries in both Date Created Range boxes.

5. Key *11122010* in both Date From Range boxes.

6. Click the box to show the accounts receivable totals at the end of the report.

7. Leave all other boxes blank.

8. Click the OK button.

9. The patient day sheet report is displayed on-screen.

10. Close the Preview Report window.

Creating a Procedure Day Sheet Report

1. On the Reports menu, click Day Sheets and then Procedure Day Sheet.

2. Select the option to preview the report on-screen. Click the Start button.

3. Leave the Procedure Code Range boxes blank.

4. Delete both entries in the Date Created Range boxes.

5. Key *11122010* in both Date From Range boxes.

6. Click the box to show the accounts receivable totals at the end of the report.

7. Leave the Attending Provider boxes blank.

8. Click the OK button.

9. The procedure day sheet report appears on-screen.

10. Close the Preview Report window.

EXERCISE 14-4: CREATING A PATIENT AGING REPORT

Print a patient aging report as a first step in the billing process. The aging report shows which accounts are overdue and how long they have been overdue.

NDCMedisoft Program Date: November 30, 2010

1. On the Reports menu, click Aging Reports and then Patient Aging.

2. Select the option to preview the report on-screen. Click the Start button.

3. Enter *11302010* in the second Date From Range box.

4. Leave all other data selection fields blank.

5. Click the OK button.

6. View the report.

7. Close the Preview Report window.

EXERCISE 14-5: CREATING A PRACTICE ANALYSIS REPORT

Print a practice analysis report for the month of November 2010.

NDCMedisoft Program Date: November 30, 2010

1. On the Reports menu, click Analysis Reports and then Practice Analysis.

2. Select the option to preview the report on-screen. Click the Start button.

3. Enter *11302010* in the second Date From Range box.

4. Click the box to show the accounts receivable totals at the end of the report.

5. Leave all other data selection fields blank.

6. Click the OK button.

7. View the report.

8. Close the Preview Report window.

EXERCISE 14-6: STEWART ROBERTSON

You need Source Documents 23 and 24 for this exercise, which consists of two parts.

Part One: December 10, 2010

A new patient of Dr. Beach, Stewart Robertson, has stopped by to schedule an appointment and to fill out a patient information form. He wants an appointment in December, specifically for the third Saturday of the month, as early as possible, for a routine physical.

NDCMedisoft Program Date: December 10, 2010

1. Using Source Document 23, enter the patient information for Mr. Robertson. Complete the Patient/Guarantor dialog box and the Case dialog box. You need to create a new case.

2. In Office Hours, schedule Robertson for his appointment (sixty minutes).

Part Two: December 18, 2010

Stewart Robertson completes his office visit with Dr. Beach.

NDCMedisoft Program Date: December 18, 2010

1. Using Source Document 24, enter Robertson's diagnosis in NDCMedisoft.

2. Enter the charges and payments for Stewart Robertson's visit.

EXERCISE 14-7: MICHAEL SYZMANSKI

NDCMedisoft Program Date: December 18, 2010

1. Read the following account of Michael Syzmanski's visit to the Family Care Center on December 18, 2010.

While driving to his daughter Hannah's soccer game, Syzmanski had a minor automobile accident in Jefferson and has a cut on his eyelid. He has come in to see Dr. Banu on an emergency basis. Dr. Banu is unavailable, so he is treated by Dr. McGrath. She determines that there has been no serious damage. After an examination using a local anesthetic, Dr. McGrath stitches the cut and tells Syzmanski to come back in a week. The procedure is simple suture.

2. In NDCMedisoft, enter all the information pertaining to this visit using Source Document 25. (*Hint:* Remember to change the default entry in the Provider column in the Transaction Entry dialog box.)

3. Close the Transaction Entry dialog box.

4. Create a backup of your work, and then exit NDCMedisoft. (Save the backup file as FCC8-14.mbk.)

CHAPTER
15
Practicing Your Skills

WHAT YOU NEED TO KNOW

To complete the exercises in this chapter, you need to know how to:
- Schedule appointments.
- Create cases.
- Enter charges for procedures.
- Enter copayments from patients.
- Create claims.
- Enter payments from insurance carriers.
- Create patient statements.
- Print reports.

In this chapter, you need to use almost all the skills you have practiced throughout the exercises in the book. If you have any problems, refer back to the chapter earlier in the book that covers the material.

EXERCISE 15-1: SCHEDULING APPOINTMENTS

Note: Steps 1 through 3 are required at the beginning of each chapter. These steps start NDCMedisoft, set the path to the correct data location, and restore the data saved at the end of the last work session.

1. Hold down the F7 key and start NDCMedisoft. Enter the location of the NDCMedisoft data in the Find NDCMedisoft Directory box and click OK. (If you are unsure what to enter, ask your instructor.) When the Open Practice dialog box appears, verify that Family Care Center is highlighted and click OK.

2. Restore the data from your last work session by selecting Restore Data on the File menu. When a Warning box appears, click OK. Enter the file path and file name in the Destination File Path and Name box, or click the Find button and browse to the desired location. The file name should be FCC8-14.mbk. The file path will vary depending on your computer and network setup. Ask your instructor for the file path.

3. Click the Start Restore button. When a Confirm dialog box appears, click OK. NDCMedisoft restores the data. When it is complete, an Information box is displayed, indicating that the restore is complete. Click OK. The Restore box closes, and the main NDCMedisoft window is displayed.

4. Enter January 5, 2011, as the program date in NDCMedisoft.

5. Schedule appointments for January 5, 2011, for the following patients. Make sure they are scheduled for the right doctors.

Jackson, Luther	30 minutes	9:00 a.m.
Hsu, Diane	15 minutes	9:15 a.m.
Hsu, Edwin	15 minutes	9:15 a.m.
Simmons, Jill	15 minutes	10:15 a.m.
Stern, Nancy	1 hour	9:30 a.m.
Syzmanski, Debra	30 minutes	9:30 a.m.
Giles, Sheila	15 minutes	9:00 a.m.
Battistuta, Pauline	30 minutes	10:30 a.m.

6. Switch the appointment times for Giles and Simmons.

7. Cancel the appointments for both Hsus.

8. Print the appointment lists for January 5, 2011, for Dr. Banu, Dr. Beach, and Dr. McGrath.

EXERCISE 15-2: CREATING CASES

1. Create new cases for all patients with appointments on January 5, 2011. Fill in the following boxes on the Personal and Diagnosis tabs using the information found on Source Documents 26-31.

   Personal Tab

   Description

   Diagnosis Tab

   Diagnosis 1

EXERCISE 15-3: ENTERING TRANSACTIONS

1. Using Source Documents 26-31, record the charge and payment transactions for each of the patients who had appointments.

EXERCISE 15-4: CREATING CLAIMS

1. Create insurance claims for all transactions that have not already been placed on a claim. (*Hint:* Leave the Transaction Dates boxes blank in the Create Claims dialog box.) Change the Status for the newly created claims from Ready to Send to Sent.

EXERCISE 15-5: ENTERING INSURANCE PAYMENTS

1. Enter the insurance payments listed on Source Documents 32-37 and apply the payments to patient charges. For capitated payments, remember to open the Transaction Entry dialog box and adjust patient accounts to a zero balance. (*Hint:* Enter one write-off transaction for each charge transaction, using the WRITEOFF code.)

EXERCISE 15-6: CREATING PATIENT STATEMENTS

1. Create remainder statements as of 12/31/2010 for patients whose last names begin with letters J through T.

EXERCISE 15-7: PRINTING REPORTS

1. Print a patient aging report as of 12/31/2010.

2. Print a practice analysis report as of 12/31/2010.

3. Print a patient day sheet for 01/05/2011.

4. Create a backup of your work, and then exit NDCMedisoft. (Save the backup file as FCC8-15.mbk.)

Source Documents

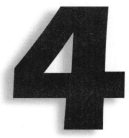

FAMILY CARE CENTER
285 Stephenson Boulevard
Stephenson, OH 60089-4000
614-555-0000

PATIENT INFORMATION FORM

Patient				
Last Name Tanaka	First Name Hiro	MI	Sex __ M _X_ F	Date of Birth 2 / 20 / 1975
Address 80 Cedar Lane	City Stephenson		State OH	Zip 60089
Home Ph # (614) 555-7373	Marital Status Single		Student Status	

SS# 812-73-6000	Allergies: penicillin			
Employment Status Full-time	Employer Name McCray Manufacturing Inc.	Work Ph # (614) 555-1001	Primary Insurance ID# 812736000 Group HJ31	
Employer Address 1311 Kings Highway	City Stephenson		State OH	Zip 60089
Referred By Dr. Bertram Brown	Ph # of Referral (614) 567-7896			

Responsible Party (Complete this section if the person responsible for the bill is not the patient)

Last Name	First Name	MI	Sex __ M __ F	Date of Birth / /
Address	City	State	Zip	SS#

Relation to Patient __ Spouse __ Parent __ Other	Employer Name	Work Phone # ( )
Spouse, or Parent (if minor):		Home Phone # ( )

Insurance (If you have multiple coverage, supply information from both carriers)

Primary Carrier Name OhioCare HMO	Price Code A	Secondary Carrier Name
Name of the Insured (Name on ID Card) Hiro Tanaka		Name of the Insured (Name on ID Card)
Patient's relationship to the insured _X_ Self __ Spouse __ Child		Patient's relationship to the insured __ Self __ Spouse __ Child
Insured ID # 812736000		Insured ID #
Group # or Company Name Group HJ31		Group # or Company Name
Insurance Address 147 Central Ave., Halevile, OH 60890		Insurance Address

Phone # 614-555-0101	Copay $ 30	Phone #	Copay $

Other Information

Is patient's condition related to:
__ Employment   _X_ Auto Accident (if yes, state in which accident occurred: <u>OH</u>)   __ Other Accident

Reason for visit: Accident - back pain

Date of Accident: 9 / 26 / 2010   Date of First Symptom of Illness: 9 / 26 / 2010

Authorization

I hereby authorize release of information necessary for my insurance company to process my claim. The above information is correct to the best of my knowledge.

Signed: <u>Hiro Tanaka</u>   Date: <u>10/4/2010</u>

I hereby authorize payment directly to FAMILY CARE CENTER insurance benefits otherwise payable to me. I understand that I am financially responsible for charges not paid in a timely manner by my insurance.

Signed: <u>Hiro Tanaka</u>   Date: <u>10/4/2010</u>

Source Document 2

ENCOUNTER FORM

10/4/2010
DATE

Dr. Katherine Yan
PROVIDER

Hiro Tanaka
PATIENT NAME

TANAKHI0
CHART #

OFFICE VISITS - SYMPTOMATIC	
99201	OF--New Patient Minimal
99202	OF--New Patient Low
99203	OF--New Patient Detailed
99204	OF--New Patient Moderate
99205	OF--New Patient High
99211	OF--Established Patient Minimal
99212	OF--Established Patient Low
99213	OF--Established Patient Detailed
99214	OF--Established Patient Moderate
99215	OF--Established Patient High

PREVENTIVE VISITS	
NEW	
99381	Under 1 Year
99382	1 - 4 Years
99383	5 - 11 Years
99384	12 - 17 Years
99385	18 - 39 Years
99386	40 - 64 Years
99387	65 Years & Up
ESTABLISHED	
99391	Under 1 Year
99392	1 - 4 Years
99393	5 - 11 Years
99394	12 - 17 Years
99395	18 - 39 Years
99396	40 - 64 Years
99397	65 Years & Up

PROCEDURES	
12011	Simple suture--face--local anes.
29125	App. of short arm splint; static
29425	App. of short leg cast, walking
45378	Colonoscopy--diagnostic
45380	Colonoscopy--with biopsy
50390	Aspiration of renal cyst by needle
71010	Chest x-ray, single view, frontal

PROCEDURES	
71020	Chest x-ray, two views, frontal & lateral
71030	Chest x-ray, complete, four views
73070	Elbow x-ray, AP & lateral views
73090	Forearm x-ray, AP & lateral views
73100	Wrist x-ray, AP & lateral views
73510	Hip x-ray, complete, two views
73600	Ankle x-ray, AP & lateral views
80048	Basic metabolic panel
80061	Lipid panel
82270	Blood screening, occult; feces
82947	Glucose screening--quantitative
82951	Glucose tolerance test, three specimens
83718	HDL cholesterol
84478	Triglycerides test
85007	Manual differential WBC
85018	Hemoglobin
85025	Complete CBC w/auto diff WBC
85651	Erythrocyte sedimentation rate--non-auto
86585	Tuberculosis, tine test
87076	Culture, anaerobic isolate
87077	Bacterial culture, aerobic isolate
87086	Urine culture and colony count
87430	Strep test
87880	Direct streptococcus screen
90471	Immunization administration
90703	Tetanus injection
90782	Injection
92516	Facial nerve function studies
93000	Electrocardiogram--ECG with interpretation
93015	Treadmill stress test, with physician...
96900	Ultraviolet light treatment
99070	Supplies and materials provided

FAMILY CARE CENTER

REFERRING PHYSICIAN
Dr. Bertram Brown

UPIN
A0011

AUTHORIZATION #

DIAGNOSIS
724.2

PAYMENT AMOUNT
$30 copay, check #123

NOTES

FAMILY CARE CENTER
285 Stephenson Boulevard
Stephenson, OH 60089-4000
614-555-0000

KATHERINE YAN, M.D.
PHYSICIAN'S NOTES

PATIENT NAME	Hiro Tanaka

CHART NUMBER	TANAKHI0

DATE	10/4/10

CASE	Accident - Back Pain

NOTES

Condition related to auto accident in Stephenson, Ohio that occurred on 9/26/10.

Patient was hospitalized from 9/26/10 to 9/27/10

Patient was totally disabled from 9/26/10 to 9/27/10

Patient was partially disabled from 9/28/10 to 10/4/10

Patient was unable to work from 9/26/10 to 10/4/10

Source Document 4

ENCOUNTER FORM

10/4/2010
DATE

Elizabeth Jones
PATIENT NAME

Dr. Katherine Yan
PROVIDER

JONESEL0
CHART #

OFFICE VISITS - SYMPTOMATIC	
99201	OF--New Patient Minimal
99202	OF--New Patient Low
99203	OF--New Patient Detailed
99204	OF--New Patient Moderate
99205	OF--New Patient High
99211	OF--Established Patient Minimal
99212	OF--Established Patient Low
99213	OF--Established Patient Detailed
99214	OF--Established Patient Moderate
99215	OF--Established Patient High
PREVENTIVE VISITS	
NEW	
99381	Under 1 Year
99382	1 - 4 Years
99383	5 - 11 Years
99384	12 - 17 Years
99385	18 - 39 Years
99386	40 - 64 Years
99387	65 Years & Up
ESTABLISHED	
99391	Under 1 Year
99392	1 - 4 Years
99393	5 - 11 Years
99394	12 - 17 Years
99395	18 - 39 Years
99396	40 - 64 Years
99397	65 Years & Up
PROCEDURES	
12011	Simple suture--face--local anes.
29125	App. of short arm splint; static
29425	App. of short leg cast, walking
45378	Colonoscopy--diagnostic
45380	Colonoscopy--with biopsy
50390	Aspiration of renal cyst by needle
71010	Chest x-ray, single view, frontal

PROCEDURES	
71020	Chest x-ray, two views, frontal & lateral
71030	Chest x-ray, complete, four views
73070	Elbow x-ray, AP & lateral views
73090	Forearm x-ray, AP & lateral views
73100	Wrist x-ray, AP & lateral views
73510	Hip x-ray, complete, two views
73600	Ankle x-ray, AP & lateral views
80048	Basic metabolic panel
80061	Lipid panel
82270	Blood screening, occult; feces
82947	Glucose screening--quantitative
82951	Glucose tolerance test, three specimens
83718	HDL cholesterol
84478	Triglycerides test
85007	Manual differential WBC
85018	Hemoglobin
85025	Complete CBC w/auto diff WBC
85651	Erythrocyte sedimentation rate--non-auto
86585	Tuberculosis, tine test
87076	Culture, anaerobic isolate
87077	Bacterial culture, aerobic isolate
87086	Urine culture and colony count
87430	Strep test
87880	Direct streptococcus screen
90471	Immunization administration
90703	Tetanus injection
90782	Injection
92516	Facial nerve function studies
93000	Electrocardiogram--ECG with interpretation
93015	Treadmill stress test, with physician...
96900	Ultraviolet light treatment
99070	Supplies and materials provided

FAMILY CARE CENTER

NOTES

REFERRING PHYSICIAN

UPIN

AUTHORIZATION #

DIAGNOSIS
250.0

PAYMENT AMOUNT

ENCOUNTER FORM

10/4/2010
DATE

Dr. John Rudner
PROVIDER

John Fitzwilliams
PATIENT NAME

FITZWJO0
CHART #

OFFICE VISITS - SYMPTOMATIC	
99201	OF--New Patient Minimal
99202	OF--New Patient Low
99203	OF--New Patient Detailed
99204	OF--New Patient Moderate
99205	OF--New Patient High
99211	OF--Established Patient Minimal
99212	OF--Established Patient Low
99213	OF--Established Patient Detailed
99214	OF--Established Patient Moderate
99215	OF--Established Patient High

PREVENTIVE VISITS
NEW

99381	Under 1 Year
99382	1 - 4 Years
99383	5 - 11 Years
99384	12 - 17 Years
99385	18 - 39 Years
99386	40 - 64 Years
99387	65 Years & Up

ESTABLISHED

99391	Under 1 Year
99392	1 - 4 Years
99393	5 - 11 Years
99394	12 - 17 Years
99395	18 - 39 Years
99396	40 - 64 Years
99397	65 Years & Up

PROCEDURES

12011	Simple suture--face--local anes.
29125	App. of short arm splint; static
29425	App. of short leg cast, walking
45378	Colonoscopy--diagnostic
45380	Colonoscopy--with biopsy
50390	Aspiration of renal cyst by needle
71010	Chest x-ray, single view, frontal

PROCEDURES	
71020	Chest x-ray, two views, frontal & lateral
71030	Chest x-ray, complete, four views
73070	Elbow x-ray, AP & lateral views
73090	Forearm x-ray, AP & lateral views
73100	Wrist x-ray, AP & lateral views
73510	Hip x-ray, complete, two views
73600	Ankle x-ray, AP & lateral views
80048	Basic metabolic panel
80061	Lipid panel
82270	Blood screening, occult; feces
82947	Glucose screening--quantitative
82951	Glucose tolerance test, three specimens
83718	HDL cholesterol
84478	Triglycerides test
85007	Manual differential WBC
85018	Hemoglobin
85025	Complete CBC w/auto diff WBC
85651	Erythrocyte sedimentation rate--non-auto
86585	Tuberculosis, tine test
87076	Culture, anaerobic isolate
87077	Bacterial culture, aerobic isolate
87086	Urine culture and colony count
87430	Strep test
87880	Direct streptococcus screen
90471	Immunization administration
90703	Tetanus injection
90782	Injection
92516	Facial nerve function studies
93000	Electrocardiogram--ECG with interpretation
93015	Treadmill stress test, with physician...
96900	Ultraviolet light treatment
99070	Supplies and materials provided

FAMILY CARE CENTER

REFERRING PHYSICIAN

UPIN

AUTHORIZATION #

DIAGNOSIS
531.30

PAYMENT AMOUNT
$15 copay, check #456

NOTES
82270 requires modifier -90

Source Document 6

CHAMPVA
240 CENTER ST.
COLUMBUS, OH 60220

PROVIDER REMITTANCE
THIS IS NOT A BILL
A PAYMENT SUMMARY AND AN EXPLANATION OF
CODES ARE AT THE END OF THIS STATEMENT

FAMILY CARE CENTER
285 STEPHENSON BLVD.
STEPHENSON, OH 60089-4000

PAGE:	1 OF 1
DATE:	10/04/2010
ID NUMBER:	214778924

PROVIDER: JOHN RUDNER, M.D.

PATIENT: FITZWILLIAMS JOHN   CLAIM: 123456789

PROC CODE	FROM DATE	THRU DATE	TREAT -MENT	STATUS CODE	AMOUNT CHRGD	AMOUNT ALLWD	COPAY/ DEDUCT	AMOUNT APPRVD	PATIENT BALANCE
84478	09/07/10	09/07/10	1	A	29.00	29.00	15.00	29.00	0.00
		CLAIM TOTALS			29.00	29.00	15.00	29.00	0.00

PROVIDER: KATHERINE YAN, M.D.

PATIENT: FITZWILLIAMS SARAH   CLAIM: 234567891

PROC CODE	FROM DATE	THRU DATE	TREAT -MENT	STATUS CODE	AMOUNT CHRGD	AMOUNT ALLWD	COPAY/ DEDUCT	AMOUNT APPRVD	PATIENT BALANCE
90471	09/07/10	09/07/10	1	A	12.00	12.00	15.00	12.00	0.00
90703	09/07/10	09/07/10	1	A	29.00	29.00	.00	29.00	0.00
		CLAIM TOTALS			41.00	41.00	15.00	41.00	0.00

******************* CHECK #214778924 IN THE AMOUNT OF $70.00 IS ATTACHED *******************

PAYMENT SUMMARY		TOTAL ALL CLAIMS	
TOTAL AMOUNT PAID	70.00	AMOUNT CHARGED	70.00
PRIOR CREDIT BALANCE	.00	AMOUNT ALLOWED	70.00
CURRENT CREDIT DEFERRED	.00	DEDUCTIBLE	.00
PRIOR CREDIT APPLIED	.00	COPAY	30.00
NEW CREDIT BALANCE	.00	OTHER REDUCTION	.00
NET DISBURSED	70.00	AMOUNT APPROVED	70.00

STATUS CODES:
A - APPROVED	AJ - ADJUSTMENT	IP - IN PROCESS	R - REJECTED	V - VOID

EAST OHIO PPO
10 CENTRAL AVENUE
HALEVILLE, OH 60890

PROVIDER REMITTANCE
THIS IS NOT A BILL
A PAYMENT SUMMARY AND AN EXPLANATION OF
CODES ARE AT THE END OF THIS STATEMENT

FAMILY CARE CENTER
285 STEPHENSON BLVD.
STEPHENSON, OH 60089-4000

PAGE: 1 OF 2
DATE: 10/04/2010
ID NUMBER: 00146972

PROVIDER: ROBERT BEACH, M.D.

PATIENT: ARLEN SUSAN   CLAIM: 123456789

PROC CODE	FROM DATE	THRU DATE	TREAT -MENT	STATUS CODE	AMOUNT CHRGD	AMOUNT ALLWD	COPAY/ DEDUCT	AMOUNT APPRVD	PATIENT BALANCE
99212	09/06/10	09/06/10	1	A	46.00	46.00	25.00	46.00	0.00
		CLAIM TOTALS			46.00	46.00	25.00	46.00	0.00

PROVIDER: JOHN RUDNER, M.D.

PATIENT: BELL HERBERT   CLAIM: 234567891

PROC CODE	FROM DATE	THRU DATE	TREAT -MENT	STATUS CODE	AMOUNT CHRGD	AMOUNT ALLWD	COPAY/ DEDUCT	AMOUNT APPRVD	PATIENT BALANCE
99211	09/06/10	09/06/10	1	A	30.00	30.00	25.00	30.00	0.00
		CLAIM TOTALS			30.00	30.00	25.00	30.00	0.00

PATIENT: BELL SAMUEL   CLAIM: 34567891

PROC CODE	FROM DATE	THRU DATE	TREAT -MENT	STATUS CODE	AMOUNT CHRGD	AMOUNT ALLWD	COPAY/ DEDUCT	AMOUNT APPRVD	PATIENT BALANCE
99212	09/06/10	09/06/10	1	A	46.00	46.00	25.00	46.00	0.00
		CLAIM TOTALS			46.00	46.00	25.00	46.00	0.00

PROVIDER: KATHERINE YAN, M.D.

PATIENT: BELL JANINE   CLAIM: 45678912

PROC CODE	FROM DATE	THRU DATE	TREAT -MENT	STATUS CODE	AMOUNT CHRGD	AMOUNT ALLWD	COPAY/ DEDUCT	AMOUNT APPRVD	PATIENT BALANCE
99213	09/06/10	09/06/10	1	A	62.00	62.00	25.00	62.00	0.00
73510	09/06/10	09/06/10	1	A	103.00	103.00	0.00	103.00	0.00
		CLAIM TOTALS			165.00	165.00	25.00	165.00	0.00

PATIENT: BELL JONATHAN   CLAIM: 56789123

PROC CODE	FROM DATE	THRU DATE	TREAT -MENT	STATUS CODE	AMOUNT CHRGD	AMOUNT ALLWD	COPAY/ DEDUCT	AMOUNT APPRVD	PATIENT BALANCE
99394	09/06/10	09/06/10	1	A	177.60	177.60	25.00	177.60	0.00
		CLAIM TOTALS			177.60	177.60	25.00	177.60	0.00

STATUS CODES:
A - APPROVED   AJ - ADJUSTMENT   IP - IN PROCESS   R - REJECTED   V - VOID

Source Document 7b

EAST OHIO PPO
10 CENTRAL AVENUE
HALEVILLE, OH 60890

PROVIDER REMITTANCE
THIS IS NOT A BILL
A PAYMENT SUMMARY AND AN EXPLANATION OF
CODES ARE AT THE END OF THIS STATEMENT

FAMILY CARE CENTER
285 STEPHENSON BLVD.
STEPHENSON, OH 60089-4000

PAGE: 2 OF 2
DATE: 10/04/2010
ID NUMBER: 00146972

PROVIDER: KATHERINE YAN, M.D.

PATIENT: BELL SARINA   CLAIM: 56789123

PROC CODE	FROM DATE	THRU DATE	TREAT-MENT	STATUS CODE	AMOUNT CHRGD	AMOUNT ALLWD	COPAY/ DEDUCT	AMOUNT APPRVD	PATIENT BALANCE
99213	09/06/10	09/06/10	1	A	62.00	62.00	25.00	62.00	0.00
		CLAIM TOTALS			62.00	62.00	25.00	62.00	0.00

PAYMENT SUMMARY		TOTAL ALL CLAIMS		EFT INFORMATION	
TOTAL AMOUNT PAID	526.60	AMOUNT CHARGED	526.60	NUMBER	1000000
PRIOR CREDIT BALANCE	.00	AMOUNT ALLOWED	526.60	DATE	10/04/10
CURRENT CREDIT DEFERRED	.00	DEDUCTIBLE	.00	AMOUNT	526.60
PRIOR CREDIT APPLIED	.00	COPAY	150.00		
NEW CREDIT BALANCE	.00	OTHER REDUCTION	.00		
NET DISBURSED	526.60	AMOUNT APPROVED	526.60		

STATUS CODES:
A - APPROVED   AJ - ADJUSTMENT   IP - IN PROCESS   R - REJECTED   V - VOID

BLUE CROSS/BLUE SHIELD
340 BOULEVARD
COLUMBUS, OH 60220

PROVIDER REMITTANCE
THIS IS NOT A BILL
A PAYMENT SUMMARY AND AN EXPLANATION OF
CODES ARE AT THE END OF THIS STATEMENT

FAMILY CARE CENTER
285 STEPHENSON BLVD.
STEPHENSON, OH 60089-4000

PAGE: 1 OF 1
DATE: 11/04/2010
ID NUMBER: 001234

PROVIDER: ROBERT BEACH, M.D.

PATIENT: GILES SHEILA   CLAIM: 123456789

PROC CODE	FROM DATE	THRU DATE	TREAT -MENT	STATUS CODE	AMOUNT CHRGD	AMOUNT ALLWD	COINS/ DEDUCT	AMOUNT APPRVD	PATIENT BALANCE
99213	10/29/10	10/29/10	1	A	72.00	72.00	14.40	57.60	14.40
71010	10/29/10	10/29/10	1	A	91.00	91.00	18.20	72.80	18.20
87430	10/29/10	10/29/10	1	R*	58.00	0.00	0.00	0.00	58.00
		CLAIM TOTALS			221.00	163.00	32.60	130.40	90.60

R* OUTSIDE LAB WORK NOT BILLABLE BY PROVIDER

PATIENT: SIMMONS JILL   CLAIM: 234567891

PROC CODE	FROM DATE	THRU DATE	TREAT -MENT	STATUS CODE	AMOUNT CHRGD	AMOUNT ALLWD	COINS/ DEDUCT	AMOUNT APPRVD	PATIENT BALANCE
99212	10/29/10	10/29/10	1	A	54.00	54.00	10.80	43.20	10.80
87086	10/29/10	10/29/10	1	A	51.00	51.00	10.20	40.80	10.20
		CLAIM TOTALS			105.00	105.00	21.00	84.00	21.00

PAYMENT SUMMARY

TOTAL AMOUNT PAID	214.40
PRIOR CREDIT BALANCE	.00
CURRENT CREDIT DEFERRED	.00
PRIOR CREDIT APPLIED	.00
NEW CREDIT BALANCE	.00
NET DISBURSED	214.40

TOTAL ALL CLAIMS

AMOUNT CHARGED	326.00
AMOUNT ALLOWED	268.00
DEDUCTIBLE	.00
COINSURANCE	53.60
OTHER REDUCTION	.00
AMOUNT APPROVED	214.40

EFT INFORMATION

NUMBER	2000000
DATE	11/04/10
AMOUNT	214.40

STATUS CODES:
A - APPROVED   AJ - ADJUSTMENT   IP - IN PROCESS   R - REJECTED   V - VOID

Source Document 9

OHIOCARE HMO
147 CENTRAL AVENUE
HALEVILLE, OH 60890

FAMILY CARE CENTER
285 STEPHENSON BLVD.
STEPHENSON, OH 60089-4000

PAGE: 1 OF 1
DATE: 10/04/2010
ID NUMBER: 001006003

OHIOCARE HMO CAPITATION STATEMENT
MONTH OF SEPTEMBER 2010

PROVIDERS
BANU DANA
BEACH ROBERT
MCGRATH PATRICIA
RUDNER JESSICA
RUDNER JOHN
YAN KATHERINE

MEMBER NUMBER	MEMBER NAME	CONTRACT NUMBER	CONTRACT STATUS
0003602149	FAMILY CARE CENTER	YG34906	APPROVED

AMOUNT OF PAYMENT $2,500.00
EFT STATUS: SENT 10/04/10 8:46AM
TRANSACTION #343434

ENCOUNTER FORM

11/4/2010
DATE

Dr. Patricia McGrath
PROVIDER

Anthony Battistuta
PATIENT NAME

BATTIAN0
CHART #

OFFICE VISITS - SYMPTOMATIC

99201	OF--New Patient Minimal
99202	OF--New Patient Low
99203	OF--New Patient Detailed
99204	OF--New Patient Moderate
99205	OF--New Patient High
99211	OF--Established Patient Minimal
99212	OF--Established Patient Low
99213	OF--Established Patient Detailed
99214	OF--Established Patient Moderate
99215	OF--Established Patient High

PREVENTIVE VISITS
NEW

99381	Under 1 Year
99382	1 - 4 Years
99383	5 - 11 Years
99384	12 - 17 Years
99385	18 - 39 Years
99386	40 - 64 Years
99387	65 Years & Up

ESTABLISHED

99391	Under 1 Year
99392	1 - 4 Years
99393	5 - 11 Years
99394	12 - 17 Years
99395	18 - 39 Years
99396	40 - 64 Years
99397	65 Years & Up

PROCEDURES

12011	Simple suture--face--local anes.
29125	App. of short arm splint; static
29425	App. of short leg cast, walking
45378	Colonoscopy--diagnostic
45380	Colonoscopy--with biopsy
50390	Aspiration of renal cyst by needle
71010	Chest x-ray, single view, frontal

PROCEDURES

71020	Chest x-ray, two views, frontal & lateral
71030	Chest x-ray, complete, four views
73070	Elbow x-ray, AP & lateral views
73090	Forearm x-ray, AP & lateral views
73100	Wrist x-ray, AP & lateral views
73510	Hip x-ray, complete, two views
73600	Ankle x-ray, AP & lateral views
80048	Basic metabolic panel
80061	Lipid panel
82270	Blood screening, occult; feces
82947	Glucose screening--quantitative
82951	Glucose tolerance test, three specimens
83718	HDL cholesterol
84478	Triglycerides test
85007	Manual differential WBC
85018	Hemoglobin
85025	Complete CBC w/auto diff WBC
85651	Erythrocyte sedimentation rate--non-auto
86585	Tuberculosis, tine test
87076	Culture, anaerobic isolate
87077	Bacterial culture, aerobic isolate
87086	Urine culture and colony count
87430	Strep test
87880	Direct streptococcus screen
90471	Immunization administration
90703	Tetanus injection
90782	Injection
92516	Facial nerve function studies
93000	Electrocardiogram--ECG with interpretation
93015	Treadmill stress test, with physician...
96900	Ultraviolet light treatment
99070	Supplies and materials provided

FAMILY CARE CENTER

REFERRING PHYSICIAN

UPIN

AUTHORIZATION #

DIAGNOSIS
diabetes

PAYMENT AMOUNT

NOTES
New address:
36 Grant Blvd.
Grandville, OH 60092

CPT 82951 requires modifier -90

Source Document 11

ENCOUNTER FORM

11/12/2010	Dr. Patricia McGrath
DATE	PROVIDER
Lawana Brooks	BROOKLA0
PATIENT NAME	CHART #

OFFICE VISITS - SYMPTOMATIC	
99201	OF--New Patient Minimal
99202	OF--New Patient Low
99203	OF--New Patient Detailed
99204	OF--New Patient Moderate
99205	OF--New Patient High
99211	OF--Established Patient Minimal
99212	OF--Established Patient Low
99213	OF--Established Patient Detailed
99214	OF--Established Patient Moderate
99215	OF--Established Patient High

PREVENTIVE VISITS	
NEW	
99381	Under 1 Year
99382	1 - 4 Years
99383	5 - 11 Years
99384	12 - 17 Years
99385	18 - 39 Years
99386	40 - 64 Years
99387	65 Years & Up
ESTABLISHED	
99391	Under 1 Year
99392	1 - 4 Years
99393	5 - 11 Years
99394	12 - 17 Years
99395	18 - 39 Years
99396	40 - 64 Years
99397	65 Years & Up

PROCEDURES	
12011	Simple suture--face--local anes.
29125	App. of short arm splint; static
29425	App. of short leg cast, walking
45378	Colonoscopy--diagnostic
45380	Colonoscopy--with biopsy
50390	Aspiration of renal cyst by needle
71010	Chest x-ray, single view, frontal

PROCEDURES	
71020	Chest x-ray, two views, frontal & lateral
71030	Chest x-ray, complete, four views
73070	Elbow x-ray, AP & lateral views
73090	Forearm x-ray, AP & lateral views
73100	Wrist x-ray, AP & lateral views
73510	Hip x-ray, complete, two views
73600	Ankle x-ray, AP & lateral views
80048	Basic metabolic panel
80061	Lipid panel
82270	Blood screening, occult; feces
82947	Glucose screening--quantitative
82951	Glucose tolerance test, three specimens
83718	HDL cholesterol
84478	Triglycerides test
85007	Manual differential WBC
85018	Hemoglobin
85025	Complete CBC w/auto diff WBC
85651	Erythrocyte sedimentation rate--non-auto
86585	Tuberculosis, tine test
87076	Culture, anerobic isolate
87077	Bacterial culture, aerobic isolate
87086	Urine culture and colony count
87430	Strep test
87880	Direct streptococcus screen
90471	Immunization administration
90703	Tetanus injection
90782	Injection
92516	Facial nerve function studies
93000	Electrocardiogram--ECG with interpretation
93015	Treadmill stress test, with physician...
96900	Ultraviolet light treatment
99070	Supplies and materials provided

FAMILY CARE CENTER

REFERRING PHYSICIAN	UPIN
AUTHORIZATION #	

DIAGNOSIS

841.0   E885   E849.3

PAYMENT AMOUNT

NOTES

Accidental fall at work

copayment not collected

FAMILY CARE CENTER
285 Stephenson Boulevard
Stephenson, OH 60089-4000
614-555-0000

CASE NOTES

PATIENT NAME	Lawana Brooks
CHART NUMBER	BROOKLA0
DATE	11/12/10
CASE	Fall at work - Worker's Compensation

NOTES

Emergency visit for injuries sustained due to a fall at work on 11/12/10.

This is classified as a work injury - non-collision.

Source Document 13

ENCOUNTER FORM

11/12/2010
DATE

Dr. Patricia McGrath
PROVIDER

Edwin Hsu
PATIENT NAME

HSUEDWI0
CHART #

OFFICE VISITS - SYMPTOMATIC	
99201	OF--New Patient Minimal
99202	OF--New Patient Low
99203	OF--New Patient Detailed
99204	OF--New Patient Moderate
99205	OF--New Patient High
99211	OF--Established Patient Minimal
99212	OF--Established Patient Low
99213	OF--Established Patient Detailed
99214	OF--Established Patient Moderate
99215	OF--Established Patient High
PREVENTIVE VISITS	
NEW	
99381	Under 1 Year
99382	1 - 4 Years
99383	5 - 11 Years
99384	12 - 17 Years
99385	18 - 39 Years
99386	40 - 64 Years
99387	65 Years & Up
ESTABLISHED	
99391	Under 1 Year
99392	1 - 4 Years
99393	5 - 11 Years
99394	12 - 17 Years
99395	18 - 39 Years
99396	40 - 64 Years
99397	65 Years & Up
PROCEDURES	
12011	Simple suture--face--local anes.
29125	App. of short arm splint; static
29425	App. of short leg cast, walking
45378	Colonoscopy--diagnostic
45380	Colonoscopy--with biopsy
50390	Aspiration of renal cyst by needle
71010	Chest x-ray, single view, frontal

PROCEDURES	
71020	Chest x-ray, two views, frontal & lateral
71030	Chest x-ray, complete, four views
73070	Elbow x-ray, AP & lateral views
73090	Forearm x-ray, AP & lateral views
73100	Wrist x-ray, AP & lateral views
73510	Hip x-ray, complete, two views
73600	Ankle x-ray, AP & lateral views
80048	Basic metabolic panel
80061	Lipid panel
82270	Blood screening, occult; feces
82947	Glucose screening--quantitative
82951	Glucose tolerance test, three specimens
83718	HDL cholesterol
84478	Triglycerides test
85007	Manual differential WBC
85018	Hemoglobin
85025	Complete CBC w/auto diff WBC
85651	Erythrocyte sedimentation rate--non-auto
86585	Tuberculosis, tine test
87076	Culture, anaerobic isolate
87077	Bacterial culture, aerobic isolate
87086	Urine culture and colony count
87430	Strep test
87880	Direct streptococcus screen
90471	Immunization administration
90703	Tetanus injection
90782	Injection
92516	Facial nerve function studies
93000	Electrocardiogram--ECG with interpretation
93015	Treadmill stress test, with physician...
96900	Ultraviolet light treatment
99070	Supplies and materials provided

FAMILY CARE CENTER

REFERRING PHYSICIAN

UPIN

NOTES
see case notes

AUTHORIZATION #

DIAGNOSIS
461.9 acute sinusitis

PAYMENT AMOUNT
$30 copay, check #1066

FAMILY CARE CENTER
285 Stephenson Boulevard
Stephenson, OH 60089-4000
614-555-0000

PATIENT NAME	Edwin Hsu
CHART NUMBER	HSUEDWI0
DATE	11/12/10
CASE	Acute sinusitis

NOTES

Patient has moved--new address is:
56 Reynolds St.
Stephenson, OH 60089
614-034-6729

Patient has new insurance coverage; company not in database so must be added.

Address Tab
Code: 16
Name: Midwest Select HMO
Address: 1245 Mohawk Lane
                               Columbus, OH 60625
Phone: 614-555-1211
Practice ID: 12345678

Options Tab
Plan Name: Midwest Select HMO
Type: HMO
Procedure Code Set: 1
Diagnosis Code Set: 1
Patient Signature on File: Signature on File
Insured Signature on File: Signature on File
Physician Signature on File: Signature on File
Print PINS on Forms: Provider name and PIN
Default Billing Method: Electronic

EDI, Codes Tab
EDI Receiver: 0000 - NDC Corporation
EDI Payor Number: 50678
EDI Sub ID: 5034

Source Document 14b

FAMILY CARE CENTER
285 Stephenson Boulevard
Stephenson, OH 60089-4000
614-555-0000

PATIENT NAME	Edwin Hsu
CHART NUMBER	HSUEDWI0
DATE	11/12/10
CASE	Acute sinusitis

NOTES

EDI, Codes Tab (continued)
NDC Record Code: 01
EDI Max Transactions: 100
Payment: MIDPAY Midwest Select Payment
Adjustment: MIDADJ Midwest Select Adjustment
Withhold: MIDWIT Midwest Select Withhold
Deductible: MIDDED Midwest Select Deductible
Take Back   MIDTBK Midwest Select Take Back

Allowed Tab
No entries

PINs Tab
McGrath PIN/Group ID: 1234 / 5560
Beach PIN/Group ID: 5678 / 5560
Banu PIN/Group ID: 9012 / 5560

A new case must be created for Edwin Hsu.

Personal Tab
Description: Acute sinusitis

Account Tab
Price Code: A

Diagnosis Tab
Default Diagnosis 1:   461.9

FAMILY CARE CENTER
285 Stephenson Boulevard
Stephenson, OH 60089-4000
614-555-0000

PATIENT NAME	Edwin Hsu
CHART NUMBER	HSUEDWI0
DATE	11/12/10
CASE	Acute sinusitis

NOTES

Policy 1 Tab
Insurance 1:	16 - Midwest Select HMO
Policy Holder 1:	HSUEDWI0
Relationship to Insured:	Self
Policy Number:	51249
Group Number:	256
Accept Assignment:	Yes
Capitated Plan:	Yes
Copayment Amount:	$30
Insurance Coverage by Service Classification	100% in all boxes

Source Document 15

FAMILY CARE CENTER
285 Stephenson Boulevard
Stephenson, OH 60089-4000
614-555-0000

PATIENT INFORMATION FORM

Patient				
Last Name Syzmanski	First Name Hannah	MI	Sex __ M _X_ F	Date of Birth 2 / 26 / 2000
Address 3 Broadbrook Lane	City Stephenson	State OH		Zip 60089
Home Ph # (614) 086-4444	Marital Status Single		Student Status Full-time	

SS# 907-66-0003	Allergies: Bee stings			
Employment Status	Employer Name		Work Ph # ( )	Primary Insurance ID# 812736000 Group HJ31
Employer Address	City		State	Zip
Referred By Harold Gearhart, M.D.		Ph # of Referral (614) 556-2450		

Responsible Party (Complete this section if the person responsible for the bill is not the patient)

Last Name Syzmanski	First Name Michael	MI	Sex _X_ M __ F	Date of Birth 6 / 5 / 1970
Address 3 Broadbrook Lane	City Stephenson	State OH	Zip 60089	SS# 022-45-6789
Relation to Patient __ Spouse _X_ Parent __ Other	Employer Name Nichol's Hardware		Work Phone # ( )	
Spouse, or Parent (if minor):			Home Phone # (614) 086-4444	

Insurance (If you have multiple coverage, supply information from both carriers)

Primary Carrier Name	Secondary Carrier Name
Name of the Insured (Name on ID Card)	Name of the Insured (Name on ID Card)
Patient's relationship to the insured __ Self __ Spouse __ Child	Patient's relationship to the insured __ Self __ Spouse __ Child
Insured ID #	Insured ID #
Group # or Company Name	Group # or Company Name
Insurance Address	Insurance Address
Phone # Copay $	Phone # Copay $

Other Information

Is patient's condition related to:	Reason for visit: Preventive exam
__ Employment __ Auto Accident (if yes, state in which accident occurred: ___) __ Other Accident	
Date of Accident: / / Date of First Symptom of Illness: / /	

Authorization

I hereby authorize release of information necessary for my insurance company to process my claim. The above information is correct to the best of my knowledge. Signed: _Michael Syzmanski_ Date: _11/12/2010_	I hereby authorize payment directly to FAMILY CARE CENTER insurance benefits otherwise payable to me. I understand that I am financially responsible for charges not paid in a timely manner by my insurance. Signed: _Michael Syzmanski_ Date: _11/12/2010_

ENCOUNTER FORM

11/12/2010
DATE

Dr. Dana Banu
PROVIDER

Hannah Syzmanski
PATIENT NAME

SYZMANHA0
CHART #

OFFICE VISITS - SYMPTOMATIC	
99201	OF--New Patient Minimal
99202	OF--New Patient Low
99203	OF--New Patient Detailed
99204	OF--New Patient Moderate
99205	OF--New Patient High
99211	OF--Established Patient Minimal
99212	OF--Established Patient Low
99213	OF--Established Patient Detailed
99214	OF--Established Patient Moderate
99215	OF--Established Patient High
PREVENTIVE VISITS	
NEW	
99381	Under 1 Year
99382	1 - 4 Years
99383	5 - 11 Years
99384	12 - 17 Years
99385	18 - 39 Years
99386	40 - 64 Years
99387	65 Years & Up
ESTABLISHED	
99391	Under 1 Year
99392	1 - 4 Years
99393	5 - 11 Years
99394	12 - 17 Years
99395	18 - 39 Years
99396	40 - 64 Years
99397	65 Years & Up
PROCEDURES	
12011	Simple suture--face--local anes.
29125	App. of short arm splint; static
29425	App. of short leg cast, walking
45378	Colonoscopy--diagnostic
45380	Colonoscopy--with biopsy
50390	Aspiration of renal cyst by needle
71010	Chest x-ray, single view, frontal

PROCEDURES	
71020	Chest x-ray, two views, frontal & lateral
71030	Chest x-ray, complete, four views
73070	Elbow x-ray, AP & lateral views
73090	Forearm x-ray, AP & lateral views
73100	Wrist x-ray, AP & lateral views
73510	Hip x-ray, complete, two views
73600	Ankle x-ray, AP & lateral views
80048	Basic metabolic panel
80061	Lipid panel
82270	Blood screening, occult; feces
82947	Glucose screening--quantitative
82951	Glucose tolerance test, three specimens
83718	HDL cholesterol
84478	Triglycerides test
85007	Manual differential WBC
85018	Hemoglobin
85025	Complete CBC w/auto diff WBC
85651	Erythrocyte sedimentation rate--non-auto
86585	Tuberculosis, tine test
87076	Culture, anaerobic isolate
87077	Bacterial culture, aerobic isolate
87086	Urine culture and colony count
87430	Strep test
87880	Direct streptococcus screen
90471	Immunization administration
90703	Tetanus injection
90782	Injection
92516	Facial nerve function studies
93000	Electrocardiogram--ECG with interpretation
93015	Treadmill stress test, with physician...
96900	Ultraviolet light treatment
99070	Supplies and materials provided

FAMILY CARE CENTER

REFERRING PHYSICIAN
Harold Gearhart, M.D.

UPIN

AUTHORIZATION #

DIAGNOSIS
v20.2

PAYMENT AMOUNT
$25 copay, check #3019

NOTES

Source Document 17

ENCOUNTER FORM

11/15/2010
DATE

Dr. Patricia McGrath
PROVIDER

Carlos Lopez
PATIENT NAME

LOPEZCA0
CHART #

OFFICE VISITS - SYMPTOMATIC	
99201	OF--New Patient Minimal
99202	OF--New Patient Low
99203	OF--New Patient Detailed
99204	OF--New Patient Moderate
99205	OF--New Patient High
99211	OF--Established Patient Minimal
99212	OF--Established Patient Low
99213	OF--Established Patient Detailed
99214	OF--Established Patient Moderate
99215	OF--Established Patient High

PREVENTIVE VISITS	
NEW	
99381	Under 1 Year
99382	1 - 4 Years
99383	5 - 11 Years
99384	12 - 17 Years
99385	18 - 39 Years
99386	40 - 64 Years
99387	65 Years & Up
ESTABLISHED	
99391	Under 1 Year
99392	1 - 4 Years
99393	5 - 11 Years
99394	12 - 17 Years
99395	18 - 39 Years
99396	40 - 64 Years
99397	65 Years & Up

PROCEDURES	
12011	Simple suture--face--local anes.
29125	App. of short arm splint; static
29425	App. of short leg cast, walking
45378	Colonoscopy--diagnostic
45380	Colonoscopy--with biopsy
50390	Aspiration of renal cyst by needle
71010	Chest x-ray, single view, frontal

PROCEDURES	
71020	Chest x-ray, two views, frontal & lateral
71030	Chest x-ray, complete, four views
73070	Elbow x-ray, AP & lateral views
73090	Forearm x-ray, AP & lateral views
73100	Wrist x-ray, AP & lateral views
73510	Hip x-ray, complete, two views
73600	Ankle x-ray, AP & lateral views
80048	Basic metabolic panel
80061	Lipid panel
82270	Blood screening, occult; feces
82947	Glucose screening--quantitative
82951	Glucose tolerance test, three specimens
83718	HDL cholesterol
84478	Triglycerides test
85007	Manual differential WBC
85018	Hemoglobin
85025	Complete CBC w/auto diff WBC
85651	Erythrocyte sedimentation rate--non-auto
86585	Tuberculosis, tine test
87076	Culture, anaerobic isolate
87077	Bacterial culture, aerobic isolate
87086	Urine culture and colony count
87430	Strep test
87880	Direct streptococcus screen
90471	Immunization administration
90703	Tetanus injection
90782	Injection
92516	Facial nerve function studies
93000	Electrocardiogram--ECG with interpretation
93015	Treadmill stress test, with physician...
96900	Ultraviolet light treatment
99070	Supplies and materials provided

FAMILY CARE CENTER

REFERRING PHYSICIAN

UPIN

AUTHORIZATION #

DIAGNOSIS
v65.5

PAYMENT AMOUNT
$30 copay, check #1001

NOTES
patient had palpitations

FAMILY CARE CENTER
285 Stephenson Boulevard
Stephenson, OH 60089-4000
614-555-0000

PATIENT INFORMATION FORM

Patient				
Last Name Palmer	First Name Christopher	MI	Sex X M __ F	Date of Birth 1 /5 / 1954
Address 17 Red Oak Lane	City Jefferson		State OH	Zip 60093
Home Ph # (614) 077-2249	Marital Status Single		Student Status	

SS# 607-50-7620	Allergies:		
Employment Status Not employed	Employer Name	Work Ph # ( )	Primary Insurance ID# 607507620
Employer Address	City	State	Zip

Referred By Dr. Marion Davis	Ph # of Referral (614) 444-3200

Responsible Party (Complete this section if the person responsible for the bill is not the patient)

Last Name	First Name	MI	Sex __ M __ F	Date of Birth / /
Address	City	State Zip	SS#	

Relation to Patient __ Spouse __ Parent __ Other	Employer Name	Work Phone # ( )
Spouse, or Parent (if minor):		Home Phone # ( )

Insurance (If you have multiple coverage, supply information from both carriers)

Primary Carrier Name Medicaid	Price Code D	Secondary Carrier Name
Name of the Insured (Name on ID Card) Christopher Palmer		Name of the Insured (Name on ID Card)
Patient's relationship to the insured X Self __ Spouse __ Child		Patient's relationship to the insured __ Self __ Spouse __ Child
Insured ID # 607507620		Insured ID #
Group # or Company Name		Group # or Company Name
Insurance Address 248 West Main St., Cleveland, OH 60120		Insurance Address
Phone # 614-599-6000	Copay $ 10	Phone #	Copay $

Other Information

Is patient's condition related to:	Reason for visit:
__ Employment __ Auto Accident (if yes, state in which accident occurred: ___) __ Other Accident	
Date of Accident: / / Date of First Symptom of Illness: / /	

Authorization

I hereby authorize release of information necessary for my insurance company to process my claim. The above information is correct to the best of my knowledge. Signed: Christopher Palmer Date: 11/12/2010	I hereby authorize payment directly to FAMILY CARE CENTER insurance benefits otherwise payable to me. I understand that I am financially responsible for charges not paid in a timely manner by my insurance. Signed: Christopher Palmer Date: 11/12/2010

Source Document 19

ENCOUNTER FORM

11/12/2010
DATE

Dr. Robert Beach
PROVIDER

Christopher Palmer
PATIENT NAME

PALMECH0
CHART #

OFFICE VISITS - SYMPTOMATIC	
99201	OF--New Patient Minimal
99202	OF--New Patient Low
99203	OF--New Patient Detailed
99204	OF--New Patient Moderate
99205	OF--New Patient High
99211	OF--Established Patient Minimal
99212	OF--Established Patient Low
99213	OF--Established Patient Detailed
99214	OF--Established Patient Moderate
99215	OF--Established Patient High
PREVENTIVE VISITS	
NEW	
99381	Under 1 Year
99382	1 - 4 Years
99383	5 - 11 Years
99384	12 - 17 Years
99385	18 - 39 Years
99386	40 - 64 Years
99387	65 Years & Up
ESTABLISHED	
99391	Under 1 Year
99392	1 - 4 Years
99393	5 - 11 Years
99394	12 - 17 Years
99395	18 - 39 Years
99396	40 - 64 Years
99397	65 Years & Up
PROCEDURES	
12011	Simple suture--face--local anes.
29125	App. of short arm splint; static
29425	App. of short leg cast, walking
45378	Colonoscopy--diagnostic
45380	Colonoscopy--with biopsy
50390	Aspiration of renal cyst by needle
71010	Chest x-ray, single view, frontal

PROCEDURES	
71020	Chest x-ray, two views, frontal & lateral
71030	Chest x-ray, complete, four views
73070	Elbow x-ray, AP & lateral views
73090	Forearm x-ray, AP & lateral views
73100	Wrist x-ray, AP & lateral views
73510	Hip x-ray, complete, two views
73600	Ankle x-ray, AP & lateral views
80048	Basic metabolic panel
80061	Lipid panel
82270	Blood screening, occult; feces
82947	Glucose screening--quantitative
82951	Glucose tolerance test, three specimens
83718	HDL cholesterol
84478	Triglycerides test
85007	Manual differential WBC
85018	Hemoglobin
85025	Complete CBC w/auto diff WBC
85651	Erythrocyte sedimentation rate--non-auto
86585	Tuberculosis, tine test
87076	Culture, anaerobic isolate
87077	Bacterial culture, aerobic isolate
87086	Urine culture and colony count
87430	Strep test
87880	Direct streptococcus screen
90471	Immunization administration
90703	Tetanus injection
90782	Injection
92516	Facial nerve function studies
93000	Electrocardiogram--ECG with interpretation
93015	Treadmill stress test, with physician...
96900	Ultraviolet light treatment
99070	Supplies and materials provided

FAMILY CARE CENTER

NOTES

REFERRING PHYSICIAN
Dr. Marion Davis

UPIN

AUTHORIZATION #

DIAGNOSIS
485 Bronchopneumonia

PAYMENT AMOUNT
$10 copay, cash

EAST OHIO PPO
10 CENTRAL AVENUE
HALEVILLE, OH 60890

PROVIDER REMITTANCE
THIS IS NOT A BILL
A PAYMENT SUMMARY AND AN EXPLANATION OF
CODES ARE AT THE END OF THIS STATEMENT

FAMILY CARE CENTER
285 STEPHENSON BLVD.
STEPHENSON, OH 60089-4000

PAGE: 1 OF 1
DATE: 11/11/2010
ID NUMBER: 4679323

PROVIDER: PATRICIA MCGRATH, M.D.

PATIENT: BROOKS LAWANA   CLAIM: 234567890

PROC CODE	FROM DATE	THRU DATE	TREAT-MENT	STATUS CODE	AMOUNT CHRGD	AMOUNT ALLWD	COPAY/ DEDUCT	AMOUNT APPRVD	PATIENT BALANCE
99212	10/29/10	10/29/10	1	A	46.00	46.00	25.00	46.00	0.00
73600	10/29/10	10/29/10	1	A	80.00	80.00	.00	80.00	0.00
	CLAIM TOTALS				126.00	126.00	25.00	126.00	0.00

PATIENT: HSU DIANE   CLAIM: 345678910

PROC CODE	FROM DATE	THRU DATE	TREAT-MENT	STATUS CODE	AMOUNT CHRGD	AMOUNT ALLWD	COPAY/ DEDUCT	AMOUNT APPRVD	PATIENT BALANCE
99213	10/29/10	10/29/10	1	A	62.00	62.00	25.00	62.00	0.00
80048	10/29/10	10/29/10	1	A	60.00	60.00	.00	60.00	0.00
	CLAIM TOTALS				122.00	122.00	25.00	122.00	0.00

PROVIDER: DANA BANU, M.D.

PATIENT: PATEL RAJI   CLAIM: 567890123

PROC CODE	FROM DATE	THRU DATE	TREAT-MENT	STATUS CODE	AMOUNT CHRGD	AMOUNT ALLWD	COPAY/ DEDUCT	AMOUNT APPRVD	PATIENT BALANCE
99212	10/29/10	10/29/10	1	A	46.00	46.00	25.00	46.00	0.00
	CLAIM TOTALS				46.00	46.00	25.00	46.00	0.00

PATIENT: SYZMANSKI MICHAEL   CLAIM: 678901234

PROC CODE	FROM DATE	THRU DATE	TREAT-MENT	STATUS CODE	AMOUNT CHRGD	AMOUNT ALLWD	COPAY/ DEDUCT	AMOUNT APPRVD	PATIENT BALANCE
99212	10/29/10	10/29/10	1	A	46.00	46.00	25.00	46.00	0.00
	CLAIM TOTALS				46.00	46.00	25.00	46.00	0.00

PAYMENT SUMMARY

		TOTAL ALL CLAIMS		EFT INFORMATION	
TOTAL AMOUNT PAID	340.00	AMOUNT CHARGED	340.00	NUMBER	4679323
PRIOR CREDIT BALANCE	.00	AMOUNT ALLOWED	340.00	DATE	11/12/10
CURRENT CREDIT DEFERRED	.00	DEDUCTIBLE	.00	AMOUNT	340.00
PRIOR CREDIT APPLIED	.00	COPAY	100.00		
NEW CREDIT BALANCE	.00	OTHER REDUCTION	.00		
NET DISBURSED	340.00	AMOUNT APPROVED	340.00		

STATUS CODES:
A - APPROVED   AJ - ADJUSTMENT   IP - IN PROCESS   R - REJECTED   V - VOID

Source Document 21

ENCOUNTER FORM

11/15/2010
DATE

Dr. Patricia McGrath
PROVIDER

Diane Hsu
PATIENT NAME

HSUDIAN0
CHART #

OFFICE VISITS - SYMPTOMATIC	
99201	OF--New Patient Minimal
99202	OF--New Patient Low
99203	OF--New Patient Detailed
99204	OF--New Patient Moderate
99205	OF--New Patient High
99211	OF--Established Patient Minimal
99212	OF--Established Patient Low
99213	OF--Established Patient Detailed
99214	OF--Established Patient Moderate
99215	OF--Established Patient High
PREVENTIVE VISITS	
NEW	
99381	Under 1 Year
99382	1 - 4 Years
99383	5 - 11 Years
99384	12 - 17 Years
99385	18 - 39 Years
99386	40 - 64 Years
99387	65 Years & Up
ESTABLISHED	
99391	Under 1 Year
99392	1 - 4 Years
99393	5 - 11 Years
99394	12 - 17 Years
99395	18 - 39 Years
99396	40 - 64 Years
99397	65 Years & Up
PROCEDURES	
12011	Simple suture--face--local anes.
29125	App. of short arm splint; static
29425	App. of short leg cast, walking
45378	Colonoscopy--diagnostic
45380	Colonoscopy--with biopsy
50390	Aspiration of renal cyst by needle
71010	Chest x-ray, single view, frontal

PROCEDURES	
71020	Chest x-ray, two views, frontal & lateral
71030	Chest x-ray, complete, four views
73070	Elbow x-ray, AP & lateral views
73090	Forearm x-ray, AP & lateral views
73100	Wrist x-ray, AP & lateral views
73510	Hip x-ray, complete, two views
73600	Ankle x-ray, AP & lateral views
80048	Basic metabolic panel
80061	Lipid panel
82270	Blood screening, occult; feces
82947	Glucose screening--quantitative
82951	Glucose tolerance test, three specimens
83718	HDL cholesterol
84478	Triglycerides test
85007	Manual differential WBC
85018	Hemoglobin
85025	Complete CBC w/auto diff WBC
85651	Erythrocyte sedimentation rate--non-auto
86585	Tuberculosis, tine test
87076	Culture, anaerobic isolate
87077	Bacterial culture, aerobic isolate
87086	Urine culture and colony count
87430	Strep test
87880	Direct streptococcus screen
90471	Immunization administration
90703	Tetanus injection
90782	Injection
92516	Facial nerve function studies
93000	Electrocardiogram--ECG with interpretation
93015	Treadmill stress test, with physician...
96900	Ultraviolet light treatment
99070	Supplies and materials provided

FAMILY CARE CENTER

REFERRING PHYSICIAN

UPIN

AUTHORIZATION #

DIAGNOSIS
487.1 Influenza

PAYMENT AMOUNT
$30 copay, check #3419

NOTES
next appt. 1 week from
today, 2:00 p.m., 15 min.

ENCOUNTER FORM

11/15/2010
DATE

Dr. Dana Banu
PROVIDER

Michael Syzmanski
PATIENT NAME

SYZMAMI0
CHART #

OFFICE VISITS - SYMPTOMATIC	
99201	OF--New Patient Minimal
99202	OF--New Patient Low
99203	OF--New Patient Detailed
99204	OF--New Patient Moderate
99205	OF--New Patient High
99211	OF--Established Patient Minimal
99212	OF--Established Patient Low
99213	OF--Established Patient Detailed
99214	OF--Established Patient Moderate
99215	OF--Established Patient High
PREVENTIVE VISITS	
NEW	
99381	Under 1 Year
99382	1 - 4 Years
99383	5 - 11 Years
99384	12 - 17 Years
99385	18 - 39 Years
99386	40 - 64 Years
99387	65 Years & Up
ESTABLISHED	
99391	Under 1 Year
99392	1 - 4 Years
99393	5 - 11 Years
99394	12 - 17 Years
99395	18 - 39 Years
99396	40 - 64 Years
99397	65 Years & Up
PROCEDURES	
12011	Simple suture--face--local anes.
29125	App. of short arm splint; static
29425	App. of short leg cast, walking
45378	Colonoscopy--diagnostic
45380	Colonoscopy--with biopsy
50390	Aspiration of renal cyst by needle
71010	Chest x-ray, single view, frontal

PROCEDURES	
71020	Chest x-ray, two views, frontal & lateral
71030	Chest x-ray, complete, four views
73070	Elbow x-ray, AP & lateral views
73090	Forearm x-ray, AP & lateral views
73100	Wrist x-ray, AP & lateral views
73510	Hip x-ray, complete, two views
73600	Ankle x-ray, AP & lateral views
80048	Basic metabolic panel
80061	Lipid panel
82270	Blood screening, occult; feces
82947	Glucose screening--quantitative
82951	Glucose tolerance test, three specimens
83718	HDL cholesterol
84478	Triglycerides test
85007	Manual differential WBC
85018	Hemoglobin
85025	Complete CBC w/auto diff WBC
85651	Erythrocyte sedimentation rate--non-auto
86585	Tuberculosis, tine test
87076	Culture, anaerobic isolate
87077	Bacterial culture, aerobic isolate
87086	Urine culture and colony count
87430	Strep test
87880	Direct streptococcus screen
90471	Immunization administration
90703	Tetanus injection
90782	Injection
92516	Facial nerve function studies
93000	Electrocardiogram--ECG with interpretation
93015	Treadmill stress test, with physician...
96900	Ultraviolet light treatment
99070	Supplies and materials provided

FAMILY CARE CENTER

REFERRING PHYSICIAN

UPIN

AUTHORIZATION #

DIAGNOSIS
455.6 Hemorrhoids

PAYMENT AMOUNT
$25 copay, check #3119

NOTES
82270 requires modifier -90

Source Document 23

FAMILY CARE CENTER
285 Stephenson Boulevard
Stephenson, OH 60089-4000
614-555-0000

PATIENT INFORMATION FORM

Patient				
Last Name **Robertson**	First Name **Stewart**	MI	Sex **X** M __ F	Date of Birth **12 / 21 / 1969**

Address **109 West Central Ave.**	City **Stephenson**	State **OH**	Zip **60089**

Home Ph # **(614)022-3111**   Marital Status **Divorced**   Student Status

SS# **920-39-4567**	Allergies:		

Employment Status **Full-time**	Employer Name **Nichols Hardware**	Work Ph # **(614) 789-0200**	Primary Insurance ID# **920394567 Group 63W**

Employer Address **12 Central Ave.**	City **Stephenson**	State **OH**	Zip **60089**

Referred By **Dr. Janet Wood**   Ph # of Referral **(614) 459-3700**

Responsible Party (Complete this section if the person responsible for the bill is not the patient)

Last Name	First Name	MI	Sex __ M __ F	Date of Birth / /

Address	City	State	Zip	SS#

Relation to Patient __ Spouse __ Parent __ Other	Employer Name	Work Phone # ( )

Spouse, or Parent (if minor):   Home Phone # ( )

Insurance (If you have multiple coverage, supply information from both carriers)

Primary Carrier Name **OhioCare HMO**	Price Code **A**	Secondary Carrier Name
Name of the Insured (Name on ID Card) . **Stewart Robertson**		Name of the Insured (Name on ID Card)
Patient's relationship to the insured **X** Self __ Spouse __ Child		Patient's relationship to the insured __ Self __ Spouse __ Child
Insured ID # **920394567**		Insured ID #
Group # or Company Name **Group 63W**		Group # or Company Name
Insurance Address **147 Central Ave., Halevile, OH 60890**		Insurance Address
Phone # **614-555-0101**	Copay $ **30**	Phone # Copay $

Other Information

Is patient's condition related to: Reason for visit: **Routine Physical**
__ Employment   __ Auto Accident (if yes, state in which accident occurred: ___)   __ Other Accident
Date of Accident: / /   Date of First Symptom of Illness: / /

Authorization

I hereby authorize release of information necessary for my insurance company to process my claim. The above information is correct to the best of my knowledge.	I hereby authorize payment directly to FAMILY CARE CENTER insurance benefits otherwise payable to me. I understand that I am financially responsible for charges not paid in a timely manner by my insurance.
Signed: **Stewart Robertson** Date: **12/10/2010**	Signed: **Stewart Robertson** Date: **12/10/2010**

ENCOUNTER FORM

12/18/2010
DATE

Dr. Robert Beach
PROVIDER

Stewart Robertson
PATIENT NAME

ROBERST0
CHART #

OFFICE VISITS - SYMPTOMATIC	
99201	OF--New Patient Minimal
99202	OF--New Patient Low
99203	OF--New Patient Detailed
99204	OF--New Patient Moderate
99205	OF--New Patient High
99211	OF--Established Patient Minimal
99212	OF--Established Patient Low
99213	OF--Established Patient Detailed
99214	OF--Established Patient Moderate
99215	OF--Established Patient High
PREVENTIVE VISITS	
NEW	
99381	Under 1 Year
99382	1 - 4 Years
99383	5 - 11 Years
99384	12 - 17 Years
99385	18 - 39 Years
99386	40 - 64 Years
99387	65 Years & Up
ESTABLISHED	
99391	Under 1 Year
99392	1 - 4 Years
99393	5 - 11 Years
99394	12 - 17 Years
99395	18 - 39 Years
99396	40 - 64 Years
99397	65 Years & Up
PROCEDURES	
12011	Simple suture--face--local anes.
29125	App. of short arm splint; static
29425	App. of short leg cast, walking
45378	Colonoscopy--diagnostic
45380	Colonoscopy--with biopsy
50390	Aspiration of renal cyst by needle
71010	Chest x-ray, single view, frontal

PROCEDURES	
71020	Chest x-ray, two views, frontal & lateral
71030	Chest x-ray, complete, four views
73070	Elbow x-ray, AP & lateral views
73090	Forearm x-ray, AP & lateral views
73100	Wrist x-ray, AP & lateral views
73510	Hip x-ray, complete, two views
73600	Ankle x-ray, AP & lateral views
80048	Basic metabolic panel
80061	Lipid panel
82270	Blood screening, occult; feces
82947	Glucose screening--quantitative
82951	Glucose tolerance test, three specimens
83718	HDL cholesterol
84478	Triglycerides test
85007	Manual differential WBC
85018	Hemoglobin
85025	Complete CBC w/auto diff WBC
85651	Erythrocyte sedimentation rate--non-auto
86585	Tuberculosis, tine test
87076	Culture, anaerobic isolate
87077	Bacterial culture, aerobic isolate
87086	Urine culture and colony count
87430	Strep test
87880	Direct streptococcus screen
90471	Immunization administration
90703	Tetanus injection
90782	Injection
92516	Facial nerve function studies
93000	Electrocardiogram--ECG with interpretation
93015	Treadmill stress test, with physician...
96900	Ultraviolet light treatment
99070	Supplies and materials provided

FAMILY CARE CENTER

NOTES

REFERRING PHYSICIAN
Janet Wood, M.D.

UPIN

AUTHORIZATION #

DIAGNOSIS
v70.0

PAYMENT AMOUNT
$30 copay, check #416

Source Document 25

ENCOUNTER FORM

12/18/2010
DATE

Dr. Patricia McGrath
PROVIDER

Michael Syzmanski
PATIENT NAME

SYZMAMI0
CHART #

OFFICE VISITS - SYMPTOMATIC	
99201	OF--New Patient Minimal
99202	OF--New Patient Low
99203	OF--New Patient Detailed
99204	OF--New Patient Moderate
99205	OF--New Patient High
99211	OF--Established Patient Minimal
99212	OF--Established Patient Low
99213	OF--Established Patient Detailed
99214	OF--Established Patient Moderate
99215	OF--Established Patient High
PREVENTIVE VISITS	
NEW	
99381	Under 1 Year
99382	1 - 4 Years
99383	5 - 11 Years
99384	12 - 17 Years
99385	18 - 39 Years
99386	40 - 64 Years
99387	65 Years & Up
ESTABLISHED	
99391	Under 1 Year
99392	1 - 4 Years
99393	5 - 11 Years
99394	12 - 17 Years
99395	18 - 39 Years
99396	40 - 64 Years
99397	65 Years & Up
PROCEDURES	
12011	Simple suture--face--local anes.
29125	App. of short arm splint; static
29425	App. of short leg cast, walking
45378	Colonoscopy--diagnostic
45380	Colonoscopy--with biopsy
50390	Aspiration of renal cyst by needle
71010	Chest x-ray, single view, frontal

PROCEDURES	
71020	Chest x-ray, two views, frontal & lateral
71030	Chest x-ray, complete, four views
73070	Elbow x-ray, AP & lateral views
73090	Forearm x-ray, AP & lateral views
73100	Wrist x-ray, AP & lateral views
73510	Hip x-ray, complete, two views
73600	Ankle x-ray, AP & lateral views
80048	Basic metabolic panel
80061	Lipid panel
82270	Blood screening, occult; feces
82947	Glucose screening--quantitative
82951	Glucose tolerance test, three specimens
83718	HDL cholesterol
84478	Triglycerides test
85007	Manual differential WBC
85018	Hemoglobin
85025	Complete CBC w/auto diff WBC
85651	Erythrocyte sedimentation rate--non-auto
86585	Tuberculosis, tine test
87076	Culture, anaerobic isolate
87077	Bacterial culture, aerobic isolate
87086	Urine culture and colony count
87430	Strep test
87880	Direct streptococcus screen
90471	Immunization administration
90703	Tetanus injection
90782	Injection
92516	Facial nerve function studies
93000	Electrocardiogram--ECG with interpretation
93015	Treadmill stress test, with physician...
96900	Ultraviolet light treatment
99070	Supplies and materials provided

FAMILY CARE CENTER

REFERRING PHYSICIAN

UPIN

NOTES

AUTHORIZATION #

DIAGNOSIS
870.8

PAYMENT AMOUNT
$25 copay, check #3139

ENCOUNTER FORM

1/5/2011
DATE

Dr. Dana Banu
PROVIDER

Luther Jackson
PATIENT NAME

JACKSLU0
CHART #

OFFICE VISITS - SYMPTOMATIC	
99201	OF--New Patient Minimal
99202	OF--New Patient Low
99203	OF--New Patient Detailed
99204	OF--New Patient Moderate
99205	OF--New Patient High
99211	OF--Established Patient Minimal
99212	OF--Established Patient Low
99213	OF--Established Patient Detailed
99214	OF--Established Patient Moderate
99215	OF--Established Patient High

PREVENTIVE VISITS	
NEW	
99381	Under 1 Year
99382	1 - 4 Years
99383	5 - 11 Years
99384	12 - 17 Years
99385	18 - 39 Years
99386	40 - 64 Years
99387	65 Years & Up
ESTABLISHED	
99391	Under 1 Year
99392	1 - 4 Years
99393	5 - 11 Years
99394	12 - 17 Years
99395	18 - 39 Years
99396	40 - 64 Years
99397	65 Years & Up

PROCEDURES	
12011	Simple suture--face--local anes.
29125	App. of short arm splint; static
29425	App. of short leg cast, walking
45378	Colonoscopy--diagnostic
45380	Colonoscopy--with biopsy
50390	Aspiration of renal cyst by needle
71010	Chest x-ray, single view, frontal

PROCEDURES	
71020	Chest x-ray, two views, frontal & lateral
71030	Chest x-ray, complete, four views
73070	Elbow x-ray, AP & lateral views
73090	Forearm x-ray, AP & lateral views
73100	Wrist x-ray, AP & lateral views
73510	Hip x-ray, complete, two views
73600	Ankle x-ray, AP & lateral views
80048	Basic metabolic panel
80061	Lipid panel
82270	Blood screening, occult; feces
82947	Glucose screening--quantitative
82951	Glucose tolerance test, three specimens
83718	HDL cholesterol
84478	Triglycerides test
85007	Manual differential WBC
85018	Hemoglobin
85025	Complete CBC w/auto diff WBC
85651	Erythrocyte sedimentation rate--non-auto
86585	Tuberculosis, tine test
87076	Culture, anaerobic isolate
87077	Bacterial culture, aerobic isolate
87086	Urine culture and colony count
87430	Strep test
87880	Direct streptococcus screen
90471	Immunization administration
90703	Tetanus injection
90782	Injection
92516	Facial nerve function studies
93000	Electrocardiogram--ECG with interpretation
93015	Treadmill stress test, with physician...
96900	Ultraviolet light treatment
99070	Supplies and materials provided

FAMILY CARE CENTER

NOTES
Difficulty breathing

REFERRING PHYSICIAN

UPIN

AUTHORIZATION #

DIAGNOSIS
485

PAYMENT AMOUNT
$30 copay, check #1291

Source Document 27

ENCOUNTER FORM

1/5/2011	Dr. Robert Beach
DATE	PROVIDER
Jill Simmons	SIMMOJI0
PATIENT NAME	CHART #

OFFICE VISITS - SYMPTOMATIC	
99201	OF--New Patient Minimal
99202	OF--New Patient Low
99203	OF--New Patient Detailed
99204	OF--New Patient Moderate
99205	OF--New Patient High
99211	OF--Established Patient Minimal
99212	OF--Established Patient Low
99213	OF--Established Patient Detailed
99214	OF--Established Patient Moderate
99215	OF--Established Patient High
PREVENTIVE VISITS	
NEW	
99381	Under 1 Year
99382	1 - 4 Years
99383	5 - 11 Years
99384	12 - 17 Years
99385	18 - 39 Years
99386	40 - 64 Years
99387	65 Years & Up
ESTABLISHED	
99391	Under 1 Year
99392	1 - 4 Years
99393	5 - 11 Years
99394	12 - 17 Years
99395	18 - 39 Years
99396	40 - 64 Years
99397	65 Years & Up
PROCEDURES	
12011	Simple suture--face--local anes.
29125	App. of short arm splint; static
29425	App. of short leg cast, walking
45378	Colonoscopy--diagnostic
45380	Colonoscopy--with biopsy
50390	Aspiration of renal cyst by needle
71010	Chest x-ray, single view, frontal

PROCEDURES	
71020	Chest x-ray, two views, frontal & lateral
71030	Chest x-ray, complete, four views
73070	Elbow x-ray, AP & lateral views
73090	Forearm x-ray, AP & lateral views
73100	Wrist x-ray, AP & lateral views
73510	Hip x-ray, complete, two views
73600	Ankle x-ray, AP & lateral views
80048	Basic metabolic panel
80061	Lipid panel
82270	Blood screening, occult; feces
82947	Glucose screening--quantitative
82951	Glucose tolerance test, three specimens
83718	HDL cholesterol
84478	Triglycerides test
85007	Manual differential WBC
85018	Hemoglobin
85025	Complete CBC w/auto diff WBC
85651	Erythrocyte sedimentation rate--non-auto
86585	Tuberculosis, tine test
87076	Culture, anaerobic isolate
87077	Bacterial culture, aerobic isolate
87086	Urine culture and colony count
87430	Strep test
87880	Direct streptococcus screen
90471	Immunization administration
90703	Tetanus injection
90782	Injection
92516	Facial nerve function studies
93000	Electrocardiogram--ECG with interpretation
93015	Treadmill stress test, with physician...
96900	Ultraviolet light treatment
99070	Supplies and materials provided

FAMILY CARE CENTER

NOTES

REFERRING PHYSICIAN	UPIN

AUTHORIZATION #

DIAGNOSIS

034.0 Strep sore throat

PAYMENT AMOUNT

ENCOUNTER FORM

1/5/2011
DATE

Dr. Patricia McGrath
PROVIDER

Nancy Stern
PATIENT NAME

STERNNA0
CHART #

OFFICE VISITS - SYMPTOMATIC	
99201	OF--New Patient Minimal
99202	OF--New Patient Low
99203	OF--New Patient Detailed
99204	OF--New Patient Moderate
99205	OF--New Patient High
99211	OF--Established Patient Minimal
99212	OF--Established Patient Low
99213	OF--Established Patient Detailed
99214	OF--Established Patient Moderate
99215	OF--Established Patient High
PREVENTIVE VISITS	
NEW	
99381	Under 1 Year
99382	1 - 4 Years
99383	5 - 11 Years
99384	12 - 17 Years
99385	18 - 39 Years
99386	40 - 64 Years
99387	65 Years & Up
ESTABLISHED	
99391	Under 1 Year
99392	1 - 4 Years
99393	5 - 11 Years
99394	12 - 17 Years
99395	18 - 39 Years
99396	40 - 64 Years
99397	65 Years & Up
PROCEDURES	
12011	Simple suture--face--local anes.
29125	App. of short arm splint; static
29425	App. of short leg cast, walking
45378	Colonoscopy--diagnostic
45380	Colonoscopy--with biopsy
50390	Aspiration of renal cyst by needle
71010	Chest x-ray, single view, frontal

PROCEDURES	
71020	Chest x-ray, two views, frontal & lateral
71030	Chest x-ray, complete, four views
73070	Elbow x-ray, AP & lateral views
73090	Forearm x-ray, AP & lateral views
73100	Wrist x-ray, AP & lateral views
73510	Hip x-ray, complete, two views
73600	Ankle x-ray, AP & lateral views
80048	Basic metabolic panel
80061	Lipid panel
82270	Blood screening, occult; feces
82947	Glucose screening--quantitative
82951	Glucose tolerance test, three specimens
83718	HDL cholesterol
84478	Triglycerides test
85007	Manual differential WBC
85018	Hemoglobin
85025	Complete CBC w/auto diff WBC
85651	Erythrocyte sedimentation rate--non-auto
86585	Tuberculosis, tine test
87076	Culture, anaerobic isolate
87077	Bacterial culture, aerobic isolate
87086	Urine culture and colony count
87430	Strep test
87880	Direct streptococcus screen
90471	Immunization administration
90703	Tetanus injection
90782	Injection
92516	Facial nerve function studies
93000	Electrocardiogram--ECG with interpretation
93015	Treadmill stress test, with physician...
96900	Ultraviolet light treatment
99070	Supplies and materials provided

FAMILY CARE CENTER

REFERRING PHYSICIAN

UPIN

AUTHORIZATION #

DIAGNOSIS
v70.0

PAYMENT AMOUNT
$30 copay, check #1022

NOTES

Source Document 29

ENCOUNTER FORM

1/5/2011	Dr. Dana Banu
DATE	PROVIDER
Deborah Syzmanski	SYZMADE0
PATIENT NAME	CHART #

OFFICE VISITS - SYMPTOMATIC	
99201	OF--New Patient Minimal
99202	OF--New Patient Low
99203	OF--New Patient Detailed
99204	OF--New Patient Moderate
99205	OF--New Patient High
99211	OF--Established Patient Minimal
99212	OF--Established Patient Low
99213	OF--Established Patient Detailed
99214	OF--Established Patient Moderate
99215	OF--Established Patient High

PREVENTIVE VISITS	
NEW	
99381	Under 1 Year
99382	1 - 4 Years
99383	5 - 11 Years
99384	12 - 17 Years
99385	18 - 39 Years
99386	40 - 64 Years
99387	65 Years & Up
ESTABLISHED	
99391	Under 1 Year
99392	1 - 4 Years
99393	5 - 11 Years
99394	12 - 17 Years
99395	18 - 39 Years
99396	40 - 64 Years
99397	65 Years & Up

PROCEDURES	
12011	Simple suture--face--local anes.
29125	App. of short arm splint; static
29425	App. of short leg cast, walking
45378	Colonoscopy--diagnostic
45380	Colonoscopy--with biopsy
50390	Aspiration of renal cyst by needle
71010	Chest x-ray, single view, frontal

PROCEDURES	
71020	Chest x-ray, two views, frontal & lateral
71030	Chest x-ray, complete, four views
73070	Elbow x-ray, AP & lateral views
73090	Forearm x-ray, AP & lateral views
73100	Wrist x-ray, AP & lateral views
73510	Hip x-ray, complete, two views
73600	Ankle x-ray, AP & lateral views
80048	Basic metabolic panel
80061	Lipid panel
82270	Blood screening, occult; feces
82947	Glucose screening--quantitative
82951	Glucose tolerance test, three specimens
83718	HDL cholesterol
84478	Triglycerides test
85007	Manual differential WBC
85018	Hemoglobin
85025	Complete CBC w/auto diff WBC
85651	Erythrocyte sedimentation rate--non-auto
86585	Tuberculosis, tine test
87076	Culture, anerobic isolate
87077	Bacterial culture, aerobic isolate
87086	Urine culture and colony count
87430	Strep test
87880	Direct streptococcus screen
90471	Immunization administration
90703	Tetanus injection
90782	Injection
92516	Facial nerve function studies
93000	Electrocardiogram--ECG with interpretation
93015	Treadmill stress test, with physician...
96900	Ultraviolet light treatment
99070	Supplies and materials provided

FAMILY CARE CENTER		NOTES
REFERRING PHYSICIAN	UPIN	
AUTHORIZATION #		
DIAGNOSIS		
v70.0		
PAYMENT AMOUNT		
$25 copay, check #3219		

ENCOUNTER FORM

1/5/2011
DATE

Dr. Robert Beach
PROVIDER

Sheila Giles
PATIENT NAME

GILESSH0
CHART #

OFFICE VISITS - SYMPTOMATIC	
99201	OF--New Patient Minimal
99202	OF--New Patient Low
99203	OF--New Patient Detailed
99204	OF--New Patient Moderate
99205	OF--New Patient High
99211	OF--Established Patient Minimal
99212	OF--Established Patient Low
99213	OF--Established Patient Detailed
99214	OF--Established Patient Moderate
99215	OF--Established Patient High

PREVENTIVE VISITS	
NEW	
99381	Under 1 Year
99382	1 - 4 Years
99383	5 - 11 Years
99384	12 - 17 Years
99385	18 - 39 Years
99386	40 - 64 Years
99387	65 Years & Up
ESTABLISHED	
99391	Under 1 Year
99392	1 - 4 Years
99393	5 - 11 Years
99394	12 - 17 Years
99395	18 - 39 Years
99396	40 - 64 Years
99397	65 Years & Up

PROCEDURES	
12011	Simple suture--face--local anes.
29125	App. of short arm splint; static
29425	App. of short leg cast, walking
45378	Colonoscopy--diagnostic
45380	Colonoscopy--with biopsy
50390	Aspiration of renal cyst by needle
71010	Chest x-ray, single view, frontal

PROCEDURES	
71020	Chest x-ray, two views, frontal & lateral
71030	Chest x-ray, complete, four views
73070	Elbow x-ray, AP & lateral views
73090	Forearm x-ray, AP & lateral views
73100	Wrist x-ray, AP & lateral views
73510	Hip x-ray, complete, two views
73600	Ankle x-ray, AP & lateral views
80048	Basic metabolic panel
80061	Lipid panel
82270	Blood screening, occult; feces
82947	Glucose screening--quantitative
82951	Glucose tolerance test, three specimens
83718	HDL cholesterol
84478	Triglycerides test
85007	Manual differential WBC
85018	Hemoglobin
85025	Complete CBC w/auto diff WBC
85651	Erythrocyte sedimentation rate--non-auto
86585	Tuberculosis, tine test
87076	Culture, anaerobic isolate
87077	Bacterial culture, aerobic isolate
87086	Urine culture and colony count
87430	Strep test
87880	Direct streptococcus screen
90471	Immunization administration
90703	Tetanus injection
90782	Injection
92516	Facial nerve function studies
93000	Electrocardiogram--ECG with interpretation
93015	Treadmill stress test, with physician...
96900	Ultraviolet light treatment
99070	Supplies and materials provided

FAMILY CARE CENTER

REFERRING PHYSICIAN

UPIN

AUTHORIZATION #

DIAGNOSIS
v03.7

PAYMENT AMOUNT
$30 copay, check #1022

NOTES

Source Document 31

ENCOUNTER FORM

1/5/2011	Dr. Patricia McGrath
DATE	PROVIDER
Pauline Battistuta	BATTIPA0
PATIENT NAME	CHART #

OFFICE VISITS - SYMPTOMATIC	
99201	OF--New Patient Minimal
99202	OF--New Patient Low
99203	OF--New Patient Detailed
99204	OF--New Patient Moderate
99205	OF--New Patient High
99211	OF--Established Patient Minimal
99212	OF--Established Patient Low
99213	OF--Established Patient Detailed
99214	OF--Established Patient Moderate
99215	OF--Established Patient High
PREVENTIVE VISITS	
NEW	
99381	Under 1 Year
99382	1 - 4 Years
99383	5 - 11 Years
99384	12 - 17 Years
99385	18 - 39 Years
99386	40 - 64 Years
99387	65 Years & Up
ESTABLISHED	
99391	Under 1 Year
99392	1 - 4 Years
99393	5 - 11 Years
99394	12 - 17 Years
99395	18 - 39 Years
99396	40 - 64 Years
99397	65 Years & Up
PROCEDURES	
12011	Simple suture--face--local anes.
29125	App. of short arm splint; static
29425	App. of short leg cast, walking
45378	Colonoscopy--diagnostic
45380	Colonoscopy--with biopsy
50390	Aspiration of renal cyst by needle
71010	Chest x-ray, single view, frontal

PROCEDURES	
71020	Chest x-ray, two views, frontal & lateral
71030	Chest x-ray, complete, four views
73070	Elbow x-ray, AP & lateral views
73090	Forearm x-ray, AP & lateral views
73100	Wrist x-ray, AP & lateral views
73510	Hip x-ray, complete, two views
73600	Ankle x-ray, AP & lateral views
80048	Basic metabolic panel
80061	Lipid panel
82270	Blood screening, occult; feces
82947	Glucose screening--quantitative
82951	Glucose tolerance test, three specimens
83718	HDL cholesterol
84478	Triglycerides test
85007	Manual differential WBC
85018	Hemoglobin
85025	Complete CBC w/auto diff WBC
85651	Erythrocyte sedimentation rate--non-auto
86585	Tuberculosis, tine test
87076	Culture, anaerobic isolate
87077	Bacterial culture, aerobic isolate
87086	Urine culture and colony count
87430	Strep test
87880	Direct streptococcus screen
90471	Immunization administration
90703	Tetanus injection
90782	Injection
92516	Facial nerve function studies
93000	Electrocardiogram--ECG with interpretation
93015	Treadmill stress test, with physician...
96900	Ultraviolet light treatment
99070	Supplies and materials provided

FAMILY CARE CENTER		NOTES
		Upper respiratory infection
REFERRING PHYSICIAN	UPIN	
AUTHORIZATION #		
DIAGNOSIS 465.9		
PAYMENT AMOUNT		

MEDICARE
246 WEST MAIN ST.
CLEVELAND, OH 60120

PROVIDER REMITTANCE
THIS IS NOT A BILL
A PAYMENT SUMMARY AND AN EXPLANATION OF
CODES ARE AT THE END OF THIS STATEMENT

FAMILY CARE CENTER
285 STEPHENSON BLVD.
STEPHENSON, OH 60089-4000

PAGE:	1 OF 1
DATE:	12/31/2010
ID NUMBER:	3470629

PROVIDER: PATRICIA MCGRATH, M.D.

PATIENT: BATTISTUTA ANTHONY   CLAIM: 234567890

PROC CODE	FROM DATE	THRU DATE	TREAT -MENT	STATUS CODE	AMOUNT CHRGD	AMOUNT ALLWD	COPAY/ DEDUCT	AMOUNT APPRVD	PATIENT BALANCE
99212	10/28/10	10/28/10	1	A	28.00	28.00	.00	22.40	5.60
82947	10/28/10	10/28/10	1	A	25.00	25.00	.00	20.00	5.00
99212	11/12/10	11/12/10	1	A	28.00	28.00	.00	22.40	5.60
82951	11/12/10	11/12/10	1	A	30.40	30.40	.00	24.32	6.08
87086	11/12/10	11/12/10	1	A	24.00	24.00	.00	19.20	4.80
	CLAIM TOTALS				135.40	135.40	.00	108.32	27.08

PROVIDER: KATHERINE YAN, M.D.

PATIENT: JONES ELIZABETH   CLAIM: 345678901

PROC CODE	FROM DATE	THRU DATE	TREAT -MENT	STATUS CODE	AMOUNT CHRGD	AMOUNT ALLWD	COPAY/ DEDUCT	AMOUNT APPRVD	PATIENT BALANCE
99213	10/04/10	10/04/10	1	A	39.00	39.00	.00	31.20	7.80
99212	10/28/10	10/28/10	1	A	28.00	28.00	.00	22.40	5.60
99214	11/05/10	11/05/10	1	A	59.00	59.00	.00	47.20	11.80
93000	11/05/10	11/05/10	1	A	29.00	29.00	.00	23.20	5.80
	CLAIM TOTALS				155.00	155.00	.00	124.00	31.00

PAYMENT SUMMARY		TOTAL ALL CLAIMS		EFT INFORMATION	
TOTAL AMOUNT PAID	232.32	AMOUNT CHARGED	290.40	NUMBER	3470629
PRIOR CREDIT BALANCE	.00	AMOUNT ALLOWED	290.40	DATE	12/31/10
CURRENT CREDIT DEFERRED	.00	DEDUCTIBLE	.00	AMOUNT	232.32
PRIOR CREDIT APPLIED	.00	COPAY	.00		
NEW CREDIT BALANCE	.00	OTHER REDUCTION	.00		
NET DISBURSED	232.32	AMOUNT APPROVED	232.32		

STATUS CODES:
A - APPROVED   AJ - ADJUSTMENT   IP - IN PROCESS   R - REJECTED   V - VOID

Source Document 33

CHAMPVA
240 CENTER ST.
COLUMBUS, OH 60220

PROVIDER REMITTANCE
THIS IS NOT A BILL
A PAYMENT SUMMARY AND AN EXPLANATION OF
CODES ARE AT THE END OF THIS STATEMENT

FAMILY CARE CENTER
285 STEPHENSON BLVD.
STEPHENSON, OH 60089-4000

PAGE: 1 OF 1
DATE: 12/31/2010
ID NUMBER: 76374021

PROVIDER: JOHN RUDNER, M.D.

PATIENT: FITZWILLIAMS JOHN   CLAIM: 123456789

PROC CODE	FROM DATE	THRU DATE	TREAT -MENT	STATUS CODE	AMOUNT CHRGD	AMOUNT ALLWD	COPAY/ DEDUCT	AMOUNT APPRVD	PATIENT BALANCE
99213	10/04/10	10/04/10	1	A	39.00	39.00	15.00	39.00	.00
82270	10/04/10	10/04/10	1	A	8.00	8.00	.00	8.00	.00
		CLAIM TOTALS			47.00	47.00	15.00	47.00	0.00

******************** CHECK #76374021 IN THE AMOUNT OF $47.00 IS ATTACHED ********************

PAYMENT SUMMARY

		TOTAL ALL CLAIMS	
TOTAL AMOUNT PAID	47.00	AMOUNT CHARGED	47.00
PRIOR CREDIT BALANCE	.00	AMOUNT ALLOWED	47.00
CURRENT CREDIT DEFERRED	.00	DEDUCTIBLE	.00
PRIOR CREDIT APPLIED	.00	COPAY	15.00
NEW CREDIT BALANCE	.00	OTHER REDUCTION	.00
NET DISBURSED	47.00	AMOUNT APPROVED	47.00

STATUS CODES:
A - APPROVED   AJ - ADJUSTMENT   IP - IN PROCESS   R - REJECTED   V - VOID

MEDICAID
246 WEST MAIN ST.
CLEVELAND, OH 60120

PROVIDER REMITTANCE
THIS IS NOT A BILL
A PAYMENT SUMMARY AND AN EXPLANATION OF
CODES ARE AT THE END OF THIS STATEMENT

FAMILY CARE CENTER
285 STEPHENSON BLVD.
STEPHENSON, OH 60089-4000

PAGE:	1 OF 1
DATE:	12/31/2010
ID NUMBER:	137291449

PROVIDER: ROBERT BEACH, M.D.

PATIENT: PALMER CHRISTOPHER   CLAIM: 56789012

PROC CODE	FROM DATE	THRU DATE	TREAT -MENT	STATUS CODE	AMOUNT CHRGD	AMOUNT ALLWD	COPAY/ DEDUCT	AMOUNT APPRVD	PATIENT BALANCE
99201	11/12/10	11/12/10	1	A	32.00	32.00	10.00	32.00	.00
71020	11/12/10	11/12/10	1	A	35.00	35.00	.00	35.00	.00
87430	11/12/10	11/12/10	1	a	23.20	23.20	.00	23.20	.00
	CLAIM TOTALS				90.20	90.20	10.00	90.20	.00

PAYMENT SUMMARY

TOTAL AMOUNT PAID	90.20
PRIOR CREDIT BALANCE	.00
CURRENT CREDIT DEFERRED	.00
PRIOR CREDIT APPLIED	.00
NEW CREDIT BALANCE	.00
NET DISBURSED	90.20

TOTAL ALL CLAIMS

AMOUNT CHARGED	90.20
AMOUNT ALLOWED	90.20
DEDUCTIBLE	.00
COPAY	10.00
OTHER REDUCTION	.00
AMOUNT APPROVED	90.20

EFT INFORMATION

NUMBER	137291449
DATE	12/31/10
AMOUNT	90.20

STATUS CODES:
A - APPROVED   AJ - ADJUSTMENT   IP - IN PROCESS   R - REJECTED   V - VOID

Source Document 35

EAST OHIO PPO
10 CENTRAL AVENUE
HALEVILLE, OH 60890

PROVIDER REMITTANCE
THIS IS NOT A BILL
A PAYMENT SUMMARY AND AN EXPLANATION OF
CODES ARE AT THE END OF THIS STATEMENT

FAMILY CARE CENTER
285 STEPHENSON BLVD.
STEPHENSON, OH 60089-4000

PAGE: 1 OF 1
DATE: 12/31/2010
ID NUMBER: 376490713

PROVIDER: JESSICA RUDNER, M.D.

PATIENT: SMITH SARABETH   CLAIM: 67891023

PROC CODE	FROM DATE	THRU DATE	TREAT -MENT	STATUS CODE	AMOUNT CHRGD	AMOUNT ALLWD	COPAY/ DEDUCT	AMOUNT APPRVD	PATIENT BALANCE
99212	09/09/10	09/09/10	1	A	46.00	46.00	25.00	46.00	0.00
		CLAIM TOTALS			46.00	46.00	25.00	46.00	0.00

PROVIDER: DANA BANU, M.D.

PATIENT: SYZMANSKI HANNAH   CLAIM: 78901234

PROC CODE	FROM DATE	THRU DATE	TREAT -MENT	STATUS CODE	AMOUNT CHRGD	AMOUNT ALLWD	COPAY/ DEDUCT	AMOUNT APPRVD	PATIENT BALANCE
99393	11/12/10	11/12/10	1	A	153.60	153.60	25.00	153.60	.00
		CLAIM TOTALS			153.60	153.60	25.00	153.60	0.00

PATIENT: SYZMANSKI MICHAEL   CLAIM: 89012345

PROC CODE	FROM DATE	THRU DATE	TREAT -MENT	STATUS CODE	AMOUNT CHRGD	AMOUNT ALLWD	COPAY/ DEDUCT	AMOUNT APPRVD	PATIENT BALANCE
99215	11/15/10	11/15/10	1	A	140.00	140.00	25.00	140.00	.00
82270	11/15/10	11/15/10	1	A	15.00	15.00	.00	15.00	.00
		CLAIM TOTALS			155.00	155.00	25.00	155.00	0.00

PROVIDER: PATRICIA MCGRATH, M.D.

PATIENT: SYZMANSKI MICHAEL   CLAIM: 90123456

PROC CODE	FROM DATE	THRU DATE	TREAT -MENT	STATUS CODE	AMOUNT CHRGD	AMOUNT ALLWD	COPAY/ DEDUCT	AMOUNT APPRVD	PATIENT BALANCE
99212	12/18/10	12/18/10	1	A	46.00	46.00	25.00	46.00	.00
12011	12/18/10	12/18/10	1	A	171.00	171.00	.00	171.00	.00
		CLAIM TOTALS			217.00	217.00	25.00	217.00	0.00

PAYMENT SUMMARY		TOTAL ALL CLAIMS		EFT INFORMATION	
TOTAL AMOUNT PAID	571.60	AMOUNT CHARGED	571.60	NUMBER	376490713
PRIOR CREDIT BALANCE	.00	AMOUNT ALLOWED	571.60	DATE	12/31/10
CURRENT CREDIT DEFERRED	.00	DEDUCTIBLE	.00	AMOUNT	571.60
PRIOR CREDIT APPLIED	.00	COPAY	100.00		
NEW CREDIT BALANCE	.00	OTHER REDUCTION	.00		
NET DISBURSED	571.60	AMOUNT APPROVED	571.60		

STATUS CODES:
A - APPROVED   AJ - ADJUSTMENT   IP - IN PROCESS   R - REJECTED   V - VOID

MIDWEST SELECT HMO
1245 MOHAWK LANE
COLUMBUS, OH 60625

FAMILY CARE CENTER
285 STEPHENSON BLVD.
STEPHENSON, OH 60089-4000

PAGE: 1 OF 1
DATE: 12/31/2010
ID NUMBER: 10694214

MIDWEST SELECT HMO CAPITATION STATEMENT
MONTH OF NOVEMBER 2010

PROVIDERS
BANU DANA
BEACH ROBERT
MCGRATH PATRICIA
RUDNER JESSICA
RUDNER JOHN
YAN KATHERINE

MEMBER NUMBER	MEMBER NAME	CONTRACT NUMBER	CONTRACT STATUS
000457396	FAMILY CARE CENTER	HMO3146	APPROVED

AMOUNT OF PAYMENT $1,500.00
EFT STATUS: SENT 12/31/10 10:46AM
TRANSACTION #10694214

Source Document 37

OHIOCARE HMO
147 CENTRAL AVENUE
HALEVILLE, OH 60890

FAMILY CARE CENTER
285 STEPHENSON BLVD.
STEPHENSON, OH 60089-4000

PAGE: 1 OF 1
DATE: 12/31/2010
ID NUMBER: 767729

OHIOCARE HMO CAPITATION STATEMENT
MONTH OF NOVEMBER 2010

PROVIDERS
BANU DANA
BEACH ROBERT
MCGRATH PATRICIA
RUDNER JESSICA
RUDNER JOHN
YAN KATHERINE

MEMBER NUMBER	MEMBER NAME	CONTRACT NUMBER	CONTRACT STATUS
0003602149	FAMILY CARE CENTER	YG34906	APPROVED

AMOUNT OF PAYMENT $2,500.00
EFT STATUS: SENT 12/31/10 2:46PM
TRANSACTION #767729

Glossary

accounting cycle   The flow of financial transactions in a business—from making a sale to collecting payment for the goods or services delivered. In a medical practice, this is the cycle between treating the patient and receiving payments for services provided

accounts receivable (AR)   Accounting software can be used to track accounts receivable (AR)—monies that are coming into the practice—and to produce financial reports

Acknowledgment of Receipt of Notice of Privacy Practices   Under the HIPAA Privacy Rule, medical practices must have a written Notice of Privacy Practices that describes the medical office's practices regarding the use and disclosure of Private Health Information (PHI). Patients must be given a copy of the notice and must sign an Acknowledgment of Receipt form.

Adjustments   Changes to patients' accounts, such as returned check fees, insurance write-offs, capitation adjustments, and changes in treatment

aging report   A report that lists the amount of money owed to the practice, organized by the amount of time the money has been owed

audit/edit report   A report used to communicate problems with insurance claims that must be corrected by the practice

backup data   A copy of data files made at a specific time that can be used to restore data in the event they are accidentally lost or destroyed

billing code   A user-defined one- or two-character sorting key (0-9 or A-Z) which can be used to divide the patients into various groups for billing purposes

business associates   Billing services or other outside professional services with whom a medical office has a contract

capitated plan   A type of insurance plan in which payments are made to physicians from managed care companies for patients who select the physician as their primary care provider, regardless of whether they visit the physician or not

capitation   In a *capitated plan*, the fixed amount paid to a provider on a regular basis

capitation payments   Payments made to physicians on a regular basis (such as monthly) for providing services to patients in a managed care insurance plan

case   A grouping of transactions for visits to a physician's office organized around a condition

case-based accounting   A method of accounting that helps keep track of transactions of a common nature

charges   Amounts that a provider bills for services performed

chart   A folder that contains all records pertaining to a patient

chart number   A unique number that identifies a patient

clearinghouse   A service bureau that collects electronic insurance claims from medical practices and forwards the claims to the appropriate health plans

CMS (Claim Management Services)   The new name for the former Health Care Finance Administration (HCFA)

coinsurance   The portion of charges that an insured person must pay

copayment   A small fixed fee, such as $30, paid by the patient at the time of the office visit

cycle billing   A method of billing in which patients are divided into groups and statement printing and mailing is staggered throughout the month

databases   Collections of related facts

day sheet   A report that provides information on practice activities for a twenty-four-hour period

default   A preset value in a field

diagnosis code   A code found in the *International Classification of Diseases* (ICD) that provides very specific information about the patient's illness(es), sign(s), and symptom(s)

edit A computer check of a claim, performed by a clearinghouse, to determine if all necessary information is included

electronic data interchange (EDI) The transfer of data from one computer to another using a network such as the Internet

electronic funds transfer (EFT) The electronic transfer of funds from one account to another

electronic medical record (EMR) Computer-based systems that record clinical data about a patient

encounter form A form that is used to record information about the procedures performed during a patient's visit

explanation of benefits (EOB) A document sent by an insurance carrier that lists services obtained and the reimbursements, or reasons for lack of reimbursement. Also known as a remittance advice (RA).

fee-for-service A type of insurance plan in which policyholders are repaid for costs for health care obtained because of illnesses and accidents

filter A condition that data must meet to be included in a selection

guarantor The person who is the holder of the insurance policy that covers the patient, and is responsible for payments on the account

health maintenance organization (HMO) A common type of managed care system in which patients pay fixed rates at regular intervals, such as monthly, that cover whatever services they need for that period

health plan Any plan, program, or organization that provides health benefits

HIPAA (Health Insurance Portability and Accountability Act of 1996) A federal law governing many aspects of health care, such as electronic transmission standards and the security of health care records

HIPAA Privacy Rule Legislation that protects individually identifiable health information

HIPAA Security Rule Legislation that outlines the administrative, technical, and physical safeguards required to prevent unauthorized access to protected health care information

HIPAA Transaction and Code Sets Standards Standards that describe a particular electronic format that providers and payers must use to send and receive health care transactions. They also establish standard medical code sets, such as *ICD* and *CPT-4*, for use in health care transactions

Indicator A code used to sort patients according to user-defined criteria

Information technology Computer hardware and software information systems used to handle administrative tasks in a medical practice

knowledge base A searchable collection of up-to-date technical information about a given subject

managed care A type of insurance in which physicians, hospitals, and other health care professionals are organized into a group or "network" in order to manage the cost, quality, and access to health care

MMDDCCYY format A specific way in which dates must be entered, in which "MM" stands for the month, "DD" stands for the day, "CC" represents century, and "YY" stands for the year

modifiers Two-digit codes that are used with procedure codes to allow more-specific descriptions to be entered for the services the physician performed

MultiLink codes Groups of procedure code entries that relate to a single activity and save time by eliminating multiple transaction entries

National Provider Identifier (NPI) A unique identifier assigned to a health care provider that is used in standard transactions, such as health care claims

navigator buttons Buttons that simplify the task of moving from one data field to another

Office Hours break A block of time when a physician is unavailable for appointments with patients

Office Hours schedule A listing of time slots for a particular day for a specific provider

once-a-month billing A billing method in which all patient statements are printed and mailed once-a-month on the same day

packing data The deletion of vacant slots from a database

patient day sheet A summary of patient activity on a given day, organized by patient

patient information form A form filled out by a patient that contains the personal, employment, and medical insurance information needed to collect payment for the provider's services

patient ledger A report that lists the financial activity in each patient's account, including charges, payments, and adjustments

patient statement A report that lists the amount of money a patient owes, organized by the amount of time the money has been owed, the procedures performed, and the dates the procedures were performed

payer   An agency, insurer, or health plan that pays for health care services and is responsible for the costs of those services, such as the government or a commercial insurance carrier

payment day sheet   A report that lists all payments received on a particular day, organized by provider

Payments   Monies that the practice receives from patients and insurance carriers

policyholder   An individual who pays a premium to an insurance company in exchange for the insurance protection provided by a policy

practice analysis report   A report that analyzes the revenue of a practice for a specified period of time, usually a month or a year

preferred provider organization (PPO)   A managed care plan with an established provider network that pays maximum benefit coverage when using its own contracted physicians and hospitals, and lesser benefits when using providers outside of the network

premium   The policyholder's payments to the insurance company in exchange for insurance coverage

procedure code   A standardized five-digit code that specifies which medical procedures and tests were performed. The most commonly used system of procedure codes is found in *Current Procedural Terminology*, Fourth Edition, also known as the *CPT*, or *CPT-4*

procedure day sheet   A report that lists all the procedures performed on a particular day, listed in numerical order by procedure code

Provider   A licensed individual in the health care field who provides services to a patient

purging data   The process of deleting files of patients who are no longer patients of the practice

rebuilding indexes   A process that checks and verifies a database and corrects any internal problems with the data

record of treatment and progress   A record that contains the physician's notes about a patient's condition and diagnosis

referring provider   A physician who recommends that a patient see another physician.

remainder statements   Patient statements that list only those charges that are not paid in full after all insurance carrier payments have been received

remittance advice (RA)   A document sent by an insurance carrier that lists services obtained and the reimbursements, or reasons for lack of reimbursement. Also known as an explanation of benefits (EOB).

restoring data   The process of retrieving data from backup storage devices

sponsor   The active-duty military service member through which other family members obtain health insurance coverage under TRICARE

standard statements   Patient statements that list all available charges, regardless of whether the insurance has paid on the transactions

tertiary   Third in rank order

walkout statement   A report that lists the charges and the amount paid by the patient, which is given to the patient at the conclusion of the visit

X12-837 Health Care Claim   The electronic claim format that is used to bill for a physician's services. Also known as *837P*.

837P   The electronic claim format that is used to bill for a physician's services

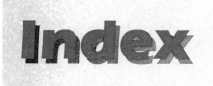

Index